The White House Physician

ALSO BY LUDWIG M. DEPPISCH, M.D.
AND FROM MCFARLAND

Women in the Life of Andrew Jackson (2021)

*The Health of the First Ladies: Medical Histories
from Martha Washington to Michelle Obama* (2015)

*The White House Physician: A History from
Washington to George W. Bush* (2007)

The White House Physician

A History from George Washington to Joe Biden

SECOND EDITION

LUDWIG M. DEPPISCH, M.D.

Foreword by Connie Mariano, M.D.

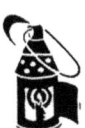

McFarland & Company, Inc., Publishers
Jefferson, North Carolina

ISBN (print) 978-1-4766-8700-1
ISBN (ebook) 978-1-4766-5476-8

Library of Congress and cataloging data are available

Library of Congress Control Number 2025002048

© 2025 Ludwig M. Deppisch, M.D.. All rights reserved

No part of this book may be reproduced or transmitted in any form or by any means, electronic or mechanical, including photocopying or recording, or by any information storage and retrieval system, without permission in writing from the publisher.

Front cover images: *left to right* Navy Rear Admiral Dr. E. Connie Mariano (courtesy of E. Connie Mariano, M.D.), Admiral Cary Grayson (National Library of Medicine), Dr. Janet Travell (National Library of Medicine). White House photograph © Allen.G/Shutterstock.

Printed in the United States of America

*McFarland & Company, Inc., Publishers
Box 611, Jefferson, North Carolina 28640
www.mcfarlandpub.com*

To Rosemarie,
whose confidence and love
made this possible

For all those Presidential and White House Physicians
who endeavored to keep America's presidents
safe and healthy through the years.

Acknowledgments

The publication of this book is the final destination of a journey that began in 1990 with an invitation to present a lecture, "The Health of Ohio's Presidents," to the medical students and faculty of the Northeastern Ohio University Colleges of Medicine (NEOUCOM). Martin Kohn, Director of NEOUCOM's Human Values in Medicine program, is owed a special thank you for his decade-long support and encouragement of my efforts, since this lecture evolved both into an annual event and into a recurring seminar for senior medical students, "The Health of Presidents and Its Effect Upon Foreign and Domestic Policy." Patty Augustine, Janet White, and Rose Guerriere, staff librarians of the Western Reserve Care System and NEOUCOM, were ever resourceful in locating the innumerable references, however obscure, that I demanded, often inappropriately, for my research. For them, a belated thank you for their generous assistance over the years. In addition, special recognition is owed to Ingrid Ebner, former librarian at the Dittrick Medical Museum, Cleveland, Ohio. No one was more persistent or more tireless in locating obscure references and medical biographies of physicians. About this time, my focus meandered and I became more interested in the physicians to the presidents than in their presidential patients.

My itinerary reached Tucson and the University of Arizona in mid–2000 as I started graduate courses in its department of history. Special thanks are due to the members of my thesis committee, doctors Michael Schaller, Roger Nichols, and Katherine Morrissey, who pointed this "nontraditional" and often wayward student in the proper direction. I owe a special debt to Katherine Morrissey, who was unsparing of her time and her encouragement as I proceeded toward completion of my thesis: "The Origins, Evolution and Present Organization of the White House Physician." It was Katherine who first suggested that my thesis was worthy of transformation into a book.

After graduation, travel became onerous. The past few years were a tough slog involving many libraries, both local and remote, government document hunts, and Internet searches. Legion were the librarians, archivists, historians, and others who courteously helped me through this period. Although too numerous to mention, I hope that this simple acknowledgment of their help will be a sufficient token of my gratitude. However, Andre Sobicinski, historian at the Department of the Navy's Bureau of Medicine and Surgery, deserves special recognition for his advice, support, and enthusiasm. Andre is a great government employee whose service makes this citizen a little less reluctant to pay federal taxes.

Doctors John Hutton, Burton Lee III, Robert Darling, and Gerry Cox, all former White House physicians, graciously answered my questions during telephone interviews, and sometimes in follow-up correspondence. Moreover, I owe a special appreciation to Dr. Connie Mariano, who over many months patiently offered her insights and reflections on her experience as presidential physician to Bill Clinton.

Good friend Dr. Jeanne Clarke was a copy editor *par excellence* who spent many hours giving my text whatever grace and fluency it might possess. Ms. Dani Dubois, Curricular Affairs, University of Arizona School of Medicine, used her wizardry with all things informatic to process my disks, e-mails, electronic files, and images into a presentable product. To both, my sincere thanks.

I wish to acknowledge the best wishes of my family during this all too long journey. Thanks to Carl, Barbara, Rich, Nick, Joey, and Jake for their unswerving support. Finally, my wife, Rosemarie, deserves my deepest gratitude for her love, patience, and encouragement during this journey. Without her support, this destination was unreachable. Now that the journey is complete, I can finally get to those many, many household chores I was able to avoid for so long.

The second edition has been enriched and updated through conversations with WHMU physicians Drs. Connie Mariano, Rob Darling, Dick Tubb, Lew Hofmann, Jeff Kuhlman, Jennifer Pena, Joanna Jackson, Francesca Cimino, Denise Whitfield, Ronny Jackson, Sean Conley, and Kevin O'Connor. I thank them for their time and supportive comments as I reviewed and appended the original manuscript. Additionally, I thank Jordan Brittain for her helpful editorial assistance. Any errors in either the original or the second edition are the responsibility of the author.

My wife, Rosemarie Deppisch, is owed my deepest gratitude for continuing to patiently and generously support me in my post-retirement attachment to historical nonfiction.

Table of Contents

Acknowledgments	vii
Foreword by Connie Mariano, M.D.	1
Preface	3
Introduction	5
1. Samuel Bard: The First Presidential Physician	9
2. The Pillars of the Profession: Presidential Physicians, 1812–1865	20
3. The Military Steps In, Part I: The Early Days, 1823–1865	29
4. The Military Steps In, Part II: Conflicts and Cooperation, 1865–1898	37
5. Admiral Presley Rixey: The First Authentic White House Physician	54
6. Captain Joel Boone and the Institutionalization of the Office of the White House Physician	64
7. The Military Keepers of the Stethoscope: Doctors Cary Grayson, Ross McIntire and Howard Snyder	73
8. Physician Anecdotes: The Returnee, the Academic, the Consultant and the Defendant, 1953–1981	92
9. Civilian Interlude, Part I: Medical Chaos in Camelot	102
10. Civilian Interlude, Part II: The Specialist Physicians of Presidents Reagan and George H. Bush	115
11. Twenty First Century Presidential: The Doctors Who Treated George W. Bush, Barack Obama, Donald Trump and Joe Biden	123
12. The White House Medical Unit Continues to Evolve	134
13. The Twenty-fifth Amendment and Its Impact on the White House Medical Unit	143
14. Psychiatry and the Presidency	151
15. The Medical Care of Vice Presidents	161

16. Presidential Physicians After Their Tenures	172
17. Final Thoughts	181
Chapter Notes	187
Bibliography	220
Index	233

Foreword

by Connie Mariano, M.D.

When medical historian and friend Dr. Lud Deppisch asked me to write the foreword to the second edition of his scholarly work, *The White House Physician: A History from Washington to George W. Bush*, I was a bit reluctant at first. Why?

To prepare this foreword, I would be forced to go backward in time, to when I served as White House Physician for nine years. I would need to relive those challenges once again: the highest of highs, the lowest of lows, the constant travel, and most of all, the pressure of knowing the health and life of the First Patient was in my hands. But throughout my life I made it a goal to learn from my struggles and to pass on the lessons to others with my saying, "may my pain become someone's gain." May another physician learn not to make the same mistakes and to find a better way to solve a problem because of what I've taught them. This rings true for White House doctors. Can the lessons I've learned from serving nine years at the White House under three sitting presidents be a way to help current and future White House doctors do their job more effectively? I hope so. The first lesson would be to read and know about the past by reading Dr. Deppisch's book. This book outlines the evolution of the White House Physician and their role in presidential health and its impact on American history.

Dr. Deppisch's second edition picks up after my tour at the White House, with extensive interviews with my successors Drs. Richard Tubb, Jeff Kuhlman, Ronny Jackson, Sean Conley, and Kevin O'Connor.

I have met and know personally all these physicians except Dr. Kevin O'Connor. I believe White House doctors should have an unwritten agreement to never openly criticize or comment about each other in the media. Instead, they should be trusted sounding boards to each other in difficult times not only regarding medical decisions but those that have significant political impact. Only very few physicians know what it is like treating the president of the United States in their private doctor's office on the ground floor of the Residence of the White House. It is very small "club." It is lonely at the "top" as president; it's even more lonely to be the president's doctor.

In this second edition, Dr. Deppisch updates the current role of the White House Physician and this physician's role in the 25th Amendment to the Constitution, a topic that has been repeatedly discussed in the media regarding presidential age and disability during the approach to the 2024 presidential election.

As White House Physician, you take care of the president as your primary patient, but you also take care of the first family, visiting dignitaries, and often at certain times, members of the press pool who travel with the president. You get to see the "talking heads" often and are subject to questions from the press. But you know as a physician, you never answer those questions without consent of your patient. And in the case of the First Patient, you never respond without talking first with both the president and his press secretary. When it comes to media inquiries, I have taught White House doctors during my term to learn from the mistakes of our predecessors at the While House. White House doctors have inherited a sad legacy when it comes to the media of engaging in what I call the "three deadly D's: deception, delusion and denial." Dr. Deppisch's book outlines these examples with Grover Cleveland's oral cancer, Woodrow Wilson's stroke, Franklin Delano Roosevelt's advanced heart disease, Dwight Eisenhower's heart attack, and John F. Kennedy's Addison disease, among others. These lessons from history teach us that not all secrets remain secrets forever. Eventually someone leaks. And if that is discovered, the White House Physician's reputation is over.

The final lesson to White House doctors is thus: remember you are the doctor, not the "spin doctor." Your job is to practice medicine, not politics. And that can be a very difficult task when you work closely with the president, the first family, and senior staff. Dr. Deppisch's well-written, extensively researched book shows how White House doctors who practice medicine based on politics can do more harm than good to their patients, as well as the health of our nation.

Connie Mariano, M.D., was a White House Physician from 1991 to 2001.

Preface

Physicians have appeared upon the landscape of the American presidency since early in the administration of George Washington. On most occasions, their presence had a salutary effect upon the president's well-being; however, at other times, their influence was harmful and even disastrous. Moreover, presidential physicians not infrequently became entangled in the web of politics that inherently enmeshes that office, with unfortunate effects upon their professional judgment and ethical conduct.

This book analyzes the changes that have occurred over time in this critical doctor-patient relationship, beginning with the first physician to treat a president, Samuel Bard, and concluding with President Joe Biden's doctor, Kevin O'Connor. Its focus will be increasingly concentrated on the White House physicians; i.e., those doctors whose sole obligation has been the health care of the occupants of the White House.

With the passage of time, the care of the president's health has evolved. The first presidential physicians made only episodic appearances to treat acute illnesses; these early doctors can be described as civilians, well educated for the times, and well respected by their professional peers. Military doctors replaced civilian practitioners in this role after the Civil War, and, with only uncommon exceptions, have managed the chief executive's medical care ever since. Interestingly, Dr. O'Connor, formerly a military physician who treated Vice President Biden, who retired from the military for a civilian academic practice, has returned to the White House as a civilian. Presently, the White House Medical Unit, the organization responsible for the chief executive's health, has grown in both number and complexity. It contains up to nine physicians and more than twenty ancillary medical personnel. It is a permanent military organization, emphasizes health maintenance and preventive care, and has continually expanding responsibilities, including the implementation of the Twenty-fifth Amendment to the Constitution on presidential disability.

Stories of the presidential doctors will help to explain this evolution. Many of the changes have been logical, but some have been serendipitous and accidental. An accounting of all the presidential physicians is replete with conflicts: civilian versus military, homeopaths versus orthodox practitioners, and the ethical commitment to maintain patient confidentiality versus the demands of the press and the public for medical information.

Additionally, this book will explore the ways in which the care of the president did or did not reflect the 200-year narrative of American medicine. Medical education, the rise of specialization, the advent and growth of hospitals, payment for health care, the role of women in medicine, and the influence of osteopathy will be examined from the perspective of these doctors' experiences.

Libraries contain many books that describe the illnesses of presidents and the treatments of selected physicians. This book is the first to examine all the presidents' physicians, their stories, their careers, and their variable relationships with their presidential patients.

Editorial necessity concluded both this edition's research and narration at the end of 2023, which precluded discussion of President Biden's 2024 cognitive decline.

Secondly Presidential Physician Ronny Jackson, designated as Rear Admiral in the text, was reduced in rank to Captain, probably for political reasons. The demotion only became public in 2024.

Introduction

From the First Edition

Of the presidents of the United States, eight have died during their presidential tenure, while a number of others have become disabled while in office, as a result of either significant surgical operations (Grover Cleveland, Ronald Reagan), severe medical illnesses (James Monroe, Woodrow Wilson, Franklin Roosevelt), or mental depression (John Adams, Calvin Coolidge).[1] In fact, almost all of our presidents, men of mature age, have had occasion to seek medical attention for illnesses during their presidencies. Consequently, contact between presidential patients and their physicians has been a constant in its frequency, although it has varied in its intensity depending upon the identity of the president. Moreover, the nature and complexity of this relationship has evolved significantly over the course of two hundred years.

Medical historians have published comprehensive studies of the health of presidents before, during, and after their presidencies, commencing with the seminal work of Rudolph Marx, whose *Health of the Presidents* was published in 1960.[2] A second seminal work was Kenneth R. Crispell and Carlos Gomez's *Hidden Illness in the White House*, which appeared in 1988. This book explored the cover-ups of significant presidential illnesses, often done with the complicity of the presidential physician. *Hidden Illness in the White House* initiated a series of investigative works that probed deception and deceit practiced by the White House to hide or diminish presidential sicknesses.[3]

In addition, a growing body of scholarship has explored in detail the illnesses of selected presidents. These monographs generally focus upon the health history of a single president and examine the effects of illness upon his political demeanor and policy decisions. They also incidentally provide rich insights into the treatments, character, and behavior of the pertinent White House physicians.[4]

A third subgenre in this field of study has been the memoirs of presidential physicians. Doctors Cary Grayson,[5] Ross McIntire,[6] Janet Travell[7] and Burton Smith[8] have written accounts of their intimate associations with individual presidents. These accounts not only describe their treatments, some of which were highly controversial, but also their personal and professional relationship with the president. Biographers have chronicled the lives of other eminent physicians who have had the responsibility of treating presidents in the White House.[9] For example, the first physician to take care of a sitting president was Dr. Samuel Bard, who treated the newly inaugurated George Washington in New York City. Bard is the subject of a biography by J. Brett Langstaff.[10]

Despite this extensive body of work, a book that comprehensively analyzes the 200-year experience of physicians who have treated presidents has not been written.

No history exists that focuses on this complex physician–presidential patient relationship, a relationship, that has changed significantly over time. This book is intended to fill that void.

In addition there has been no comprehensive evaluation of the qualifications, training, professional certification, and organizational relationships of the many men, and the rare women, who have provided medical care in the White House. These doctors have held many titles over the years which have confused discussion: Presidential Physician, Physician to the President, White House Physician, and White House Doctor. Specific designations have evolved with time, but, fortunately, official definitions have been adopted more recently.[11]

The White House Physician, the title of this book, was selected as the most recognizable designation that would include all the physicians who provided medical care to sitting presidents from George Washington to the present. However, it was only in the 1920s that "White House Physician" appeared as a government title (see Chapter 6), although Dr. Presley Rixey had unofficially assumed near full-time responsibilities at the White House twenty years earlier (see Chapter 5).

This work concentrates neither upon the details of presidential illnesses nor their treatments. These subjects have been well covered in the literature previously noted. Presidential illness will be covered tangentially only as it deals with the interrelationships, political pressures, and professional behaviors of the White House physicians. Nor does this work concentrate on the evolution in medical treatment or upon the disparity of care between that of the public and the president. Both of these worthy topics could be a book unto themselves.

Medical care of presidents has evolved from the episodic to the continuous, from the treatment of acute illnesses to an ongoing maintenance of the patient's health, from civilian to military to civilian and back again, from independent practitioners to government employees, from a one-on-one personal, and frequently intimate, relationship to a more complex connection with a modern semi-bureaucratic health care organization (the White House Medical Unit). In like manner the responsibilities of the White House physicians have evolved and increased. For example, contingency planning for the proper implementation of the Twenty-fifth Amendment to the Constitution, the presidential disability and succession amendment, has recently been added as a major duty. Soon thereafter, medical coverage was extended to the vice presidential family. The political pressures upon the White House physician have been many, since the president not only possesses the powers of the presidency, but also controls the reward and benefits system of his physician. Instances of political control and physician acquiescence, and misuse of the patient confidentiality privilege will be presented. Finally this book devotes special attention to issues of physician deference, as it is expressed in medical decision making by committees of physicians, in power relationships between the presidential physician and his subordinates and consultants, and in conflicts, perceived or real, between civilian and military doctors who take care of an ill president.

A recounting of the 200-year history of presidential physicians may have an additional benefit. It provides a useful matrix upon which to chronicle the dramatic developments in practice, competence, organization and scope that have occurred in American medicine during the corresponding time span. During the colonial and antebellum eras, presidential physicians were the products of varied educational venues— apprenticeship with a practicing physician, European training, and attending American medical schools, with or without the attainment of a doctorate of medicine. The first American medical school was established in Philadelphia in 1765.[12] During the succeeding century and a half, the schools first developed slowly both in numbers and in the rigor of their training, then experienced a rapid and uncontrolled growth spurt for most of the nineteenth century.[13] At that point they became regulated by societal and governmental influences. As a result, the number of American medical colleges declined sharply from 162 in 1906 to 81 in 1922.[14] The educational experiences of the physicians who treated American presidents illustrate this phenomenon.

The scientific expanse and reliability of medical knowledge has changed dramatically since George Washington's era, and this trend has accelerated over the past 100 years. A corresponding inevitability in the length and complexity of the postgraduate education of physicians has resulted, with the appearance first of the hospital internship, then residency training, professional specialization, and the conferring of board certification. The training experiences of the White House physicians likewise reflect this evolution.

The Pennsylvania Hospital was founded in Philadelphia in 1751 as the first hospital in the United States.[15] Few additional American hospitals were established until the 1880s, when a period of enormous growth commenced.[16] Many sitting presidents, including Washington, William Henry Harrison, Garfield and Wilson were ill to a degree that in the modern era would have demanded hospitalization. Surprisingly, the first sitting president to be admitted to a standard hospital was Harry Truman in 1952.[17] The reasons for this apparent neglect will be examined as the evolution of the American hospital is considered in the context of presidential health.

Physician compensation has become increasingly institutionalized over the past 200 years. Many of the early presidents paid their doctors on a fee for service basis, but during the latter part of the nineteenth century payment for services rendered became bureaucratized as the treating physicians were increasingly employees of the government. In recent decades third party payment by insurance companies has been a factor in settling a president's financial liability for incurred medical expenses.

Finally, two other historical topics are of interest. They are sectarian medicine, especially the rise and fall of homeopathy during the nineteenth century, and the rise of osteopathic medicine during the twentieth. Interestingly, at least two doctors who were the principal presidential caregivers were homeopathically trained, but the only identified osteopaths served in secondary roles.

The role of women in medicine has increased dramatically during the past half-century. After a rise in the numbers of female doctors during the late nineteenth century, their prominence diminished precipitously during the first half of the twentieth, only to be reversed by cultural and equity considerations during the second half of the twentieth century. However, female representation among White House physicians lagged, and it has been only recently that the first two women have been appointed presidential physicians.

About the Second Edition

Why a second edition of *The White House Physician*? Since this book was published in 2007, four different presidents have cumulatively served eighteen years in office. During this period five different physicians have attended the president as his personal doctor.

All the recent presidential physicians have been male, although an occasional female physician has graced the White House Medical Unit (WHMU), and two have been osteopaths. Whether the composition of the presidential physicians or the WHMU in general reflect the composition either of women or of osteopathic physicians in the United States' doctor population will be updated.

The White House Medical Unit continues to evolve; the physician to the president remains focused upon the first family's care, while the responsibilities, duties, and personnel of the rest of the White House medical personnel are directed by a non-physician, either a nurse or a physician's assistant who is subject to a military command structure. Additionally, there has been increased recruitment of both physician assistants (PAs) and Emergency Room doctors into its ranks.

Recent Doctors to the President Richard Tubb, Jeff Kuhlmann, Ronny Jackson, and Sean Conley were military officers. However, for the first time in almost thirty years, a civilian doctor, Kevin O'Connor, was selected by President Joe Biden to fill this role.

Three further issues will be examined in length in the second edition:

The Twenty-fifth Amendment has been invoked at least twice more recently. Its Section 3 deals with the voluntary surrender of executive powers by the president, and its recovery by the president is deemed able to reassume his duties. The circumstances of its use will be considered at length in a revised chapter.

Twenty-fifth Amendment Section 4 was raised in political and press speculation during the Donald Trump and Joe Biden administrations. The issue was whether either Trump or Biden suffered from a cognitive impairment so severe that they were disabled from fulfilling their oath of office.

Thirdly, the treatment of the president has become so politicized that the physician has been attacked personally by a hostile press corps and its biased acolytes. Dissension and intramural conflict among members of the WHMU was rumored. As a result, former Navy Admiral Ronny Jackson resigned and commenced a political career. He was elected as a Republican from Texas to the U.S. House of Representatives in 2020. The character of the physician to the president had not been so disparaged since the tenure of Dr. Wallace Graham during the Truman administration.

After almost twenty years, new book manuscripts and recent scholarship have brought to light new information about the physician who cared for Presidents Andrew Jackson, Franklin Roosevelt and Ronald Reagan. Their chapters are updated to include the new material.

Chapter 1

Samuel Bard

The First Presidential Physician

It was on a late spring Saturday, June 13, 1789, that Dr. Samuel Bard was summoned to a home at No. 3 Cherry Street in lower Manhattan described as "the plainly but handsomely furnished residence" of the newly inaugurated first president of the United States of America, General George Washington.[1] Washington had delivered his inaugural address in New York City, the nation's first capital, on April 30, 1789, only six weeks earlier.[2] The eminent patient had been struck with a high fever and violent pains in his left thigh.[3] Thus commenced the intriguing and fluid narrative of professional contact between physicians and their presidential patients.

Doctor James Craik of Alexandria, Virginia, had been Washington's close friend, comrade-in-arms and personal physician for decades, and would have been, in the words of the president, "the man of my choice in all cases of sickness." However, recognizing the reality of the situation, Washington lamented "…how far the circumstances at present would justify his quitting his practice in Alexandria, and its vicinity to gratify his inclinations and my wishes…."[4] Instead, Samuel Bard, a mere acquaintance, was summoned to the president's residence, because, as his biographer noted, "…in those days Sam Bard was at the height of his professional career."[5]

During this illness and a second serious illness one year later, several significant precedents evolved from the Bard-Washington professional relationship. For the next seventy-five years, doctors were called to diagnose and treat presidents, episodically, for acute medical problems. These physicians were mainly, but not all, civilian practitioners without any formal connection to the government, and they were compensated on a fee for service basis by the respective presidents. Washington's selection of the gifted Bard, the most prominent doctor present in colonial New York City despite the latter's known Tory sympathies was a wise decision. Unfortunately, some of Washington's successors neglected to follow his example and chose their physicians for reasons other than excellence.

In addition, recurring themes emanated from Washington's second illness, namely management by committee in times of medical crisis, a fixation upon secrecy during threatening presidential illnesses, and the imposition of political considerations upon the words and deeds of the presidential physicians. The following descriptions of the careers of doctors James Craik and Samuel Bard and of George Washington's pre-presidential and presidential medical history are described in detail in this chapter because of their precedent-setting nature. Virtually everything Washington did, or didn't do, became a precedent because he was the first.

The future president, although a hardy man who had lived an active life of farming, surveying and soldiering before he took office, suffered from a myriad of infectious diseases. In his youth he contracted smallpox in Barbados that marked his face permanently with scars. He suffered with intermittent dysentery, which was so profound that Dr. James Craik ordered him home from active military service in 1757. In 1761 and again in 1786, Washington experienced attacks of ague and fever, most likely due to malaria. As treatment, Dr. Craik administered quinine, in the form of Jesuit bark derived from the cinchona tree. Rheumatism of the shoulder, quinsy, and extreme dental decay were a few of the other maladies that plagued the man.[6]

James Craik, Scottish by birth, received his academic and medical education at the University of Edinburgh, which at the time was not only the premier site for educating English-speaking students in medicine, but also a primary resource in the training of other future presidential physicians. Craik left Scotland in the 1750s, apparently, as was common, without obtaining a medical degree. He joined the British army and was posted as a physician, first to the West Indies, and then to General Braddock's British-Virginian Army in Pennsylvania. This was where he became, first, the physician to George Washington, and secondly, his good friend. Craik subsequently served with distinction in the colonial army's medical department. Craik was awarded an honorary medical degree from the University of Pennsylvania in 1782 for his services to the new nation. After the Revolution, Washington, persuaded his physician and friend to settle in Alexandria, Virginia, in order to be close to Mount Vernon. When the retired president became ill with his terminal throat infection in December 1799, it was to Craik that he turned for medical assistance. Craik responded immediately, and was one of three physicians who attended the ex-president on his deathbed.[7]

Samuel Bard, the son of respected New York physician John Bard, had the advantage of an excellent education. He attended King's College, now Columbia University,

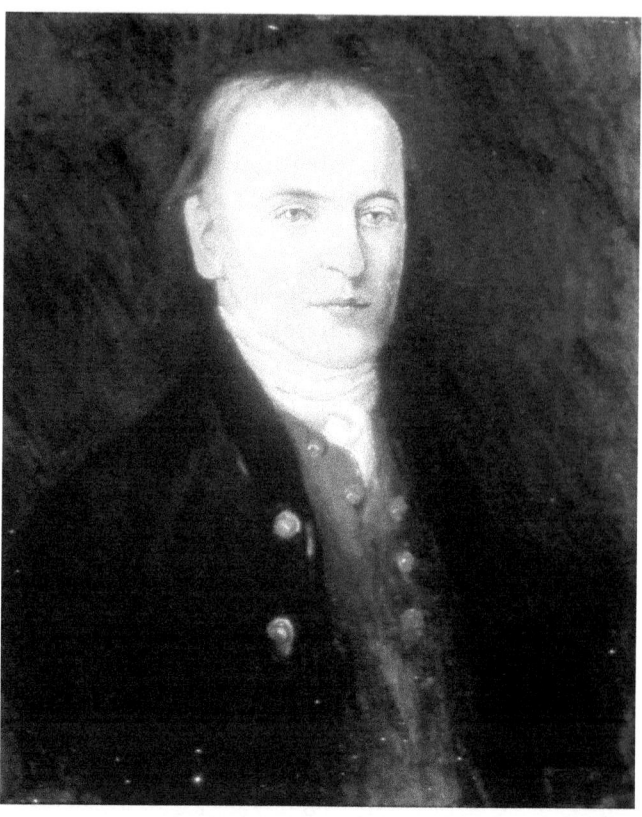

James Craik. Oil painting of Dr. Craik. Edinburgh-trained physician and longtime doctor to George Washington. Craik was unable to relinquish his Virginia medical practice to care for the first American president in the capital cities of New York and Philadelphia. (National Library of Medicine)

and then traveled to Europe for his formal medical training. A prior college education was unusual for an eighteenth-century medical student; it would not become a prerequisite for medical school admission until the twentieth century.

Bard subsequently graduated from the prestigious University of Edinburgh medical school where he spent the greater part of three years in the 1760s. The medical school of the University of Edinburgh was the institution of choice for those Americans of wit, ambition, and means who strove to achieve a doctorate of medicine during this country's colonial and early national periods.[8] It was only in 1765 that the first American medical school was established in Philadelphia, with a second founded in New York City in 1768. It was not until near the turn of the nineteenth century that America's third and fourth medical schools were opened.[9] As a consequence, although colonial Americans might visit London hospitals to learn practical medicine, it was only the Edinburgh school, with its complement of excellent professors and its integration with a teaching hospital, that enabled Americans to return home with an M.D. degree.[10]

The University of Edinburgh had been founded in the late sixteenth century,[11] and its medical school had its antecedents as early as 1685.[12] Alexander Monro was appointed Professor of Anatomy in January 1720, but it was only in 1726, with the appointment of four additional professors who like Monro had studied at Leiden University under the tutelage of the famous medical educator Herman Boerhaave, that the Edinburgh School of medicine was officially chartered.[13] At the onset of the eighteenth century, the University of Leiden school of medicine and Boerhaave, its eminent professor of botany, chemistry, and medicine, attracted medical students and physicians from all over Europe.[14]

The new medical school in the Scottish capital was innovative, including both the disciplines of medicine and surgery in its curriculum, and providing practical exposure in a teaching hospital. The Edinburgh Infirmary opened in 1741 with

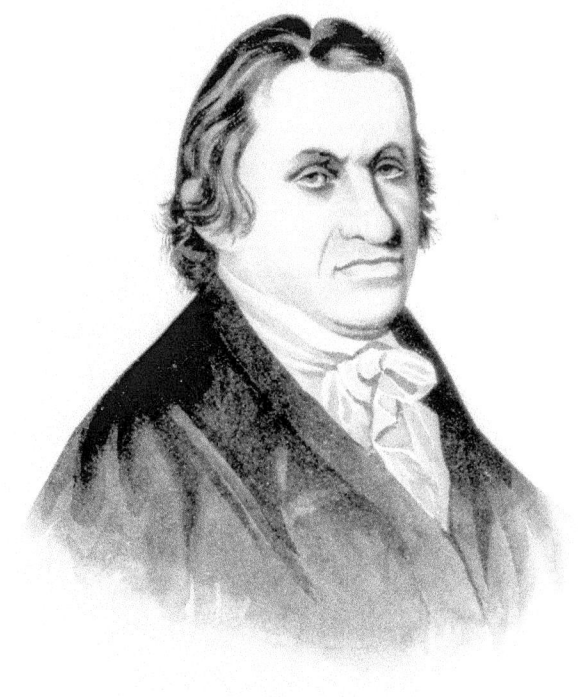

DR. SAMUEL BARD.

Samuel Bard. Edinburgh-educated Samuel Bard of New York became the first presidential physician when he treated President George Washington on two occasions in New York for life-threatening illnesses. (National Library of Medicine) accommodations for 228 beds, additional facilities for the insane, consulting and waiting rooms for physicians and patients, and, significantly, a surgical amphitheater with viewing room for upwards of 200 medical students.[15]

During the last half of the seventeenth century, from 1749 to 1799, 117 Americans received medical degrees from Edinburgh. Many others, both American and British, attended a variety of courses without formal graduation. Scotsman James Craik was a notable example of the latter; the average number of medical students attending each year (1776–1783) was 400 but only 22 students graduated annually with a medical degree.[16] The medical school in Edinburgh, then a city of 80,000 inhabitants, had become the ancestral source for the professional formation not only of America's first physician-educators, but also of many who would heal its presidents.[17]

Prominent American medical graduates of Edinburgh included John Morgan (M.D. 1763), a founder of the first American medical school in Philadelphia; William Shippen, Jr., (M.D. 1761), charter professor of anatomy, surgery and midwifery at the same school; Adam Kuhn (M.D. 1767), this school's charter professor of Materia medica and botany; John Witherspoon (M.A. 1739), a signer of the Declaration of Independence, and Benjamin Rush (M.D. 1765), also a signer of the Declaration of Independence. Rush went on to become a friend of presidents; but his professional influence surpassed any political standing. Not only did Rush, together with fellow Edinburgh alumni Morgan, Shippen and Kuhn, form the charter faculty of the first American medical school, but

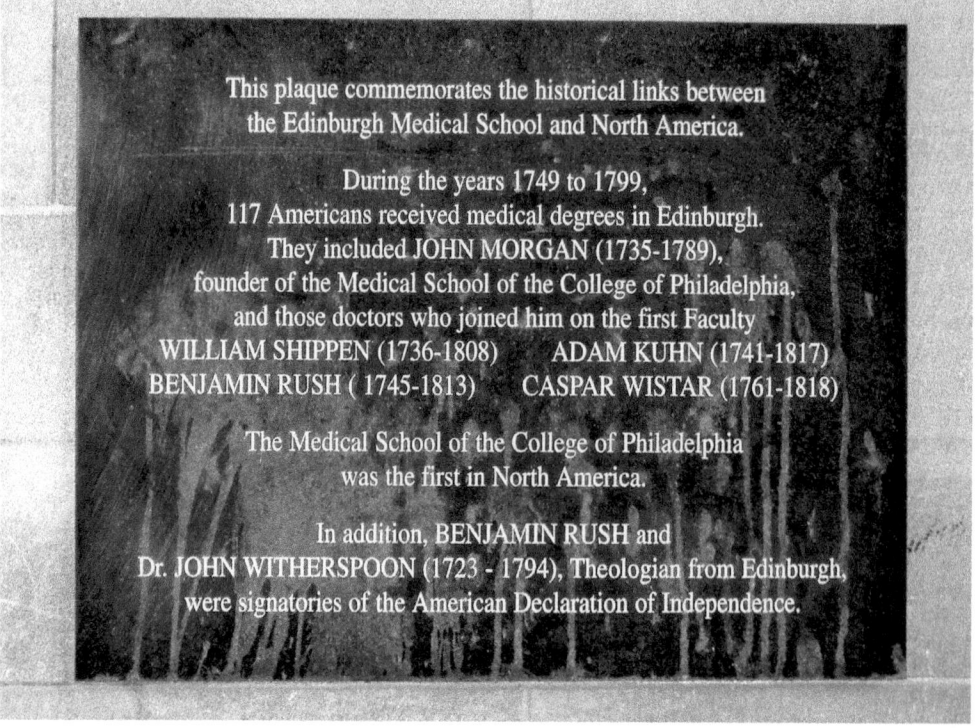

University of Edinburgh Plaque. Plaque at the gate of Edinburgh medical school quadrangle honoring graduates who founded the first medical school in America, the Medical School of the College of Philadelphia. (Courtesy of Jim Edmondson)

his long tenure there also allowed him to become the most influential teacher of future American physicians during the late eighteenth and early nineteenth centuries. Today a plaque at the courtyard entrance to the University of Edinburgh commemorates its alumni who had founded the Philadelphia medical school. The future presidential physician, Samuel Bard, received his medical degree from Edinburgh in 1765, the same year as Rush.[18]

Thomas Tudor Tucker was another future presidential physician, attending Edinburgh between 1765 and 1770 and receiving his medical degree in 1770. Tucker, a future Treasurer of the United States, was one of the physicians who attended President James Madison during his 1813 illness.[19] In 1833 President Andrew Jackson consulted with the appropriately named Dr. Philip Syng Physick in Philadelphia for injuries caused by an old bullet wound. Dr. Physick was a 1792 graduate of the University of Edinburgh.[20] That same year another Edinburgh alumnus Dr. John Collins Warren (M.D. 1801), treated Jackson when he became seriously ill in Boston.[21]

In addition to establishing the first (Pennsylvania) and second (Columbia) American medical colleges, Edinburgh's academic progeny were involved in the formation of still others. Dr. Gustavus Richard Brown (M.D. 1768) was one of the 101 cofounders of the Medical and Chirurgical Faculty of Maryland in 1799. In 1802 this organization appointed a committee to establish a college of physicians in Maryland; this effort achieved the establishment in 1807 of the University of Maryland School of Medicine, the nation's first public and fifth oldest medical college. The Edinburgh alumnus did not live to witness the school's foundation, since he died in 1804. Dr. Brown was also one of the two doctors to assist James Craik during George Washington's mortal illness.[22]

Samuel Latham Mitchill (M.D. 1786) of New York decided to pursue the paradoxical careers of scientist, medical educator and politician. He served in both the United States House of Representatives and the Senate from 1801 to 1813, but his pertinence to

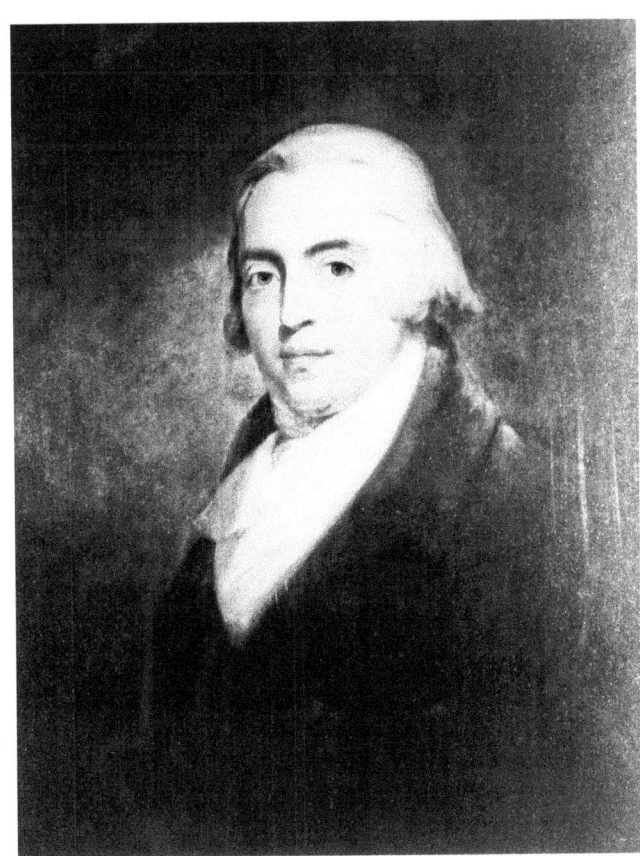

Philip Syng Physick. Philip Syng Physick received his medical degree from Edinburgh. Many years later President Andrew Jackson sought his medical opinion in Philadelphia. (National Library of Medicine)

this story is dependent upon the following biographical gleaning: "In 1826 he helped found Rutgers Medical College and served as its Vice President during the four years of its existence."[23]

Doctor John Bard, Samuel's father, had sought advice about his son's medical education from William Samuel Johnson, the president of King's College, New York. They agreed that Sam should go abroad for his studies since "he could have no hospital experience equal to that of London," and that Edinburgh's faculty had a high reputation.[24] Consequently young Bard, like other Americans of his era, commenced his European studies in London. As a start he read the Materia medica, witnessed operations at the Saint Thomas and Guy's hospitals, and attended medical lectures.[25] In September 1762 he commenced the required three years of education at Edinburgh. According to the prerequisites for graduation, Bard submitted his thesis, titled *Testamen medicum inaugurale de veribus opii,* a description of the effects of opium on the human system. After approval of his thesis, he passed an oral examination in Latin by two professors, and received his M.D. degree.[26]

Bard returned to the colonies and embarked on his career, which was composed partially of clinical practice in concert with his father, and partially of medical education and organization. The younger Bard was one of the five founding physicians of the medical school of King's College, now Columbia, the second American medical college. He held its chair of theory and practice of physic. In addition, he was one of the founding physicians of a prominent hospital. The cornerstone of this hospital, the New York Hospital, was laid in 1773.[27]

Bard's attitude towards the American Revolution was at best ambivalent. His cousin, William Bard, was a British officer who died at the Battle of Bunker Hill,[28] while his brother, John, served in the Colonial Army.[29] Bard described his stance as nonpartisan, but there was undoubted sympathy for the mother country where he had been educated. He remained in New York City after its occupation by the British, but his political position, according to his biographer, "was diminishing his medical

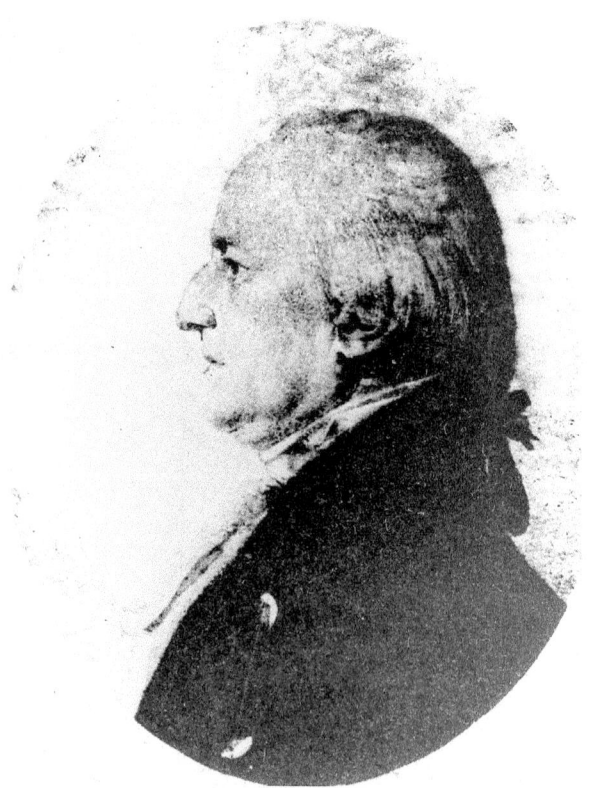

Thomas Tudor Tucker. Dr. Thomas Tudor Tucker, a 1770 graduate from the University of Edinburgh, attended President James Madison during Madison's 1813 illness. (Library of Congress)

practice in the city," and the loss of patients had led to financial embarrassment.[30] After leaving New York, he moved to his father's estate in New Hyde Park, New York, and then to New Jersey. Subsequently, through the use of his important contacts, Bard returned to British-occupied New York City, and rebuilt a substantial practice.[31] He had refused to take an oath of loyalty to the Continental Congress,[32] and at the conclusion of the Revolutionary War he and his family evacuated the city with the Loyalists to the English crown. However, in 1784 Dr. Bard returned once again to New York City, drawn by his involvement with the King's College medical school.[33]

Bard's ambivalent political past certainly did not disqualify him from serving the president. He was cho-

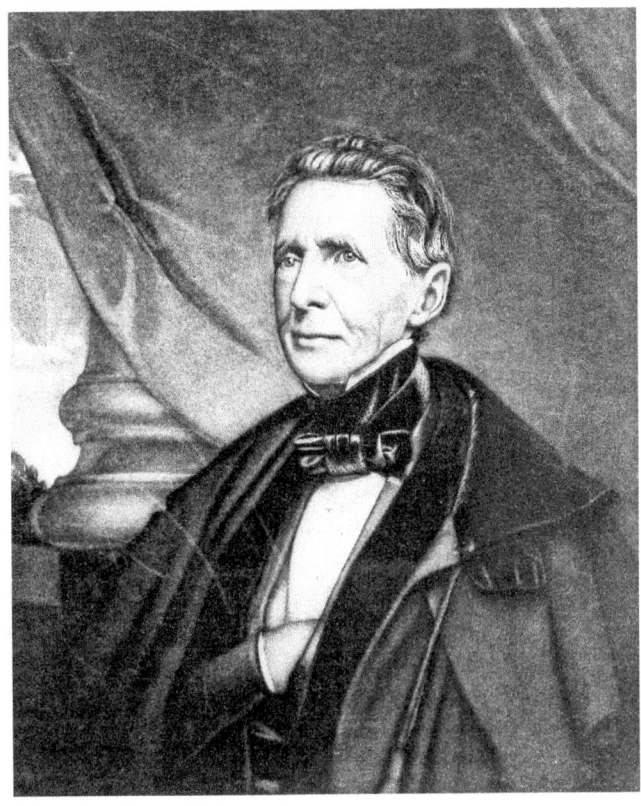

John Collins Warren. The prominent Boston physician Dr. John Collins Warren bled the ailing President Andrew Jackson during Jackson's trip to New England. (National Library of Medicine)

sen, as several have written, "because there never was a medical man in the city of New York, so much beloved and esteemed as a practitioner."[34] Bard examined Washington and detected a tumor of his left thigh that was described as one "that grew fast and took on a fiery hue; soreness spread to such an extent that he could not sit down except in acute pain."[35] Tobias Lear, the president's secretary, classified the swelling as a malignant carbuncle, or anthrax.[36] In retrospect, Washington's condition has been diagnosed as a bacterial abscess. Bard accurately perceived that the abscess required immediate incision and drainage, and advised his patient that although an operation might not prevent his death there was no alternative. Several days later, under the wise counsel of his experienced father, Dr. John Bard, the younger Bard lanced and cut away the abscessed swelling. Washington's recovery was slow, and several unrelated minor illnesses intervened that required 109 days of clinical attendance by the two doctors Bard.[37]

Samuel and John Bard submitted a bill for professional services rendered during the period June 15 to October 2, 1789, for 84 pounds, 3 shillings. In so doing, they established the precedent of fee for service for the medical care of a president. When this bill was paid by George Washington, he thereby assumed personal, and not public sector, responsibility for payment.[38] These physicians had charged Washington a princely sum for their medical services. In comparison, at this time, the average annual income for skilled artisans, like carpenters and craftsmen, in London and in Wales was between 55 and 60 pounds.[39]

Washington suffered a second serious, potentially fatal illness in New York City during May and June 1790. The president's diary entry for May 9 read: "Indisposed with a bad cold." The next entry ominously did not appear until June 24, 1790.[40] The cold progressed to a life-threatening pneumonia. The circumstances of the stricken president's medical attendance during this episode are somewhat unclear, but Major William Jackson, in the absence of Washington's faithful assistant, Tobias Lear, assumed control of the situation. Jackson apparently summoned Samuel Bard first, and when Washington demonstrated no improvement, he engaged both doctors Charles MacNight, a friend and military colleague of the president, and John Charlton. The nature of the interaction between these physicians has not been recorded, other than they cooperated in the traditional behavior of physicians when confronted with serious medical challenges, which is, *management by committee*. This activity, whether employed to seek out the best advice or to diffuse responsibility or blame if the outcome was untoward, is magnified whenever the patient in distress is very important (VIP Medicine). VIP Medicine for a president would be practiced many times during future crises.

When the patient was *in extremis* on May 12, his physicians wished to enlarge their committee, and so sent for Dr. John Jones from Philadelphia.[41] The honor and responsibility of treating a president frequently attracts the most eminent and renowned physicians. Jones certainly qualified for this description. At the time, he served as the physician to Benjamin Franklin, and had authored the first American text in surgery. Jones had received his medical education, both as an apprentice to Dr. Thomas Calwalader in the United States and as a student at the premier European medical centers of Edinburgh, London, Paris and Leyden. His medical degree was from the University of Rheims. He probably was known to Washington for his medical service in

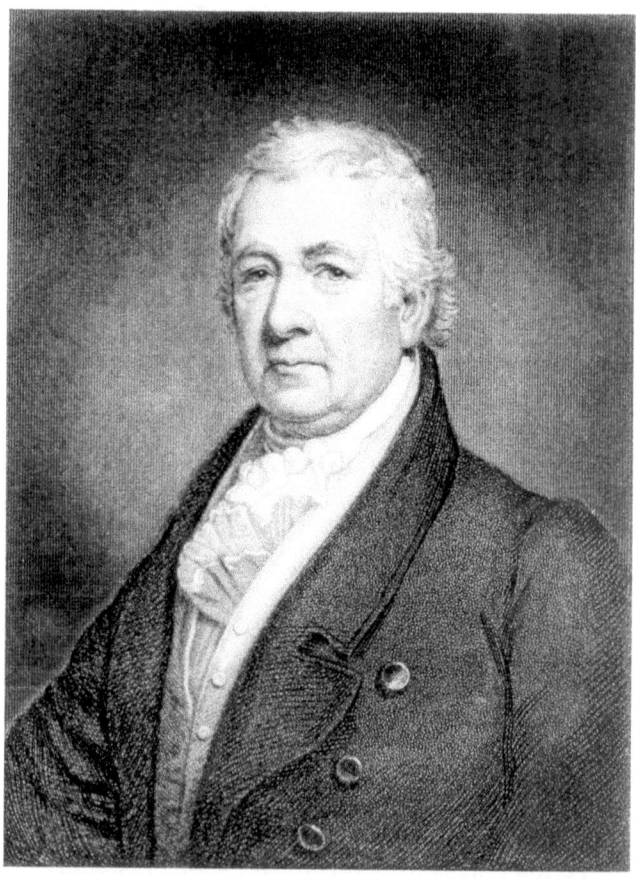

Samuel Mitchill. Samuel Mitchill, another American who graduated from the University of Edinburgh medical school, also played a significant role in early American medical education. (National Library of Medicine)

both the French and Indian and Revolutionary wars. He certainly was well known to Bard, since Jones had been a colleague in establishing both the King's College School of Medicine and the New York Hospital.[42]

Secrecy and political considerations are both introduced into this narrative by the summoning of Jones. Jackson dispatched a coach to Philadelphia and extended every effort to ensure that Jones' consultation remained clandestine.[43] Jackson wrote a letter to Clement Biddle in Philadelphia which in turn contained an enclosed letter for Jones. Within, in addition to an urgent request for Jones' services in New York, Jackson suggested, "The Doctor's presence will suggest the propriety of setting out as privately as possible, perhaps it may be well to assign a personal reason for visiting New York, or going into the Country."[44] The collection of these physicians, whether deliberately or inadvertently, was successful in curing their patient, since Washington recovered completely from the pneumonia.

Images of contemporary presidential medical care usually include technologically advanced spaces occupied by sophisticated teams of health care specialists. Such images are unknown in the context of eighteenth and nineteenth-century medical care of sick United States chief executives. It is only in recent times that a sitting president has been treated in a hospital, even for a life-threatening emergency. There was no hospital in New York City at the time of George Washington's 1789 and 1790 illnesses.

Even the few existing hospitals were woefully inadequate. The first hospital on American soil, for example, was the Pennsylvania Hospital in Philadelphia, founded in 1751. Although beds were available for patients in 1755, the hospital was not fully functional until 1805 due to lags in fund-raising and the uncertainties of the Revolutionary War.[45]

Samuel Bard, interestingly, was one of the founders of the second American hospital, the New York Hospital on Manhattan Island. This hospital had been chartered by King George III on June 13, 1771. Its cornerstone was laid on July 23, 1773, and at the outbreak of the War of Independence, it was almost completed. However, the building remained practically idle for many years thereafter and was only opened for patients on January 3, 1791, after the seat of the United States government had moved to Philadelphia.[46] The only New York institution that remotely resembled a hospital at the time of Washington's illnesses was a room set aside for the indigent. A single room, thirty-five by twenty-three feet, had been set aside as an infirmary, in the building known as the Publick Workhouse and House of Correction of the City of New York.[47]

The 1790 removal of the capital to Philadelphia severed the president's association with the first presidential physician. Samuel Bard continued his productive associations with King's, which shortly became Columbia School of Medicine and the New York Hospital. He became dean of the medical faculty at the former and senior attending physician at the latter. His medical practice continued to be active, and one of his patients was Alexander Hamilton. Moreover, Bard was active in fighting the New York yellow fever epidemics of 1795 and 1798. He contracted the disease himself during the 1798 epidemic and almost died. At age 56, Bard retired to New Hyde Park to be near his family and to pursue his interest in botany.[48]

In Philadelphia, George Washington's medical history was not as dramatic. Doctor John Jones became the family physician there, but the extent and circumstances of any care rendered to the president are not recorded. Upon Jones' death in 1791, Dr. Adam Kuhn, then professor of the theory and practice of medicine at the Philadelphia school, became the family physician and treated George Washington Custis' measles. Custis was the son of the president's stepson. Kuhn was identified as "now generally considered the leading physician in the city."[49] No health crises confronted the first president during his tenure in Philadelphia. Thomas Jefferson, in a letter to James Madison, described "little lingering fevers hanging around him for a week or ten days."[50] A skin lesion may have been excised from the president's face in 1794.[51] Furthermore, the president wrenched his back while horseback riding to inspect the new federal city on the banks of the Potomac.[52] However there is no evidence that Kuhn actually treated the first president.

Samuel Bard, the first presidential physician, attended the first president during two serious medical emergencies. From these encounters several traditions began, including the manner of selection, fee for service, management by committee, the maintenance of secrecy, and political interference.

Neither of Washington's immediate successors, John Adams and Thomas Jefferson, suffered from significant acute illnesses while president. Consequently, professional medical care was not sought either by Adams in Philadelphia or by Jefferson in Washington, D.C., which had become the nation's third and permanent capital in 1800. President Jefferson frequently sought out the company of physicians, but the nature of his contacts was principally philosophical and intellectual rather than medical or therapeutic. However, he occasionally consulted with his friend and cosigner of the Declaration of Independence, doctor Benjamin Rush of Philadelphia, on health matters. But Jefferson seldom accepted his friend's advice. His opinion of Rush's "heroic treatments" was expressed in an 1814 letter, in which Jefferson wrote, "In his theory of bleeding.... I was ever opposed to my friend Rush, whom I greatly loved; but who has done much harm."[53] Jefferson's attitude towards contemporary medicine was summed up in this famous opinion expressed to Dr. Robley Dunglison: "That whenever he saw three physicians together, he looked upward to discover whether there

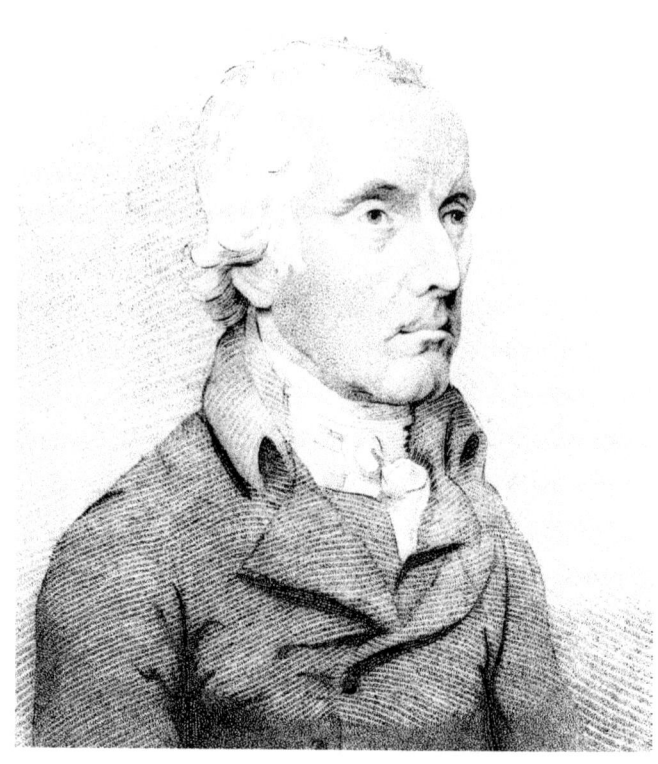

Benjamin Rush. Benjamin Rush, a member of the charter faculty of the first American medical school, was the preeminent medical educator during the later 18th and early 19th centuries. (National Library of Medicine)

was not a turkey buzzard in the neighborhood."[54] In his daily habits, Jefferson emphasized the importance of health maintenance rather than the treatment of acute illness, thereby anticipating the thinking of White House physicians by nearly 200 years.[55]

It is not an easy matter to discard Dr. Rush from this narrative even though any direct care of a president is lacking. However, as a result of his long professorial tenure at the University of Pennsylvania, he became a major influence that shaped the medical philosophy of hundreds of physicians, including some who did become the doctors of presidents.[56] Rush also was the first American practitioner to develop theories of the causes and treatment of mental diseases.[57] Finally Rush was a political and personal friend to both John Adams and Thomas Jefferson. President Adams, at a time when the doctor had suffered financial reverses, appointed Rush to the directorship of the United States mint. It was Benjamin Rush who initiated the epistolary reconciliation of the two ex-presidents in their retirement. Both Adams and Jefferson issued extremely laudatory comments at the time of Rush's death in 1813.[58]

Chapter 2

The Pillars of the Profession
Presidential Physicians, 1812–1865

On the morning of September 26, 1817, in a small hotel or tavern called Tennison's, situated on Pennsylvania Avenue near Fourteenth Street in the still-infant city of Washington, D.C., sixteen physicians, including nearly all those practicing in Washington and Georgetown, gathered to discuss the formation of a medical society. On the following January 5 its officers were elected. The articles of incorporation of the newly formed Medical Society of the District of Columbia were submitted for government approval later in 1818; on February 16, 1819, President James Monroe signed his approval. Presidential physicians Arnold Elzey, John Thomas Shaff, Nicholas Worthington, Frederick May, Henry Huntt and Thomas Sim were among the organizers of the new society.[1] Two other eminent doctors of the city, James Crowdhill Hall and Thomas Miller later held important positions with this organization; both served as its president.[2] Robert King Stone, the Lincoln family's physician, was a member of the Society's Board of Examiners from 1855 to 1857,[3] and at its May 3, 1865, meeting, he read an account of the death of President Lincoln and the results of the autopsy.[4]

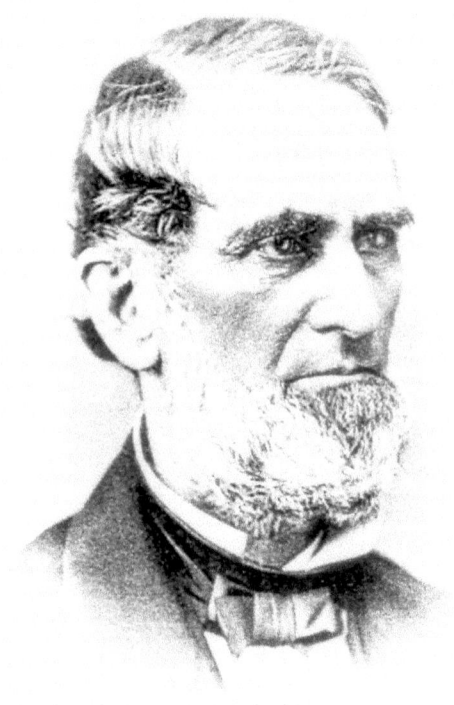

James Crowdhill Hall. James Crowdhill Hall was a Pillar of the Profession, one of an elite group of Washington physicians whose prestigious medical practice included presidents of the United States. (National Library of Medicine)

20

Chapter 2. The Pillars of the Profession

The story of the medical care provided to presidents, commencing with the inauguration of James Madison and terminating with the death of Abraham Lincoln, is dominated by five prominent leaders of the District's Medical Society: Huntt, Sim, Hall, Miller and Stone. Their historical significance and professional contributions entitle them to the designation Pillars of the Profession, and this chapter, so titled as an acknowledgment of them, will consider the contributions of these elite civilian physicians. Of the thirteen United States presidents who served during this period, six contracted serious illnesses and three of them died while in office. Charles Roos, a previous reference librarian of the National Library of Medicine, lists thirty-two physicians, excluding those present during Lincoln's death watch, for these thirteen leaders; in this survey several doctors appear multiple times because of service to more than one chief executive. Civilians dominated the presidents' medical care throughout the period; only seven of the enumerated doctors were military.[5]

An examination of the educational histories of the Pillars of the Profession illustrates the state of American medical education during the national and antebellum eras.[6] For Americans, the paradigm of educational excellence had shifted from an Edinburgh doctorate during the colonial period to a medical degree from an institution located on American soil, specifically the University of Pennsylvania. The physician-educator-public citizen Benjamin Rush serves as a convenient nexus between these two chapters of history. Rush, a signer of the Declaration of Independence, was a close friend of both John Adams and Thomas Jefferson, although he was a doctor to neither. He received his M.D. degree from the University of Edinburgh in 1768 and soon after he was appointed as one of the founding faculty of the institution that would become the Medical School of the University of Pennsylvania. As a renowned professor for over forty years, he was instrumental in the medical education of several thousand medical students, several of whom later treated American presidents.[7]

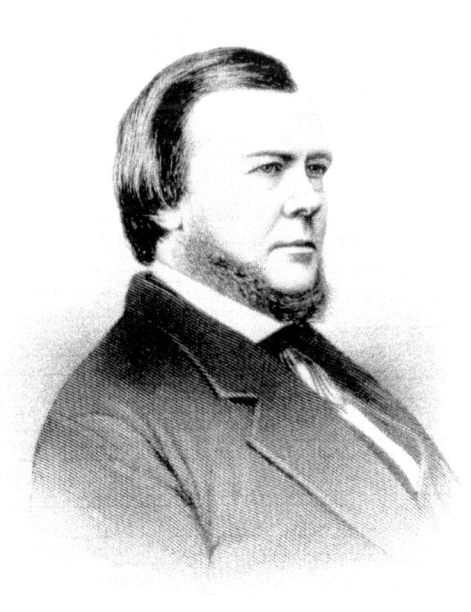

Robert King Stone. Dr. Robert King Stone was another of the Pillars of the Profession. He was the Lincoln family physician and a pioneer medical specialist who had an interest in ophthalmology. (National Library of Medicine)

Then as now, American presidents were served by doctors who were among the most educationally qualified, albeit, unfortunately, not always the most successful. At a time when most medical doctors were without extensive, or even any, formal didactic training, the early and mid-nineteenth-century presidents, with a rare exception, were under the care of a medical school graduate. In contrast, most doctors of this era were products of a frequently inadequate apprenticeship. The character and frequency of a medical apprenticeship will be examined later in this chapter. Postgraduate training and medical specialization would not become commonplace until the twentieth century. The experiences of Pillars James Hall and Robert Stone foreshadowed these trends by many years.

Prestigious members of the District of Columbia medical society were the physicians most often called upon when a president was acutely ill. Since the time span of their professional eminence usually exceeded the tenures of their presidential patients, these physicians often served more than one president: Henry Huntt (two), Thomas Sim (two), Thomas Miller (three), and James Crowdhill Hall (at least five). Care for the president and his extended family was but a part of busy practices that included many Washington families. For example, Dr. James Crowdhill Hall, who attended at least five different presidents, was also the physician during this era to the families of every justice of the Supreme Court, every cabinet member, every foreign legation, and every prominent senator and representative![8] These physicians were independent practitioners who engaged in episodic care and charged the patients a fee for their services. When a medical disaster struck, the Pillars were wise or cautious enough to draw in their fellows for consultation. Finally, two additional precedents were set during this period: overnight stays in the White House to provide continuous care to an ill president, and the publication by the treating physician of an *apologia* to explain the reasons for a disastrous outcome from his treatment.[9]

President James Monroe's presidential tenure (1817–1825) was marked by two serious illnesses: malaria in 1818,[10] and an episode in August 1823, when he was described as "suddenly seized ... with cramps or convulsions of such extreme violence that he was at one time believed dying...."[11] Monroe's intimate friend and personal physician of long duration, Charles Everett, a 1795 graduate of the University of Pennsylvania medical school,[12] unfortunately was not available for either illness. Everett had elected to continue his practice in rural Virginia and, following in the tradition of James Craik, did not relocate to the nation's capital city to care for his famous patient. Monroe's regard for Everett extended even to the political sphere, as revealed in a letter penned by the former to the latter in which Secretary of State Monroe described his working relationship with Everett to President Madison: "On publick [sic] affairs we confer without reserve, each party expressing his own sentiments and viewing dispassionate the existing state, animated by a sincere desire to promote the public welfare. I have full confidence that this relation will be always preserved in future...."[13]

Monroe's medical attendants in Washington during his 1818 illness are unnamed. However, the president returned to his Virginia home to convalesce from his bout with malaria and one might speculate that Dr. Everett attended him during his return.[14] Monroe continued to view Everett as a family physician, as is shown by several letters written to the doctor, solicitous of advice over his wife's, the first lady's, chronic ill health.[15] In an 1820 letter written in Highland, Virginia, Monroe requested his assistance: "It would be very gratifying to us, if you could make her an early visit, and after examining fully all the circumstances of her case, give your advice, as to the remedy to be pursued systematically thereafter."[16]

Navy physician Bailey Washington treated Monroe during his 1823 episode[17] and probably served as the Monroe family physician in Washington. In a November 1823 letter to Everett, the president wrote, "It has been thought by Dr. Huntt, who has attended her (Elizabeth Monroe, his wife) in the absence of Dr. Washington that the Erysipelas by fixing on her stomach, was her complaint...."[18] Doctor Thomas Sim also attended this president in the nation's capital.[19]

The Pillars established and promoted other important Washington health organizations. Doctors Huntt and Sim were charter members of the district's board of health, and afterward Huntt served as its president from 1822 to 1833. Miller and Stone were also its presidents, and Miller commenced the record keeping of Washington births during his tenure. Dr. Miller was active in the establishment of St. Elizabeth's Asylum, while Dr. Hall was named a trustee of the Washington City Orphan Asylum and was one of the incorporators of its Children's Hospital. Miller also was the physician to the district's jail for many years.[20]

Medical education and emergency care for the community also were pursued by these distinguished doctors. Hall had been the chairman of the department of surgery at Columbian College and, later, Stone was named professor of anatomy, physiology and microscopic anatomy and subsequently professor of ophthalmic and aural surgery at the National Medical College, Columbian College's successor.[21] Additionally, during the district's devastating cholera epidemic of 1832, Sim, Hall, Huntt, and Miller worked tirelessly and with distinction. During his service Thomas Sim contracted the infection and died.[22] James Hall's commitment to his community extended beyond medicine. He was one of the founding trustees of the Corcoran Art Gallery[23] and one of the directors of the society for the construction of the Washington Monument.[24]

Andrew Jackson was already sixty-two years of age when he was first inaugurated, but he served as president for two complete terms (1829–1837). Jackson's medical difficulties had been frequent, and of infectious, traumatic, and physician origins. For example, he suffered from retained bullets, within his left shoulder joint and his left lung, acquired during a gunfight and a duel. He also had survived both smallpox and malaria, and was weakened by a persistent diarrheal illness contracted during his military campaigns. In addition, he continued to experience the ill effects of the mercury, lead, and bloodletting therapies of his many physicians.[25]

President Jackson was as profligate in his selection of physicians as he was in his temperament. At least seven different doctors cared for him during his presidency. Old Hickory had a definite predilection for civilian physicians; on only a single occasion did a military doctor treat him. Thomas Harris, a navy surgeon, removed the bullet from Jackson's left shoulder in 1832.[26]

Neither Henry Huntt, one of Old Hickory's presidential physicians, nor doctors Francis May and John Esselman, who treated Jackson in Tennessee, possessed medical degrees. Instead, their training had been obtained by means of a medical apprenticeship.[27]

The standard of medical expertise in the urban centers along the Atlantic coast, including Washington, probably exceeded that which was available in the rural and interior sections of the country. Apprenticeship was the principal form of physician training during the colonial, national, and even the early antebellum periods. At the time of the Revolutionary War, 3,500 to 4,000 was the estimated number of practicing physicians in America. Only 400 had any formal medical education, and perhaps only about 200 had received a medical doctorate.[28] As late as 1850 in eastern Tennessee, only 35 of 201 (17 percent) doctors were medical school graduates; 42 of the remainder claimed to have taken medical courses or lectures. Presumably the majority of this sample had been trained as medical apprentices.[29]

The apprenticeship system commenced early in colonial America, and became more common after 1700. It prevailed during the eighteenth century; even during the early nineteenth century the great majority of American physicians had been trained as apprentices. Apprenticeship seemed to be reserved for males only; the only comparable opportunity that remained for women was midwifery.[30]

A male between the ages of fourteen and eighteen would be accepted into the office of a doctor who served as preceptor. Any physician could serve as preceptor; the limiting factor was his ability to attract willing apprentices. It was likely, but not certain, that the more reputable and accomplished would be the strongest magnets for drawing apprentices. The apprenticeship length was variable and the minimum length required for subsequent licensing was three years in most states. Although a three-year tenure was typical, lengths of up to seven years have been reported.[31]

A formal contract often was entered into between the apprentice and his preceptor, which detailed the reciprocal responsibilities of each. Occasionally its terms were so restrictive as to make the apprentice an indentured servant. Generally, a fee of $100 per annum was paid depending upon the renown of the preceptor. For this fee, the doctor provided medical instruction, food, drink, clothing, lodging, washing and mending. The apprentice would have access to the physician's library and would shadow his preceptor, first in the doctor's office, and later, when he was more experienced and competent, he would accompany the preceptor on his rounds. On occasion an advanced apprentice would substitute for his preceptor on a house call. Not surprisingly, an apprentice tended the sick slaves at Mount Vernon when the physician was unavailable.[32]

In return the apprentice would mix the doctor's chemicals, clean his office, and "even perform household chores."[33] The apprentice would gradually learn to bleed patients, prepare drugs, extract teeth, apply cupping, and in general assist his preceptor. In Virginia, the contract was written as "binding the apprentice to absolute obedience, forbidding him to divulge his master's secrets, or to marry, gamble, frequent alehouses, taverns, and play-houses."[34]

The quality of apprenticeship training was, unsurprisingly, extremely variable. There was no standardization, although apprenticeship over time came under the loose purview of state licensing laws. Unfortunately, this oversight was nominal, and all commentators have viewed the apprenticeship system as deeply flawed. As an example, the only access that an apprentice had to anatomical study was the chance arm or leg that had been traumatically amputated by an accident.[35]

The preceptor's principal commitment to his students was the provision of a certificate of completion at the conclusion of the apprenticeship. The certificate attested to the bearer's service and proficiency and was registered in a court of record. Its registration legally qualified the former apprentice as a practitioner of medicine.[36]

For some, medical apprenticeship in a modified form became a supplement rather than an alternative to formal medical school education. Many American medical schools required an apprenticeship of some sort prior to admission, since these schools provided little or no clinical training.[37] James Hall, after graduating from Jefferson College, Pennsylvania, in 1823, returned to Washington, D.C., and began the study of medicine with Dr. Thomas Henderson. After "having sufficiently grounded himself in the principles of medicine to make it profitable to attend lectures, in 1825 he attended the University of Pennsylvania."[38] Thomas Miller, as his daughter Virginia explained, also followed this track: "After completing his course of study at Gonzaga, my father began the study of medicine, studying chemistry and pharmacy practically with a druggist as a preparation. He studied medicine with both Dr. Cutbush and Dr. Henry Huntt, finally going to Philadelphia, where he graduated with much distinction in 1829."[39]

Apprenticeship disappeared as the requirements for medical licensing deteriorated between 1820 and 1870, contemporaneous with the rise of many poor quality American medical schools. A medical novice found that he could obtain a diploma in less than two years from these institutions, rather than indenturing himself to a medical master for three.[40] Thomas Sim was an example. He was the family physician during Jackson's term as a U.S. Senator from Tennessee from 1823 to 1825, and he resumed care when Jackson returned to Washington as the newly elected president in 1829. In his selection of Sim, Jackson probably deviated from President Washington's wise precedent of choosing the most qualified physician available regardless of personal or political attachments. Sim had been politically active during Jackson's successful 1828 campaign and is identified in Parton's biography as "an old friend." However, Sim's professional reputation was suspect. During his senatorial term, Jackson developed a severe infection at the site of a retained bullet in his left arm. Several of Old Hickory's friends appealed to his wife, Rachel, "in the hope that through her influence, the general might be prevailed upon to call in another physician." Mrs. Jackson so entreated her husband, but was rebuffed with the following rejoinder: "Dr. Sim(s) is my friend—an old and valued friend. His professional reputation, his standing as a physician, his feelings as a man, as a friend, are all at stake in this matter.... He shall cure me, or he shall kill me. I entreat you never to speak to me upon the subject."[41]

After Sim's 1832 cholera death from treating patients, doctors Huntt and Hall were called to treat Jackson and his family. They charged the president for the privilege. In a letter, the president refers to paying Huntt $175 for medical services during 1836, and a further review of his correspondence discloses the payment of more than $400 for unspecified care for him and his family during the years 1833–37.[42] James Hall likewise charged Jackson for services rendered. In the president's correspondence there is a receipted bill, dated January 1, 1832, "to operating for hydrocele and subsequent attendance, $30.00." It is uncertain who was the surgical patient, but presumably it was the president. In addition, Hall charged Jackson an additional $70 for various minor surgical treatments of the Jackson family between 1832 and 1835.[43]

In June 1833, an ailing President Jackson embarked on a political trip to New England. Before the standardization of continuous presidential care that occurred at the end of the nineteenth century, regular medical attendance on presidential trips away from Washington was nonexistent. Jackson became sick while in Boston. His nephew Donelson recorded that "…he began hemorrhaging. It started with a cold, and abscess formed and then ruptured." Dr. John Warren was summoned to the president's bedside, and Donelson further related, "…and the first thing he did was to bleed the President. When that procedure failed to gain results the good doctor bled his patient a second time…."[44]

Warren was far from a struggling doctor who needed to supplement his income by making house calls. Instead, he was the 55-year-old leader of the Boston medical community. He was then the professor of anatomy and surgery at Harvard School of Medicine. His accomplishments included the founding of the Massachusetts General Hospital, the introduction of ether anesthesia, and leadership in establishing both *The New England Journal of Medicine* and the American Medical Association.[45] Warren, the scion of a distinguished Boston family, had obtained his formal medical education in Europe with studies in London and Paris and a medical degree from Edinburgh.[46] Earlier on the same trip, before arriving in Boston, the president had consulted with the prestigious Philadelphia surgeon Philip Synge Physick for the same complaint of pulmonary hemorrhage. Physick advised cupping and provided encouragement. The surgeon also had studied medicine in London and had received his medical degree from Edinburgh in 1792.[47]

Four years after Jackson's retirement, another general, William Henry Harrison, was elected the ninth president of the United States in 1840. His election was due to his success in both the Indian Wars of the early 1800s and the War of 1812. Harrison had been remarkably healthy during his long life and had escaped the traumatic injuries and infectious illnesses that usually accompanied a military career. Consequently, he had developed no long-term relationship with any physician at the time of his inauguration.[48] When he became acutely ill after his inauguration in 1841, he followed the practice of the two illustrious generals, Washington and Jackson, who preceded him as president. He chose the most qualified civilian practitioner available.[49]

His choice of a physician was Dr. Thomas Miller, who was presumably selected because of his reputation in the Washington medical community. Shortly after his inauguration, Harrison developed an upper respiratory infection, which progressed to pneumonia. When the president's condition worsened despite his initial treatments, Miller resorted to a common strategy of the medical profession, one that had been previously employed by Samuel Bard when his patient George Washington was severely ill, and by James Madison's doctors when their patient was slow to recover from a severe case of malaria—the employment in consultation of as many prestigious practitioners as possible.[50] In the case of recovery, the diverse skills and experience of those assembled would be tapped, and in the case of therapeutic misfortune, accountability, blame and responsibility could be diluted and shared. Miller called upon his distinguished Washington colleagues, James C. Hall, Nicholas Worthington, and Frederick May, and upon Ashton Alexander, a prominent physician from Baltimore.[51]

During this episode Miller and Hall became the first physicians to remain overnight in the White House during the serious illness of a president.[52] When Harrison died, these physicians established another precedent. They published a statement explaining and justifying their medical care. It was in the form of a letter dated April 4, 1841, addressed to Daniel Webster, the secretary of state, and signed by all five attending physicians.[53] Miller subsequently authored a seven-page description of his medical care that was published in the June 2, 1841, issue of the *Boston Medical and Surgical Journal*. Therein this doctor appeared to blame his patient, rather than the physicians, for his rapid death. "The change which occurred in all his habits, in consequence of his political relations, and the fatigues and anxieties incident to his official duties after his arrival in Washington, tended to interrupt and disturb the repose of body and mind necessary for the healthful operations of his constitution."[54]

It is unknown whether or how these physicians were compensated for their presidential care. The Congressional Record does not contain an appropriation for Harrison's medical expenses, although Congress did pass statutes that paid for the deceased president's funeral expenses and provided a payment of $25,000 to his widow.[55]

The presidents of this period were treated by graduates of the most esteemed medical schools. Whether deliberate or fortuitous, these chief executives were spared the ministrations of graduates from the rapidly proliferating, often inferior, institutions that had sprung up. In 1850, forty-two American medical schools were in existence; as a comparison, the entire country of France hosted only three. A second enumeration counted Twenty-six new schools that had been established between 1810 and 1840.[56]

Most new schools were proprietary ventures initiated by their faculties as a means to secure income. Usually, a group of physicians would approach a local college with a proposal to inaugurate a college of medicine. The college would lend legitimacy to the venture, while the medical college would enhance the renown of the college. Meanwhile, the founding physicians, who had become the school's professors, would receive both prestige and profit. The student fees would be divided among the lecturers. The capital costs for establishing a new medical school were low, merely requiring the rental of space, often just two rooms, and the purchase of minimal furnishing and equipment, probably including a skeleton or two for examination.[57]

Daniel Drake, the famous Western medical pioneer, proposed a second reason for this phenomenon: "The extraordinary increase may be ascribed in part to the great number of state sovereignties which make up our confederacy, each of which … is ambitious to rival its neighbors in the number, if not the excellence of its institutions."[58]

The physical facilities of many of the new schools were at best substandard. There were no laboratories, other than a room in which to study a skeleton; library facilities were minimal; and there were no affiliated hospitals where students might gain practical experience. The standard course of study was for two years, but the second year's lectures repeated the first. Each term lasted only three or four months, typically from the end of November to the beginning of March. Drake commented: "In all the medical schools of the United States, the lectures of each preceding year are as topics the same with the last and there is no classification of students according to the different stages of their studies." Finally, examinations were brief and practically no students were disqualified from continuing or graduating.[59]

It was James Crowdhill Hall's misfortune to be called in consultation to the deathbed of a second United States president. Nine years after the death of Harrison, President Zachary Taylor became terminally ill with a severe gastrointestinal ailment, possibly typhoid fever. When Taylor did not respond to the initial treatments of his military physicians, Hall was called in.[60] Again medical management by committee was unsuccessful. In 1865 Hall was present at the deathbed of a third president, Abraham Lincoln. He was one of the many doctors who responded to the emergency of Lincoln's assassination.[61] One might speculate that the hapless Dr. Hall was the turkey buzzard of Jefferson's famous description, which lurked around whenever three physicians gathered in one area.[62]

The career of James Hall is of interest to this narrative for yet another reason. At a time when graduating medical students plunged immediately into practice, Hall spent a year as resident physician at Blockley Hospital in Philadelphia.[63] As noted in his obituary, "After receiving his degree he was appointed one of the physicians … where he spent a year in attentive and laborious study."[64] Hall's specific duties at Blockley are not recorded, but it is reasonable to assume that he functioned as did future interns in public hospitals. Blockley, the ancestor of the Philadelphia General Hospital, functioned as an almshouse and a city hospital.[65] Many decades elapsed before one or more years of postgraduate in-hospital training became routine; the underdevelopment of hospitals, both in scope and in numbers, acted as a bar to postgraduate training until much later in the century.

Robert K. Stone, Lincoln's family physician, also responded to treat the dying president. Stone, a Pillar of the Profession in Washington, was probably brought to Lincoln's attention due to his considerable reputation among his contemporaries and his particularly good education. He had a Princeton College B.A., a University of Pennsylvania M.D., and a period of study at the principal European medical centers. However, Stone's political views were opposed to the president's. One of Lincoln's supporters warned the president against the selection of Stone because he was a Democrat and a bitter opponent to Republicans.[66]

In mid-century the scope of medical practice largely remained formless, in that a practitioner felt qualified to engage equally in many areas of medicine. Henry Huntt, for example, engaged at one time in rural general practice, obstetrics, pediatrics, and surgery. Medical specialties had yet to be defined, and medical specialty societies, training programs, and certificates of specialty achievement were still in the future.[67]

After graduation from the University of Pennsylvania medical school, Robert Stone spent several years in Europe where he studied with the masters of the new specialty of ophthalmology at clinics in London, Edinburgh, Paris and Vienna. Although his subsequent Washington practice encompassed many facets of general medicine, almost one quarter of his patients appeared with eye problems. Stone became professor of ophthalmic and aural surgery at the National Medical College, the predecessor of George Washington Medical School.[68] Stone's interest in diseases of the eye corresponded in time with the molding of ophthalmology as a distinct specialty. In the years 1851 to 1864, the ophthalmoscope and instruments of refraction were discovered, which provided both a technical definition and a visible demarcation for this early medical specialty. Contemporaneously, both the *American Journal of Ophthalmology* and the American Ophthalmologic Society were formed, both contributing to its members' professional identity.[69]

The death watch at Lincoln's bed was viewed by numerous physicians, the majority of whom were military.[70] His passing figuratively signaled the demise of one pattern of health care—acute care on a fee for service basis by an elite physician who considered the president-patient as just one of many in a busy practice. The medical care of United States presidents over the next century, with very rare exceptions, would be delivered by military men. And the pattern of health care would change significantly with the transition from civilian to military.

Chapter 3

The Military Steps In, Part I

The Early Days, 1823–1865

In midsummer of 1848, shortly after the conclusion of the Mexican-American War, President James Polk euphemistically asked "Doctor Foltz to accompany him to Bedford Springs, Pennsylvania…. One may imagine the delight with which he responded, for the heat in Washington was intense…." Navy surgeon Jonathan Foltz then was assigned to Washington; his previously published study of the curative effect of the waters of Bedford Springs was one reason why Polk wanted him nearby. Thus, a combination of a president seeking respite from the concerns of a war just consummated, the availability of a knowledgeable military doctor, and the oppressive heat of midsummer Washington led to the first presidential journey with medical accompaniment.[1]

A highly significant occurrence in the evolution of medical care by physicians at the White House during the nineteenth century was the replacement of civilian doctors by military officers. For these military physicians, the care of the president and the first family progressively became their major and, later, their sole responsibility. This change was most evident in the role of navy physician Dr. Presley Rixey, the White House physician to the McKinley family at the dawn of the twentieth century. Presidential health care was primarily in the hands of civilians until 1865, and then almost exclusively it became the responsibility of the military for the next 100 years, until 1961.

This chapter examines those instances in which care by military physician was countercurrent to the presidential reliance upon eminent members of the Washington medical establishment in the first half of the nineteenth century. There were several reasons for the selection of military physicians over civilians: the greater availability of military physicians for either immediate bedside consultation or for travel; the likelihood that the cost of care would be assumed by the government rather than by the patient; and the greater control exercised by the presidential patient as commander in chief over the treating military officer. The presidential patient had control over any advancement in rank and promotion, e.g., the appointment of surgeon general.[2] Each case will be analyzed to determine which, if any, of these reasons, applied.

In addition, these early military doctors established a significant precedent on two occasions—travel with the president outside Washington. A close examination of the circumstances of two early presidential journeys will be made.[3]

Three sitting presidents died in Washington between 1841 and 1865: William Henry Harrison and Zachary Taylor in the White House, and Abraham Lincoln in a private home across the street from Ford's Theater. In addition, James Monroe had two serious but nonfatal illnesses that required close medical attention in the executive mansion. No consideration was given in any of these cases to admitting the president to a Washington hospital. This chapter concludes with an examination of the status of the district's hospitals during the first two-thirds of the nineteenth century.

Naval officer Bailey Washington was the first military physician to treat a sitting president. Washington, a distant relative of the first president, was a graduate of the University of Pennsylvania School of Medicine.[4] He had been commissioned a surgeon in the U.S. Navy in 1813 and saw service in the War of 1812. Subsequently he was stationed in the capital city, where he became a member of the District's medical society and served for three years on its board of examiners.[5] Approximately one half of the society's initial incorporators were military officers.[6] At the time of his death in 1854, Bailey Washington was visiting surgeon of the navy yard and marine barracks in Washington, D.C.[7]

The circumstances of Washington's attendance during President Monroe's acute illness in August 1823 are unclear. Secretary of State John Quincy Adams made the following notation in his diary for August 2: "The President was suddenly seized this morning with cramps or convulsions, of such extreme violence that he was at one time believed dying, and he lay upward of two hours in a state of insensibility." Medical historians speculated that cerebral malaria, among other possibilities, was a cause for Monroe's sudden collapse.[8] Adams called upon Monroe that afternoon, and discussed his condition with attending physicians Bailey Washington and Professional Pillar Thomas Sim. The latter "pronounced the danger to be past, and did not apprehend a renewal of the attack."[9]

It is likely that the reason for Washington's attendance during this episode was his availability. He may have been the physician on call at the Navy Yard when the president was stricken, and responded together with Dr. Sim to this medical emergency. The Washington Navy Yard, the U.S. Navy's oldest shore establishment, had been established on October 2, 1799; twelve years later the navy founded a hospital in a rented building near the navy yard in

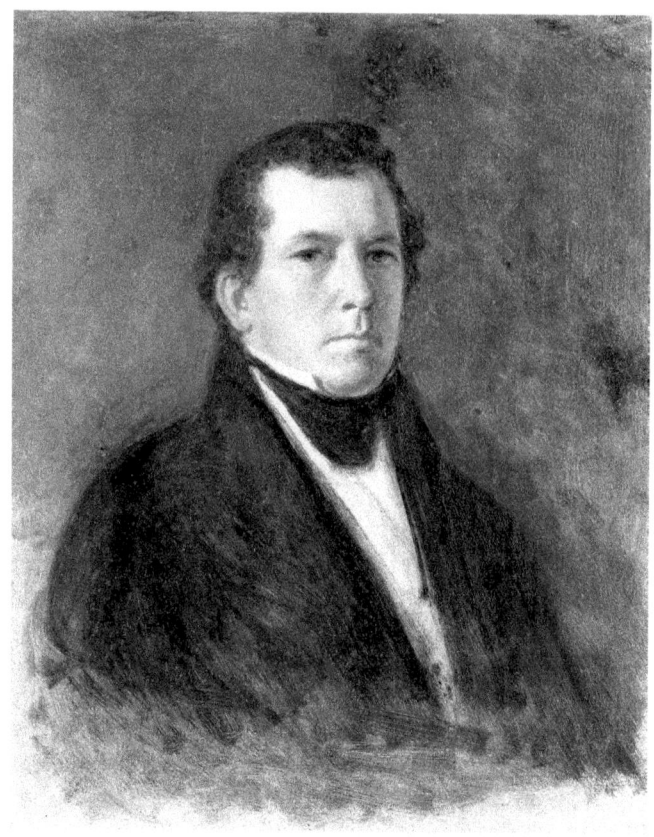

Bailey Washington. Bailey Washington was the first military physician to treat a president. (Courtesy of the Bureau of Medicine and Surgery Library and Archives)

order to provide care for its personnel.[10] Apparently Dr. Washington's medical abilities were appreciated, since a November 13, 1823, letter from the president to Charles Everett implied that Dr. Washington continued to treat the first family.[11] Perhaps more as a result of this naval surgeon's long tenure in the District than his successful treatment of President Monroe, Washington's naval career flourished. Secretary of the Navy Woodbury in 1834 selected him as his consultant in all matters connected with the naval medical corps. In this capacity Washington mistakenly recommended against the distribution of army physician Dr. William Beaumont's seminal physiologic treatise, *Experiments and Observations on the Gastric Juice and the Physiology of Digestion*.[12]

It was nearly a decade later when a president next enlisted the medical assistance of a naval physician. In 1832 Andrew Jackson took advantage of an opportunity to correct one of his chronic medical problems. In this case, an 1813 gunfight in downtown Nashville had left a debilitating bullet in his left shoulder.[13] When the accomplished navy surgeon from Philadelphia, Dr. Thomas Harris, "was casually in the city,"[14] the president requested him to remove the bullet, presumably because a military doctor would have greater experience than a civilian physician in treating gunshot wounds. Harris expertly removed a "half ball of ordinary size," whose metal coating was flattened by contusion and somewhat hackled on its edge. The surgeon dressed the wound and the president returned to work.[15]

Harris was yet another graduate of the University of Pennsylvania School of Medicine. He joined the navy as a surgeon during the War of 1812. Harris obtained combat experience during the war and was later instrumental in the organization of the Naval Medical Institute in Philadelphia. At the time of his visit to Washington, Harris was the principal navy surgeon in Philadelphia, and was a lecturer in operative and military surgery at its Naval Medical Institute.[16] Taking advantage of Harris's presence in Washington, Jackson had him remove the troublesome bullet rather than calling upon one of his coteries of civilian physicians. After this operation, Jackson's shoulder wound ceased to be a problem. There is no record in the Jackson correspondence of any payment to Harris for his services.[17]

Zachary Taylor, the country's twelfth president and the fourth army general to be elected to this office, relied almost exclusively upon the military for his medical care, probably out of habit and familiarity. Taylor was a career army officer, serving almost continuously from his commissioning as a lieutenant in 1808 until his successful presidential campaign in 1848. He was stationed in remote parts of the American republic, including Texas and Florida, where the only medical care available was dispensed by an army physician. During his military career, Taylor required treatment for yellow fever and dysentery and three times for malaria.[18]

Surgeon Robert Crooke Wood, a graduate of Columbia College of Medicine, New York, was a career army officer. He married Taylor's oldest daughter, Anne, in 1829. Subsequently Wood was frequently assigned to Taylor's command. The doctor served as Taylor's staff physician during the 1839–40 Florida campaign, and became his father-in-law's confidante, not only in medical but also in political matters.[19] During the Civil War, Colonel Wood served the Union as Assistant Surgeon General in Charge of Medical Affairs of the West and Southwest.[20]

Wood was stationed in Baltimore during Taylor's abbreviated presidency. However, he accompanied the president on his August 1849 political trip to Pennsylvania and upper New York State. In an August 1 letter to Surgeon General Thomas Lawson, his superior in Washington, Wood wrote, "I have the honor to inform you that I have been requested by the President of the United States to accompany him on his proposed visit to the North." The letter continued with a request to employ a surgeon as his replacement in Baltimore.[21] Wood thus became the second physician to accompany a president on his travels.

The trip was eventful. Taylor was struck by diarrhea in Carlisle, Pennsylvania, where Wood "prescribed for him." The symptoms first disappeared but reappeared several days later in Erie, Pennsylvania, and the president was prostrated with diarrhea and fever. His son-in-law consulted with navy surgeon W.W. Wood. The president was subsequently moved to the latter's residence where constant attention could be focused upon his illness. After nine days, Taylor recovered and his trip was resumed.[22]

But the illness recurred the following July, this time with a fatal result. In the summer of 1850 Taylor was struck by a violent diarrheal illness accompanied by fever, the

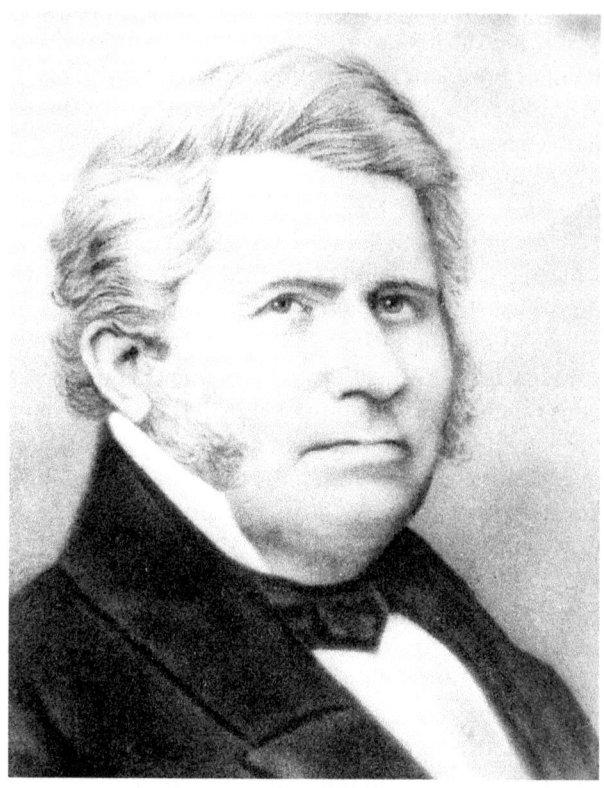

Thomas Harris. Dr. Thomas Harris, a prominent navy surgeon. He removed a bullet from Andrew Jackson's left shoulder joint. (Courtesy of the Bureau of Medicine and Surgery Library and Archives)

cause of which remains uncertain and controversial to this day. During the late afternoon or evening of the third day, "someone at the White House called in Army Surgeon Alexander S. Wotherspoon." The doctor made a diagnosis of *cholera morbus*, administered calomel and opium, and returned home.[23] At the time Wotherspoon was serving as an assistant army surgeon in Washington. He had been well educated in medicine, graduating from the Columbia College of Physicians and Surgeons and acting as a resident physician at the New York Hospital for three years before joining the army.[24]

Wotherspoon was recalled to the White House the following day since the president's condition had worsened. His response was predictable—the summoning of professional colleagues. These included army assistant surgeon Richard H. Coolidge, then on duty in the office of the army surgeon general in Washington, son-in-law Robert Crooke Wood from Baltimore, and the ubiquitous Washington Pillar James C. Hall.[25] Treatment by committee failed and Zachary Taylor became the second United States president to die in office. The faithful son-in-law, Dr. Wood, requested and received a six month leave of absence to tidy up Taylor's personal and financial affairs.[26]

It is unknown whether Wotherspoon's professional career suffered as a consequence of his unsuccessful treatment of the moribund president, since the doctor died thereafter in 1854 at an early age thirty-seven.[27] However, one event in his career presaged the consequential struggle for professional supremacy that involved later presidential physicians. Wotherspoon, an orthodox trained physician, had collaborated with the homeopathic doctor John Charles Peters in publishing a translation of Rokitansky's *Pathologic Anatomy* in 1849.[28]

The next military actor was navy surgeon Jonathan Foltz. Foltz played a starring role in the nineteenth-century drama demonstrating the evolution of presidential medical care. He served two presidents, James K. Polk (1845–49) and James Buchanan (1857–61). Foltz was the first doctor to accompany a sitting president on a trip outside the nation's capital. Additionally, he was the first physician to be assigned a bedroom in the White House. Further, he was the first, and probably the only, military physician to submit a bill to a president for medical services rendered. Finally, Foltz had a unique estrangement from his presidential patient, James Buchanan. The breach occurred over the disappearance of a promised promotion, and Foltz's criticism of Buchanan was severe and malicious.

Jonathan Foltz graduated from Jefferson Medical College in Philadelphia in 1830. Subsequently he applied for the post of assistant naval surgeon and supplied letters of recommendation in support of his candidacy from six notable citizens from Lancaster, Pennsylvania, his hometown. The most prominent supporter was James Buchanan, later secretary of state under Polk, and later president.[29] The young physician received his commission and spent most of the next twenty years on naval ships in the Mediterranean, South America, and Sumatra, and saw combat in the Mexican War.[30] Both presidential physicians Foltz and Wood served apprenticeships prior to admission to medical school. Foltz received "an academic education" from Dr. William Thompson, while Wood studied under a Dr. Warren of South Carolina.[31]

Foltz also experienced intermittent service at the Washington Navy Yard and Marine Barracks. This was the billet of naval surgeon Foltz in the summer of 1848, when a weary President James K. Polk decided to reinvigorate himself at Bedford Springs, Pennsylvania. The president, a well-known workaholic, had recently recovered from a protracted illness and had overseen the recent successful conclusion of the Mexican War. Polk's diary entry for August 17, 1848, reads, "I retired late at night, exceedingly fatigued from a most oppressive day's labour. The weather is very warm, and I greatly need rest & relaxation from business. This hope I shall have for the next few days." The basis for Polk's hope was repose in the healing waters of Bedford Springs.

Foltz's assignment to accompany the president during his August 19–28 excursion resulted from the unavailability of doctors Miller and Hall, the Polk family physicians, for this journey, and upon the commander in chief's executive ability to command a competent naval physician to minister in their stead. Moreover, his former patron, Secretary of State Buchanan, may have recommended Foltz to the president. Foltz himself attributed his selection to his previously published treatise on the curative effects of the aforementioned Pennsylvania waters.[32]

There is no record in the administration of any medical care to the president during the August 19–28, 1848, trip. Instead, Foltz acted more as a concierge, arranging for Polk's travel, food, and lodging. A Sunday August 27 diary entry reads, "...but Dr. Foltz wrote to Capt. Bowie, who was at the Springs, to engage rooms for me."[33]

Meanwhile, the casual acquaintanceship between Buchanan and Foltz developed into a personal and professional friendship. In 1847 Secretary Buchanan requested surgeon Foltz, then recuperating from an illness in Newport, Rhode Island, to treat his nasal polyps. Foltz wrote: "I proceeded to Washington without delay, and found Mr. Buchanan laboring under a severe surgical disease requiring a series of tedious and painful operations. For the convenience of treating his case, he desired me to live in the house with him, where I took up my quarters and remained with him for many months."[34] He summarized their relationship: "It was here an intimacy grew up which I had thought had grown into the warmest friendship. In our professional, confidential and constant social intercourse, every thought, every action of his life appeared thrown open to me, and I trust I never have and never shall betray it."[35] This gave rise to a subsequent warm correspondence between the two men. In honor of his famous friend, Dr. Foltz named his first born son Frederick Buchanan.[36]

Foltz accompanied the president-elect on a preinaugural trip to Washington, D.C., in January 1857, and treated Buchanan when the latter was afflicted by the mysterious *National Hotel Disease*, a name given by the press to an outbreak of virulent dysentery that affected guests staying at Washington's National Hotel in February of 1857.[37] At the president-elect's request, Foltz again accompanied Buchanan to the capital for his inauguration. Foltz described his status "as his medical attendant during the inauguration ceremonies."[38] When his patron again contracted a strange illness, Dr. Foltz "...was in constant attendance upon him ... and he was in a carriage just behind the one that conveyed the retiring President and the President-elect ... and that he had to administer remedies."[39] Buchanan requested that Foltz continue to treat him at the White House, and assigned the surgeon his own personal room which adjoined the president's.[40]

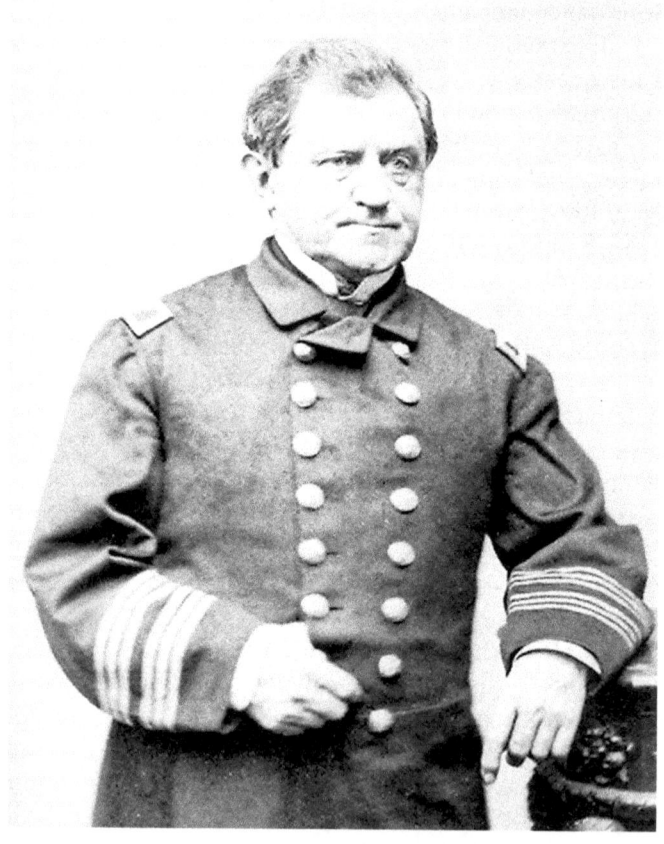

Jonathan Foltz. Dr. Jonathan Foltz cared for two presidents, James Polk and James Buchanan. Uncharacteristic of physicians to the president, Foltz feuded with Buchanan, his former patient, when he did not receive his anticipated appointment to surgeon general of the navy. (Courtesy of the Bureau of Medicine and Surgery Library and Archives)

Ross McIntire, a future White House physician, identified Jonathan Foltz as the first regular White House physician. McIntire explained that Foltz, being a family friend of Buchanan, merited his appointment because the president found him likable and companionable as well as being a competent doctor.[41]

At the request of President Buchanan, the secretary of the navy extended this physician's leave of absence while Foltz attended to the president's ills for another week.[42] Thereupon the doctor returned to his duty station at the Naval Rendezvous in Philadelphia. While in Washington on official business in April 1857, Foltz, at Buchanan's request, boarded at his assigned room in the White House. There is no record of any medical treatment during this visit.[43]

However, Foltz underwent a progressive estrangement from the president. His promised appointment as chief of the Bureau of Medicine and Surgery (surgeon general of the navy) did not materialize, and Foltz blamed Buchanan's dishonesty and irresoluteness for this "betrayal."[44] In disgust, Foltz renamed his first born Frederick Steinman, née Buchanan[45] and began to make derogatory and critical statements about his former friend.[46] In an 1872 letter to his son, Foltz wrote, "James Buchanan was born, one of the wisest and one of the worst men ever born in America. He tried to dissolve the American Union and he stabbed the Democratic Party to the heart."[47] Commenting upon Buchanan's death in a June 16, 1868, letter to his brother-in-law, he left no question as to his opinion of the former president: "He was a bad man, and his life and deeds were evil."[48] In the same letter, Foltz authorized his brother-in-law to bill Buchanan's estate for $1000 for the professional services he rendered to Buchanan over the years.[49] He finally received his long sought promotion when President Grant appointed Foltz surgeon general of the navy and chief of the Bureau of Medicine and Surgery in October 1871.[50]

The scope of medical attention provided by the aforementioned military doctors did not include in-hospital care, which may seem curious considering the broad range of hospital services available today. Yet, in 1801 there were only two hospitals in America, one in Philadelphia and the other in New York City. The third American hospital, the Massachusetts General Hospital in Boston, was not established until 1821. The development of hospitals, in the modern sense of the word, was so delayed that the first American hospital census in 1873 could identify only 178, and that included mental institutions.[51]

The initial hospitals in the nation's capital emerged from the poorhouse tradition. In 1806 the corporation of Washington established the Washington Infirmary "the more effectively to provide for the poor, disabled, and infirm persons."[52] This institution was a poorhouse or almshouse, and was perceived and utilized as one. Congress subsequently donated land for a larger institution, and in 1846 the poorhouse inmates were moved to the renamed Washington Asylum.[53] A fire completely destroyed the Asylum in 1861.[54]

Almshouses were the ancestors of general hospitals. They were a European tradition and in America almshouses were founded as early as the seventeenth century. They provided general welfare functions, and only incidentally cared for the sick. Almshouses, also known as poorhouses, cared for all classes of dependent persons, including the aged, the poor, the orphaned, the sick migrant, the insane, the syphilitic, and the impoverished who also were ill. Philadelphia General Hospital, Bellevue Hospital in New York City, and the Baltimore General Hospital all evolved from almshouses.[55] The hospitals of this period carried the stigma that was attached to almshouses.

As Rosenberg notes, "In 1800, the hospital was still an insignificant aspect of American medical care. No gentleman of property would have found himself in a hospital unless stricken with insanity or felled by an epidemic or accident in a strange city. When respectable persons or members of their family fell ill, they would be treated at home."[56] Additionally, there was little medical benefit to be gained by hospital care; the major scientific advances in medicine did not occur until later in the nineteenth century, and with them the development of the modern hospital.

In 1832 temporary cholera hospitals were organized in the District of Columbia to treat the stricken from that year's terrible epidemic. In 1866 the Columbia Hospital for Women and Lying In was founded. The oldest continually operating hospital in the nation's capital was the Providence Hospital, chartered by Abraham Lincoln in 1861 until it discontinued its inpatient operations in 2019. In 1882 the Medical Society of the District of Columbia was instrumental in organizing the Garfield Memorial Hospital.[57] Garfield eventually was merged into the Washington Hospital Center.[58] Therefore, even if an ill president was willing to expose his medical condition to the public scrutiny of a hospital admission, the choices for hospital care were limited if not altogether absent in the early days.

Although the medical care of sitting presidents for the most part remained in the hands of the District of Columbia's professional elite until after the Civil War, the attention of military physicians occasionally was required. The selection of a military practitioner was based on familiarity or kinship in the cases of presidents Buchanan and Taylor, but availability, convenience and control were the predominant reasons for summoning these doctors. Medical attention continued to be mostly episodic and reserved for acute illnesses. However, for the first time, a physician was responsible for continuous care when they accompanied a president on a journey outside the nation's capital. For many reasons, this responsibility could only be handled by a military doctor.

Chapter 4

The Military Steps In, Part II
Conflicts and Cooperation, 1865–1898

On Saturday, July 2, 1881, the day when assassin Charles Guiteau gunned down President James Garfield in a Washington, D.C., train station, Garfield's physician, army colonel Jedediah Baxter, was out of town in Pennsylvania. After Baxter expeditiously returned to Washington in order to resume the medical care of his patient, he was barred from access to Garfield by civilian doctor D.W. Bliss, who had assumed temporary control of the case in Baxter's absence. Bliss stated, "I don't see the necessity of your seeing the patient; I wish to keep him quiet,"[1] and continued: "I know your game; you wish to sneak up here and take this case out of my hands."[2] Bliss and his son angrily confronted the colonel and the ensuing altercation threatened to become physical. Baxter, concerned that such bitter acrimony could have unsalutary effects upon the dying president who was in a nearby room, backed off and made no further attempt to see his former patient.[3] This episode dramatically illustrated the conflict that occupied military and nonmilitary practitioners in Washington during the first half of this period (1865–1881).

The military, with a few exceptions, was in charge of maintaining the health of the presidents and their families during the years between the death of President Lincoln and the appointment of naval doctor Presley Rixey as the first recognizable White House physician. The latter cared for the family of William McKinley at the turn of the twentieth century. Cost may have been a primary reason for presidential reliance upon service physicians, since any medical care rendered by these doctors to the presidential patients was free of charge. However, the code of ethics of the Medical Society of the District of Columbia forbade the provision of care gratis to those who were able to pay. The ensuing conflict between civilians and military engulfed those practitioners who treated presidents Andrew Johnson, Ulysses Grant and James Garfield. Fortunately for the patient, these bitter disputes had evolved into a harmonious and deferential cooperation during the second presidency of Grover Cleveland.

When the president is the patient the customary hallowed physician-patient dynamic may be altered, resulting in a new paradigm wherein the presidential patient becomes dominant. The commander in chief may hold even greater sway when his physician is a military officer. Interestingly, several of these treating physicians were present or future army or navy surgeons general. The origins, structure, and relationship to the presidency of the Offices of the Surgeons General requires analysis.

During the latter third of the nineteenth century, the number of American medical schools rapidly expanded, women increasingly entered the practice of medicine, and the sect of homeopathy challenged orthodox medical practice. These trends also will be viewed through the lens of the presidential physicians of this period.

Military physicians were the first two responders when Abraham Lincoln was shot by John Wilkes Booth. Newly appointed Assistant Surgeon (U.S. Volunteers) Charles A. Leale entered the wounded president's box by stairway and reduced the pressure upon his cranial wound. Immediately thereafter, a second doctor, Acting Assistant Surgeon (U.S. Army) Charles S. Taft was lifted into Lincoln's balcony box from the theater stage to assist Leale.[4] For most of the nineteenth-century Congress had stipulated that there were but two ranks for most army physicians, surgeon and assistant surgeon; surgeons were entitled to the pay and emoluments of an army major, and assistant surgeons that of a captain or lieutenant.[5]

In accordance with professional ethics the Lincoln family physician, Robert K. Stone, assumed control of the president's care upon his arrival at Lincoln's bedside at the Peterson home across the street from Ford's theater.[6] Roos lists fourteen physicians in attendance during the president's final hours; of these six were military.[7] One physician who put in an appearance at the president's deathbed was the surgeon general of the army, Joseph K. Barnes. He arrived directly from a consultation at the house of Secretary of State Seward, who had just been knifed by Louis Powell, a second Confederate assassin. Sixteen years later surgeon general Barnes would make frequent visits to the bedside of assassinated president James Garfield during his protracted death agony. The specific medical measures undertaken by Barnes on any of these occasions are not recorded. Perhaps the Surgeon General considered it his responsibility to be available whenever a ranking member of the government was in a dire medical condition. Barnes, an 1838 graduate of the University of Pennsylvania School of Medicine, had continued his medical studies under the guidance of the expert military and Andrew Jackson surgeon, navy doctor Thomas Harris.[8]

Army physician Basil Norris, an 1849 graduate of the University of Maryland medical school,[9] was stationed as the attending physician of officers of the regular army and their families in the City of Washington from 1863 to 1884.[10] On the night of Lincoln's assassination, Norris was also at Secretary of State William H. Seward's bedside, treating his private patient for a double fracture of the upper jaw, when John Wilkes Booth's coconspirator, Powell, attacked the secretary. Norris treated Seward for his wounds and subsequently became the physician for President Andrew Johnson and his family, and later for President Grant and his family[11] during their terms of office (1865–1877). As a consequence, Norris became embroiled in the acrimonious debate between civilian members of the Medical Society of the District of Columbia and those army and navy members who maintained a private medical practice in Washington.[12]

President Andrew Johnson suffered from recurrent kidney stones during his abbreviated tenure. Cowan, his secretary, described his disease as follows: "Afflicted with gravel he found no cessation from pain, and but little relief in standing while at work for hours, in preference to remaining in a sitting posture, or from the variety of an occasional 'fit of the gravel' with its excruciating torture."[13] Johnson's malady was both serious and episodic, and it felled the president in the summer of 1865,[14] and again in the late winter and spring of 1867.[15] Johnson, in order to obtain relief, "had taken to working at a high desk, standing up."[16] When Andrew Johnson became extremely ill in March 1869, probably from a recurrence of renal stones, Norris expeditiously traveled to the ex-president's home in Greeneville, Tennessee, where Johnson wrote, "…In my extreme illness after my return from Washington, when my life had been despaired of, your presence at my bedside, after so short a notice, seemed almost to be the work of magic power."[17] Although his successor, President Grant, and Grant's family suffered from no significant illness during their eight years in the White House,[18] Grant, upon departing the presidency, expressed his "…gratitude and that of his family for your many acts of kindness and professional attendance in every case occurring with us for the past eight years."[19]

The District of Columbia medical society had a history of abiding by contentious ethical rules that regulated professional discourse among its members. Article VI of its code of ethics prohibited members of the society from prescribing or visiting professionally "any case gratuitously when the circumstances of the patient will justify a charge" except in the cases of fellow physicians or ministers.[20] This stricture was followed so stringently that the estimable James C. Hall was arraigned in 1850 for neglect in charging for his cases and failure in sending bills for his professional services. Hall was humbled, excused himself "with the statement that he did not need the money … and promised that he would in the future make the best effort he could to comply with the regulations of the Association."[21]

In 1877, Colonel Norris became a major figure in a protracted imbroglio over whether a military physician could ethically provide professional care to a civilian, even though that civilian was the commander in chief of the United States. The economic interests of the civilian practitioners of medicine in Washington insisted that only civilians, if available, could treat civilian members of the government. An investigating committee of the society charged that for the preceding ten or twelve years military officers had free of charge supplied civilians, including presidents of the United States and their families with "medicines and hospital supplies from the Army Dispensary."[22] Additionally, President Grant was accused of using his influence "to retain at this post the particular Medical Officer who had held such relations to his family, and who, under the rules of the Department, should have been transferred to

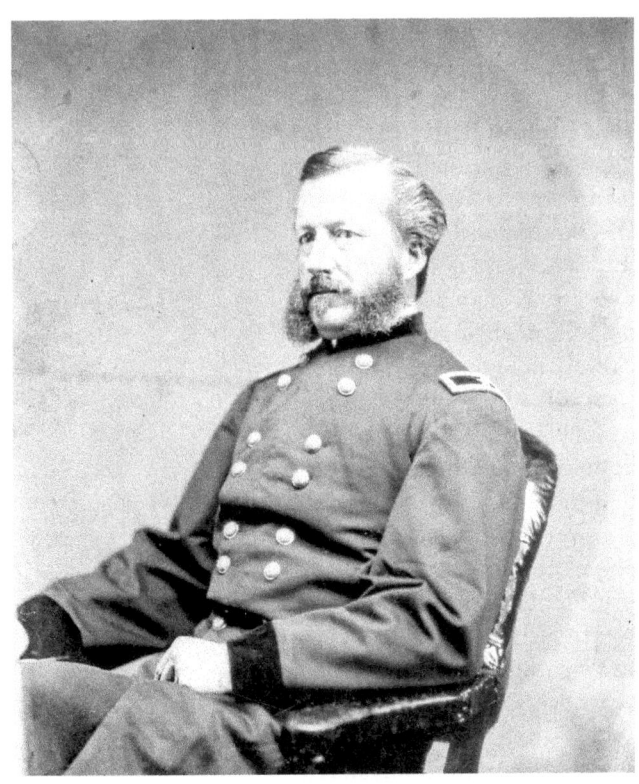

Joseph Barnes. Perennial army surgeon general Joseph K. Barnes played a minor supporting role in the treatment of the assassinated presidents Lincoln and Garfield. (National Library of Medicine)

some other post on duty."[23] A subsequent report by a second committee of the society stated that military physicians who had treated presidents without charge had committed an infringement of the code of ethics of both the District and the American Medical Association.[24] However, the offending medical officers were eventually exonerated by the society,[25] after its civilian members conceded that free medical care was a legitimate perquisite of the presidency.

For most of the nineteenth-century army and navy medical officers were able to supplement their income by treating civilians. In the United States Navy, the permission to moonlight was a prerogative of one's commanding officer and was limited to the doctor's off duty hours.[26] Military pay lagged considerably behind the earnings of civilian physicians to the extent that "most chiefs (i.e., Navy Surgeon Generals), up to and including Presley M. Rixey (1902–1910) had to maintain active civilian practices to earn a living."[27] Army Surgeon General Barnes believed that medical officers should treat local citizens. He was of the opinion that the practice enabled his physicians to provide better care for their soldier patients "by reason of the experience gained by becoming familiar with the disease present in the community." During the intensity of the Civil War, the energetic surgeon Basil Norris had applied for a transfer from his post with the Union Army of the Potomac, finding "...my duties here are not important. These duties can be performed by volunteer Surgeons, quite as well as by me. In Santa Fe I could add to my income by private practice and my appointment I believe would be agreeable...."[28]

Perhaps as an acknowledgment of his service to two presidents, Norris remained as attending army physician in Washington for twenty-one years, while also busying himself with his private practice. Local civilian physician Joseph B. Moore, taking note of Norris's professional activity, challenged the Secretary of War: "...if this surgeon ...

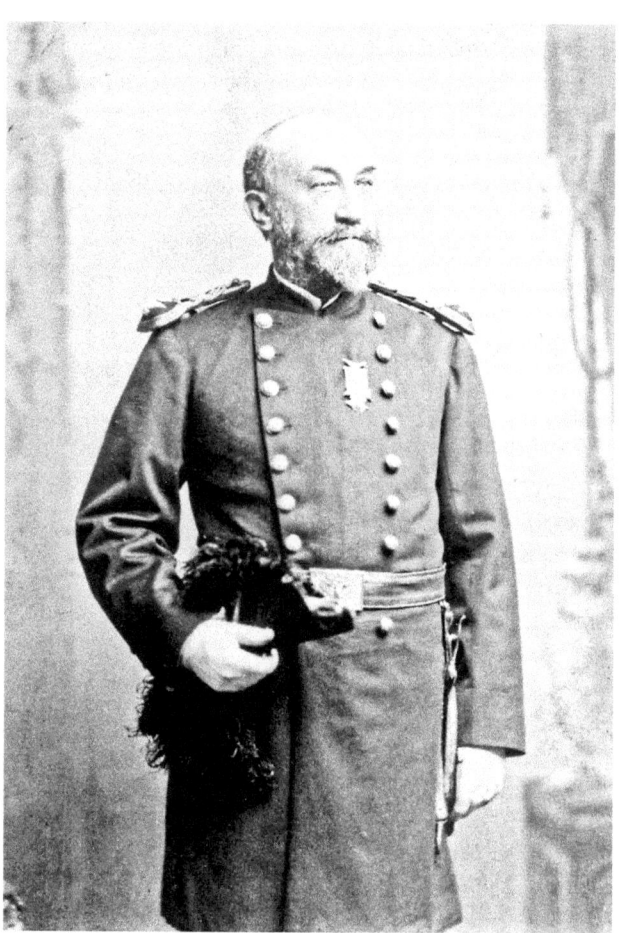

Basil Norris. Army colonel Dr. Basil Norris treated presidents Andrew Johnson and Ulysses Grant and thereby precipitated a row with the civilian members of the Medical Society of the District of Columbia over the limits of a military physician's practice. (National Library of Medicine)

possess the power and the lawful right to bestow medicines and medical attendance on any persons outside of commissioned officers and enlisted men."[29] Finally in 1892, the then army surgeon general Sutherland ordered that the tradition of civilian practice by army doctors be discontinued.[30]

Grant's successor, Rutherford B. Hayes of Ohio, selected army surgeon Jedediah Baxter as his physician.[31] Baxter, who was stationed in Washington for thirty years, was another veteran military physician who had been accused of unethical professional conduct by the District of Columbia's medical society. Civilian doctor A.Y.P. Garnett, in a May 22, 1877, complaint, accused Baxter of "a desire or willingness to visit a lady patient of mine" while "at the same time declaring a disbelief in the expressed opinion of the attending physician [Garnett] as to the nature of her malady." In blunt terms, this military doctor was accused of stealing a civilian physician's patient! Yet another standing committee of the society was impaneled; after an investigation it exonerated Baxter.[32]

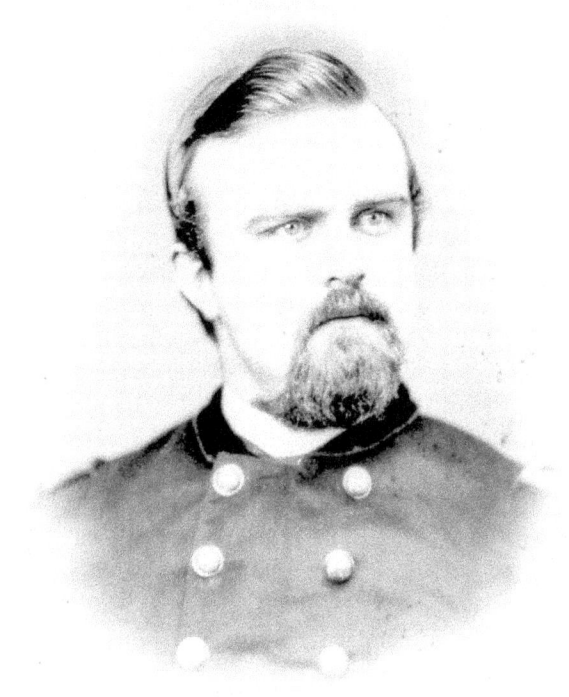

Jedediah Baxter. Army colonel Dr. Jedediah Baxter was both confrontational and entrepreneurial. He finally achieved his long-sought goal of surgeon general of the army after appointment to the position by his patient, President Benjamin Harrison. (National Library of Medicine)

Colonel Baxter held the military post of chief medical purveyor during this period. The scope of his military duties failed to satisfy the needs of this ambitious officer, since while at this post Baxter not only obtained a law degree from the Law School of the Columbian University, but also "found the time for the active practice of his profession" as a physician.[33] Baxter attended the families of presidents Hayes, James Garfield, and Benjamin Harrison. In addition, his services were extensively employed by senators, congressmen, and government officials, much to the resentment of the medical society's elites. It is likely that President Hayes, newly arrived from Ohio, selected his doctor on the basis of favorable commentary from Baxter's civilian patients.[34]

Hayes's health was excellent during his term (1877–1881), and only a few references to his physician's care exist. Hayes's diary entry for February 1, 1880, reported that "Dr. Baxter vaccinated the household on 23d January viz. Lucy, Webb, Fanny, Scott and myself—also our guests."[35] Hayes wrote to his wife on March 8, 1880, that "rheumatism is like a taste for genealogy. If it fastens on the body, it is never shaken off. Just now all of the bruised and shattered places of the war, and accidents are growling with it. Dr. Baxter gives me bad tasting and atrocious smelling compounds, but in vain."[36]

Presidential physicians still did not accompany their patients on journeys away from Washington. It was during a presidential trip to Ohio in 1879 that the versatile Baxter, remaining in Washington, took on an added duty. The presidential cat, Siam, took ill in the White House. Sadly, according to the historical record, "[despite] all the White House physician, Dr. J.H. Baxter and William T. Crump, the family steward, could do" Siam expired.[37]

Baxter's controversial and extensive civilian practice included the powerful Ohio congressman James A. Garfield. The doctor treated the congressman for "neurologic dyspepsia" during January and November 1874.[38] Garfield again required Baxter's services in 1878 and 1880.[39] On these occasions gastric distress was treated with a diet of "bread and milk and rare beefsteak."[40] The physician's medical care extended to members of the Garfield family, including his son Hal and his wife, Lucretia.[41]

When James Garfield was elected President of the United States in November 1880 to succeed fellow Ohioan Rutherford Hayes, the new president apparently was comfortable with Jedediah Baxter as his family physician, since he maintained this physician-patient relationship. In May 1881 Garfield summoned this allopathic practitioner to treat his wife's malaria and nervous exhaustion. Lucretia Garfield had a predilection for homeopathic physicians, but the president preferred the ministrations of allopathic doctors during medical crises.[42] Baxter's treatment was apparently effective, since Mrs. Garfield recovered. Meanwhile the busy Colonel Baxter maintained his military position as chief medical purveyor for the District of Columbia.[43] The term allopath was coined by Samuel Hahnemann, the founder of homeopathy, to distinguish his followers from allopaths, i.e., regular, or orthodox, practitioners of medicine.[44]

Professional conflict marred the medical aftermath of the assassination attempt upon President James Garfield. The behavior of Dr. D.W. Bliss, the principal physician attending the wounded president, underscored three controversies that embroiled the medical profession during the latter part of the nineteenth century: the competition for patients, the admission of women to medical school, and the role of homeopathic medicine.

James Garfield was mortally wounded by assassin Charles Guiteau on the morning of July 2, 1881, while awaiting a train at Washington's Baltimore and Potomac depot. Garfield's fatal abdominal wound festered for eighty-one days while as many as twenty-one different doctors unsuccessfully attempted to assuage the president's injuries.[45] Civilian physician D.W. Bliss, although he had no prior professional relationship with the president, was summoned to the scene by Secretary of War Robert Todd Lincoln.[46] Bliss aggressively assumed control of the president's case and dismissed all other physicians except military doctors Joseph K. Barnes and Joseph Woodward and local civilian practitioner Robert Reyburn.[47] When Colonel Baxter arrived at the White House in an attempt to resume care of his presidential patient, he was crudely and dismissively rebuffed by Bliss.[48] The latter maintained professional hegemony over Garfield's case until Garfield's death on September 19, 1881.

At this point in his career D.W. Bliss was very sensitive to the rules and regulations of organized medicine. Previously, in 1871, this doctor had been expelled from the District's medical society for attempting to liberalize its restrictive policies on membership and consultation. He had criticized its expulsion of black physicians from membership, but the precipitating cause for his expulsion was his overt consultation with a nonmember physician.[49]

In May 1847, the American Medical Association adopted its code of ethics. Its Consultation Clause therein stated that "no one can be considered as a regular practitioner, or a fit associate is based upon an exclusive dogma, to the rejection of the accumulated experience of the profession."[50] This language was intended to disqualify irregular physicians, especially homeopathic doctors, as respectable members of the medical profession. This clause had been instituted to prevent professional concourse with homeopathic physicians, since practitioners of this philosophy were prohibited from membership in traditional medical societies. As applied, no homeopath could consult with a regular physician, even if requested by the patient, and no regular physician could come to the aid of a patient whose doctor was a homeopath, unless the homeopath was first dismissed from the case. The professional ostracism was such that no acknowledged homeopath physician was granted an appointment as a physician in the Civil War Union Army.

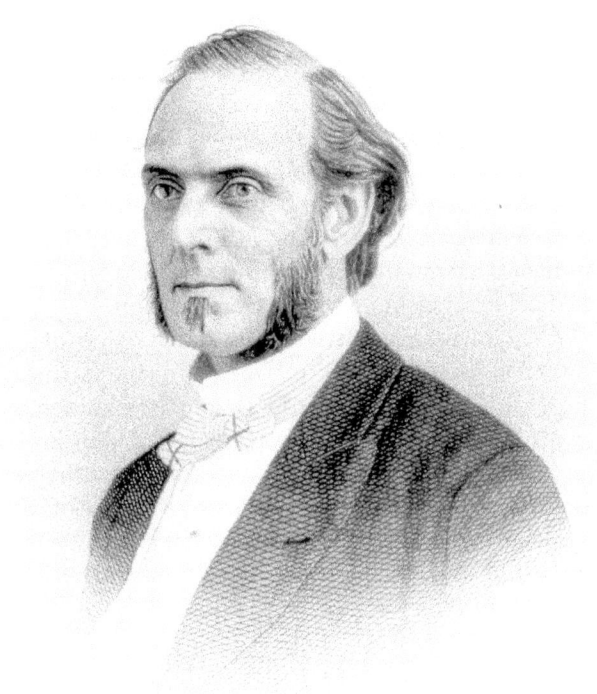

D.W. Bliss. Dr. D.W. Bliss seized control of President Garfield's case after the July 1881 assassination attempt. Bliss was in the center of the civilian-military physician and the allopathic-homeopathic controversies of the 1865–1885 period. (National Library of Medicine)

The District of Columbia medical society modeled its own consultation regulations after the AMA's (American Medical Association).[51] Bliss openly challenged the society by announcing that he would consult with a physician who was not a member. He thereupon consulted with regular physician Dr. Christopher Cox. Cox, a friend of Bliss, had previously been expelled for serving on the Washington board of health with a homeopath.[52] The homeopath in question was Dr. Tullio Suzzara Verdi, who had at least once before provoked the ire of organized medicine. Verdi, a graduate of Hahnemann Medical College of Philadelphia, was also one of Secretary of State Seward's doctors. After his patient was seriously wounded in April 1865, Verdi requested an urgent consultation from the ubiquitous surgeon general, Joseph K. Barnes. Barnes responded and Seward recovered. For his efforts, Barnes was denounced for "allowing a quack to prescribe medically while he was attending surgically."[53]

The members of the medical society disdained Bliss's appeal of his termination. According to Busey, the transgressor's violation was considered so severe that "his appeal did not bring him the success and éclat that he courted and expected. The community had no sympathy with a man under sentence of dishonor."[54] As a consequence, Bliss's medical practice suffered considerably.[55] Bliss, cowed, apologetic and remorseful, was readmitted to the society in 1876.[56] The District's medical society, a gathering of elite, cosmopolitan, community-minded physicians during the first half of the century, had become a cauldron of petty, vengeful, interpersonal and institutional conflicts in its second half. Not surprisingly, Bliss refused to acknowledge the professional status of homeopathic physicians Silas Boynton and Susan A. Edson despite their long-standing medical relationship with the Garfield family.

The antagonism between the two practices of medicine was based on their different ideas regarding effective treatment. The basic tenets of homeopathy were derived from the teachings of its founder, German physician Samuel Hahnemann (1755–1843). Homeopathy's primary principle was the law of similia, which declared that a disease would be cured by remedies that produced in a healthy person the same symptoms found in that disease. Its second principle was the law of infinitesimals. This precept held that the smaller the dose, the more effective it became in stimulating the vital curative force. According to Hahneman, a drug's potency to heal was inversely proportional to its concentration. Therefore, the more dilute the dose, the greater its potency.[57]

As a consequence, homeopathic physicians adopted a minimalist approach toward treatment, in which remedies would be administered in doses that would not produce ill effects. In contrast, physicians of the orthodox, or allopathic, school employed potent cathartics and emetics together with violent practices such as bleeding and scarification. The gentler practices of the homeopaths at least did no harm, and their professional stature was enhanced vis-à-vis the allopaths.[58]

Bliss's professional behavior was greatly criticized. Homeopathic physician Silas Boynton, the president's cousin, certified that the wounded Garfield had affirmed that Baxter had been his physician for many years and that he still considered him to be his physician. According to Boynton, the president also stated that he had no knowledge of ever having placed himself under the professional care of Dr. Bliss.[59] An editorial in *Walsh's Retrospect,* a medical journal of the era, scathingly criticized Bliss's violations of professional deference as "a scandal calculated to throw discredit upon the medical profession." The editorial emphasized that Dr. Bliss had violated that tenet of the American Medical Association's code of ethics, which stated, "When a physician is called to an urgent case, because the family attendant is not at hand, he ought, unless his assistance in consultation be desired, to resign the care of the patient to the latter immediately on his arrival."[60]

Bliss's refusal to acknowledge the long-term medical association of homeopathic doctors Silas A. Boynton and Susan A. Edson in the care of Garfield should be no surprise. Consequently, Dr. Boynton's multifarious carping upon the former's performance during this crisis is likewise not unexpected. The role relegated to the two homeopaths by Bliss was that of nurses and "watchers." Boynton frequently attended the president during the nights and was Garfield's watcher the entire night prior to the day of his death.[61] Doctor Boynton was the president's first cousin, and had been a childhood neighbor of the Garfield family. In later years Garfield frequently returned to his Ohio boyhood home site to "recapture the joys of tramping through the woods, playing with his Boynton cousins, and reading by the flickering hearth fire."[62] Garfield enjoyed an ongoing easy relationship with his cousin. There are at least seventeen references in the Garfield diaries that recount visits to the Silas Boynton home from 1867 to 1881.[63] A student at Hiram College, where Garfield was later president, Boynton graduated from the homeopathic Hospital College in Cleveland in 1862. Later he was alternatively on the faculty of the Woman's Homeopathic Medical College from 1868 until 1880 as professor of physiology, pathology, and microscopic anatomy, while engaged in the practice of homeopathic medicine in Cleveland.[64]

Boynton's medical connection with the Garfield family was not only with the president himself. In March 1875, when his mother-in-law was dying, Garfield telegraphed Boynton to come and consult with her attending physician.[65] In April and May 1881, Lucretia Garfield became severely ill, apparently from malaria, with symptoms of fever and prostration. Since there was no improvement in his wife's medical condition, the anxious president summoned his cousin from Boynton's ranch near Wichita, Kansas. In Garfield's words, "I have become satisfied that her illness is more serious than either Dr. Edson or Pope believes, and that their remedies are not of sufficient potency. I therefore put the case absolutely in Dr. Boynton's hands, who has burst the narrow boundaries of homeopathy, and gives heroic doses whenever the case requires it."[66] Boynton expeditiously returned, confirmed Dr. Edson's diagnosis of malaria, and took control of the case. He recommended a transfer of the patient to the New Jersey shore, away from the malaria swamps that reached to the backyard of the White House. The change of venue permitted a full and complete recovery.[67] Therefore, it was hardly surprising that shortly after the assassination attempt upon her husband, Mrs. Garfield telegraphed Dr. Boynton: "...pleased to have you come as soon as possible."[68]

The second homeopath intimately connected with Garfield's medical treatment was Lucretia Garfield's personal physician, Susan A. Edson. Edson, likewise a graduate of the Homeopathic Hospital College in Cleveland, received her medical degree in 1854. She practiced medicine in northeast Ohio for several years before becoming the first female physician to practice in Washington, D.C. She served the Union during the Civil War as a nurse, since homeopaths were excluded from service as physicians.[69]

Subsequently, at some undetermined time, Edson assumed the personal medical care of Lucretia Garfield and became a favorite of the entire Garfield family. Their youngest son, Abe, referred to her as "Dr. Edson, full of Med'cin."[70] Edson's personal influence may have elicited a small token of patronage from the newly formed administration with the appointment of Mrs. Webster, apparently a friend, to the Bureau of Engraving and Printing.[71] During April and May 1881 Mrs. Garfield became ill. As described above, Dr. Edson diagnosed malaria, proclaimed an optimistic prognosis, and attended Mrs. Garfield during her illness.[72]

The treatments of Bliss and his colleagues were much criticized, especially after the debilitated president expired some eighty days after the assassination attack.[73] Boynton became a prominent critic. He found fault with the allopathic usage of high maintenance doses of quinine and morphine, sips of brandy, and a single dose of calomel. Most of the attending clinicians' efforts were expended in locating the site of the assassin's bullet by frequent manipulations and probings of the entrance wound, and by several unorthodox, and unsuccessful, experiments.[74] Moreover, Boynton publicly challenged the official results of the autopsy performed upon Garfield. He correctly considered septicemia caused by the unwashed finger probings of the entrance wound to be the underlying cause of the president's death. The official autopsy report stated that Garfield had died secondary to blood loss from a traumatic rupture of the splenic artery.[75]

To counter the assaults of the critics, D.W. Bliss continued the tradition of publishing a favorable explanation of his handling of the case.[76] He and other of the president's medical and nursing attendants submitted claims for payment to Congress that totaled $91,000. Bliss claimed a sum of $25,000, of which the United States government finally approved $6,500.[77]

Susan Edson also was a recipient of government payment for services rendered during Garfield's illness. She had billed the government $10,000, and was awarded $3,000. Interestingly, Boynton, her homeopathic colleague, submitted a bill for only $4,500, and was awarded $4,000. It is easy to ascribe this differential to sexism. Moreover, the government's official document on the matter ascribed Edson's monetary award "for skillful attendance in professional capacity as physician."[78] The latter was an unintended irony, since the allopathic Bliss had demoted this homeopath to strictly nursing duties. Nevertheless, Dr. Edson (1823–1897) became the first woman physician to have a role in the medical care of a president. Many factors, including male sexism, would contribute to the rarity of women serving in the White House Physician's Office until much later in the twentieth century.

However, it is fitting the first female presidential physician was from the homeopathic school of therapy, since homeopaths in the nineteenth century were far more welcoming to women than allopaths. Kirschmann enumerated reasons why homeopathy naturally existed within a strong female culture, including a tendency for mothers to seek homeopathic practitioners for their own and their children's health problems.[79] While

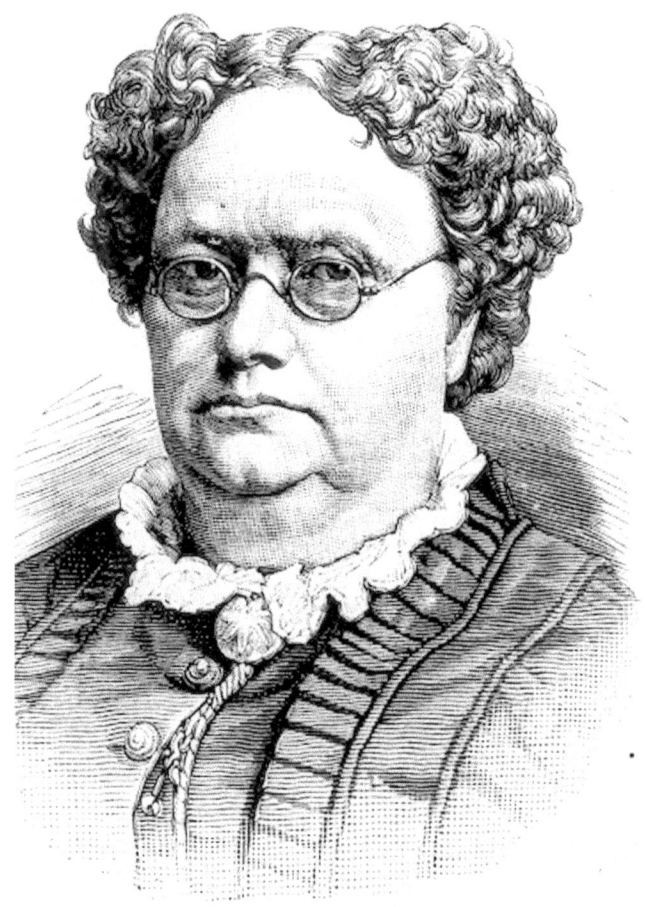

MRS. DR. SUSAN EDSON.

Susan Edson. Homeopathic physician Dr. Susan Edson, doctor to the Garfield family, was demoted to that of a "watcher" by provocative allopathic physician Dr. D.W. Bliss in the care of the dying President James Garfield. (Library of Congress) regular medical schools admitted women only with great reluctance, there was conversely an early acceptance of women in homeopathic medical colleges in Cleveland (1852), Chicago (1871), Detroit (1872), and Ann Arbor (1877).[80] Between 1890 and 1900, women constituted 18 percent of all homeopathic physicians; and in different locations and at different points in time, woman homeopaths equaled or exceeded the number of female regulars.[81] The 1870 meeting of the American Institute of Homeopathy voted to admit woman members, while the American Medical Association waited until 1915 to change its bylaws regarding the admission of women.[82]

Edson continued to practice medicine in Washington after Garfield's death. With another homeopath, Carolyn Winslow, she chartered the Homeopathic Free Dispensary that treated 2,000 patients a year—most of them women and a majority black—until the clinic was merged with the National Homeopathic Hospital in 1895.[83]

Jedediah Baxter was another victim of the prevailing homeopath-orthodox rivalry. President Benjamin Harrison (1889–1893) exhibited excellent health during his term of office. Harrison made many forays out of Washington during his presidency, but Baxter, his physician, did not accompany him on any of these trips, some of which lasted as long as five weeks.[84] This may have been simply a testament to the president's good health, or the continuance of the tradition of limited care for the nation's chief executive. Baxter previously had been consulted during Lucretia Garfield's illness; he confirmed Dr. Edson's diagnosis of malaria. When Baxter subsequently sought appointment as Surgeon General of the Army, he was criticized for his consultation with a homeopath during that episode.[85] However after three disappointments for promotion to this office, Baxter finally was rewarded for his faithful service to the presidency on August 16, 1890. Baxter's promotion "coincided with the occupancy of the War Secretary by a personal friend, the Hon. Redfield Proctor, and the incumbency of the Executive by a comrade and long-term patient, President Benjamin Harrison."[86] It is ironic that a second first lady, Caroline Harrison, also preferred the medical attention of a homeopath. Dr. Franklin A. Gardiner, a graduate of the New York Homeopathic Medical College, treated Mrs. Harrison during her final illness. Tuberculosis caused her death in the White House in October 1892.[87]

Grover Cleveland served two nonconsecutive terms as president (1885–1889 and 1893–1897). His first term was uneventful, but the medical travails of his second term contribute significantly to this narrative. The 1893 discovery of a cancer in the president's upper jaw and its subsequent surgical treatment both heralded a renewed spirit of cooperation between the president's military and civilian physicians, and exemplified the political pressures that periodically dominated presidential health care.

Cleveland followed the practice of the majority of his recent predecessors by choosing as his doctor a competent military officer serving in Washington. Robert Maitland O'Reilly contemporaneously held the post of attending army surgeon in the nation's capital city. He was a Philadelphia native who commenced his study of medicine at the University of Pennsylvania immediately upon graduation from the Philadelphia public school system. His formal medical education was interrupted by the Civil War, wherein he served as a medical cadet. After the war's conclusion, O'Reilly completed his medical school education at the University of Pennsylvania. Subsequently, in 1867, he was appointed assistant surgeon in the army and served as an army medical officer until his retirement in 1909.[88]

O'Reilly was ordered to duty as an Army surgeon to Washington, D.C., in 1882. In November 1884 he was promoted to attending surgeon of the District, a position which he held until November 1889, a period roughly corresponding to the first term of Grover Cleveland.[89] At that time, the Attending Surgeon stationed at the United States Army Dispensary in Washington was the official medical attendant for the officers of the federal government.[90] This assignment was interrupted in September 1888 when O'Reilly, according to Special Orders No. 284, was detached from Washington to Nonquitt, Massachusetts, to attend to the last illness of the general of the army, Philip Sheridan. From time to time in future years White House physicians would be temporarily detached from their primary responsibilities to care for other very important persons (VIPs).[91]

Cleveland was in general good health during his first term,[92] and there is no evidence of any specific medical care rendered to him by his military doctor.

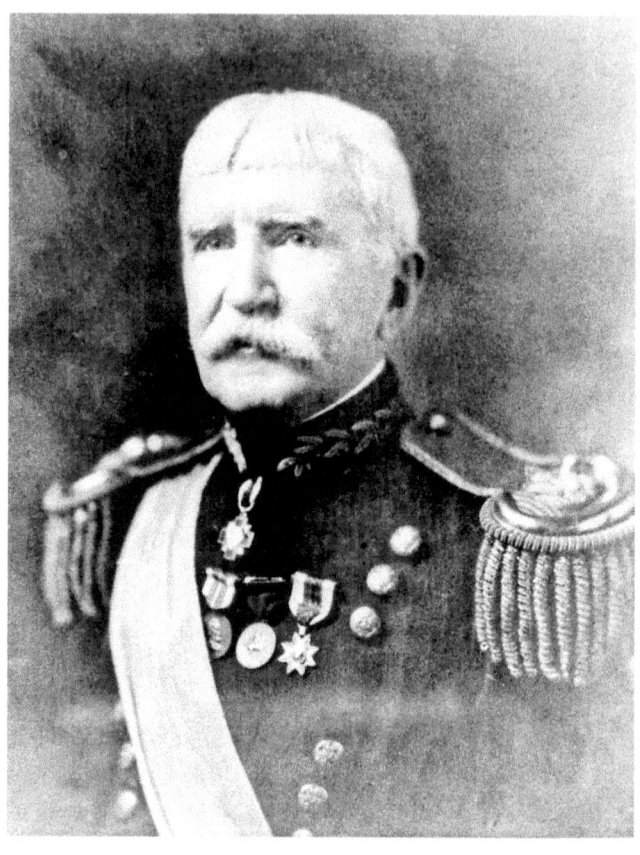

Robert O'Reilly. Dr. Robert O'Reilly worked cooperatively with civilian Dr. Joseph Bryant in the successful management of President Cleveland's cancer of the maxilla. (National Library of Medicine)

O'Reilly was detailed to Fort Logan, Colorado, in 1890, but in February 1893, just before his inauguration to his second term, Grover Cleveland exercised his presidential prerogative as commander in chief to request that O'Reilly be returned to Washington, D.C., again as attending surgeon.[93] In so doing, Grover Cleveland exercised his right to select his personal physician and thereby avoided dependence upon the unknown medical skill of whomever currently held that military post. Pilcher characterized the doctor's reputation: "O'Reilly was an exceedingly popular and acceptable medical attendant and during his tours of duty in Washington, his services were widely sought for."[94] Evidently Major O'Reilly's medical obligations extended far beyond the care of the first family. Further proof of his diverse responsibilities is located in O'Reilly's mandatory information slips submitted to the different surgeon generals of this period, in which he often recorded, "Absent on Special duty with the President of the United States."[95] Apparently, special permission was required to discharge this doctor from his professional responsibilities to the military before he could attend to the medical needs of the president.

Shortly after his second inauguration, on March 5, 1893, President Cleveland noted a rough spot on the roof of his mouth (maxilla). This lesion produced increasing discomfort, and on June 18 the president was examined by O'Reilly. The physician discovered "a malignant growth as large as a quarter of a dollar, extending from the molar teeth to within an inch of the middle line, encroaching on the soft palate, and accompanied by some diseased bone."[96] A biopsy of the lesion provided an indeterminate diagnosis, but O'Reilly, alarmed by the appearance of the tumor, either advised the president to consult with Dr. Joseph Bryant of New York City[97] or called Bryant into consultation himself.[98]

The issue of the selection of medical consultants by the presidential physician in times of diagnostic or therapeutic crises is a complex matter.[99] However, in this instance, Bryant's selection was almost inevitable, based both upon a prior personal relationship with President Cleveland and upon Bryant's impressive professional reputation. Three years previously, Bryant had addressed the Medical Society of the State of New York on "A History of Two Hundred and Fifty Cases of Excision of the Superior Maxilla," of which two cases were his own.[100] Moreover, Bryant was recognized as an accomplished surgeon and held many teaching appointments at Bellevue Hospital Medical School in New York. At various times he served as professor of general, descriptive, and surgical anatomy, professor of anatomy and clinical surgery, and Associate Professor of Orthopedic Surgery. He later wrote a standard textbook of surgery. Bryant also was active in medical politics, serving as president of the American Medical Association.[101]

Most importantly, however, Bryant enjoyed a personal relationship with Grover Cleveland. This may have developed from the doctor's prior association with the president's influential private secretary, Daniel S. Lamont. Frequent letters between Lamont and

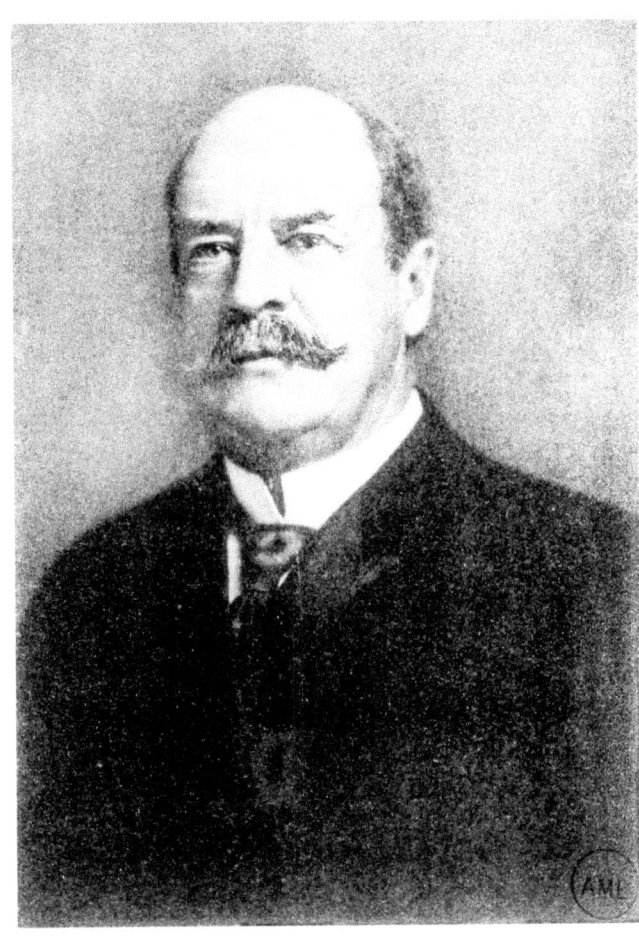

Joseph Bryant. Dr. Joseph Bryant successfully removed a malignant tumor from the mouth of his friend, President Grover Cleveland. In order to retain physician-patient confidentiality, he continued the tradition of misleading the press and the public. (National Library of Medicine)

Bryant during Cleveland's first term discussed the failing health of ex-president Ulysses S. Grant,[102] Bryant's request for library materials[103] and letters of introduction,[104] and the presentation of a gift to Lamont from Bryant.[105] The doctor also volunteered medical advice to Lamont prior to the president's departure on a trip in late September 1887 to the southern and western states. Bryant advised that Lamont stock "a few dozen bottles of lotion water (Buffalo)" and "20 grains of bromide of potassium" on the president's train, probably as a suggested treatment for Cleveland's gout.[106]

The Cleveland-Bryant friendship blossomed during the four years of the Benjamin Harrison interregnum. Many letters from this period attest to a growing close personal friendship,[107] including several letters from Cleveland thanking Bryant for his Christmas gifts,[108] and one inviting the doctor to join the then ex-president in his favorite recreation, fishing.[109] Grover Cleveland enjoyed the companionship of a small group of friends during his years out of office, and one such friend was surgeon Joseph D. Bryant.[110]

For these reasons, Major O'Reilly, the physician officially charged with the medical care of government officials in Washington, deferentially relinquished control over the president's medical emergency to Joseph Bryant. However, O'Reilly cooperated with Bryant in the management of Cleveland's case, and even administered ether anesthesia during the president's surgery.[111] Bryant advised surgery, determined the availability of a suitable discreet venue for an operation, the yacht of Commodore Benedict, and enlisted the consultative and operative support of an outstanding group of physicians. These were Professors William Williams Keen, John Erdmann and Edward Janeway.[112] Bryant himself performed the surgery that removed a sizable segment of Cleveland's maxilla.[113]

Purely political considerations dictated the time, the venue, and the attendant personnel for the president's surgery. In mid–1893, the United States was in the midst of a terrible financial panic, and its business and financial communities were dependent upon Cleveland's leadership to resolve the economic crisis. Unfortunately for Cleveland, he had succumbed to the demands of the antibusiness wing of his Democratic party and acquiesced in the selection of the Illinois populist Adlai Stevenson as his vice-presidential running mate. Cleveland's staff feared that any hint that Stevenson might succeed to the presidency would initiate an even more profound economic slide. Therefore, in order to avoid a panic that would compound the ongoing financial contraction, the president demanded the strictest secrecy for his medical plans. Bryant obeyed Cleveland's demands and delayed the surgery to correspond to the president's previously announced vacation plans. He clandestinely assembled his cast of consultants and performed the delicate surgery upon the yacht *Oneida* sailing upon the waters of New York City's East River. In an additional move to avoid disclosure, nurses were excluded from this adventure, and deckhands, sworn to secrecy, were utilized in their stead! Finally, after the successful surgery, Bryant was forced to lie to the press on two occasions in order to continue the deception.[114] As a footnote, O'Reilly was promoted to the coveted position of Surgeon General of the Army with the rank of brigadier general in September 1902.[115]

During the nineteenth and twentieth centuries, occupants of the surgeon generalship of the army and the navy figured prominently in the narrative of presidential physicians. Among nineteenth-century presidential physicians, six at some time during their career held the rank of surgeon general, and a seventh was passed over for promotion on two occasions. Doctors Thomas Harris, Jonathan Foltz, and Presley Rixey served as surgeons general of the navy, while doctors Joseph Barnes, Jedediah Baxter, and Robert O'Reilly became surgeons general of the army. The unsuccessful candidate for this office was Dr. Robert Crooke Wood.

There never has been either a statutory or an administrative connection between this office and the medical care of a president. Rather, the frequency with which present or future surgeons general held this post has been attributed to circumstance, convenience, or personality. In nineteenth-century Washington, the military medical presence consisted almost entirely of the small group of physicians who staffed the surgeon generals' offices. Thus, whenever necessary, simply convenient, or just economical, it was a physician from either of these sources who was called to minister to the health needs of the president or a member of his family.[116]

A May 1813 act of Congress established the offices and duties of the physician and surgeon general of the army, and a subsequent army reorganization by Secretary of War John Calhoun in 1818 conferred permanence to this office. Hospital surgeon Joseph Lowell was appointed its first surgeon general with the rank of brigadier general.[117]

The Department of the Navy, which was a separate cabinet department until after World War II, lagged in the reorganization of its medical personnel, despite the urgings of many of its senior surgeons, including Thomas Harris. Finally, in 1842, President John Tyler signed the naval reorganization bill that reorganized the Navy Department into five bureaus, one of which was the Bureau of Medicine and Surgery (BUMED). A navy surgeon was placed in charge with an annual compensation of $2,500 (less than the heads of the other four bureaus). Surgeon William P.C. Barton of Philadelphia was selected as the first surgeon general of the navy[118] (then designated as chief of the Bureau of Medicine and Surgery).

When Zachary Taylor was abruptly stricken with fatal dysentery in 1850, Alexander Wotherspoon and Richard Coolidge, two army surgeons from the surgeon general's office, were summoned.[119] And in 1832 future surgeon general of the navy (1844–1853) Dr. Thomas Harris traveled on official business to Washington from his post in Philadelphia; this circumstance may have motivated Andrew Jackson to take advantage of this especially qualified navy surgeon's availability. As discussed previously, Harris successfully removed the bothersome bullet impacted in Jackson's left shoulder since an 1813 gunfight,[120] but any connection with his future advancement is improbable.[121]

The surgeon generalship was the highest position to which a military medical officer might aspire. Was it possible that a professional association with the commander in chief might have political consequences for a military physician's career? Was the prestigious post of surgeon general a reward for care well given? The answer is certainly yes in the case of the ambitious Jedediah Baxter. Colonel Baxter, Chief Medical Purveyor in Washington, D.C., was promoted to Surgeon General of the Army on August 16, 1890.[122]

Military medical historians Mary Gillett and P.M. Ashburn chronicle Baxter's promotion: "Baxter benefited from the fact that the new president, Benjamin Harrison, was both a friend and a patient; thus, he triumphed over Sutherland, his longtime rival for the position of surgeon general." Doctor Charles Sutherland had served fifteen years longer in the Army Medical Department and was eight years older than Baxter.[123] Colonel Baxter, however, had been a perennial candidate for the surgeon generalship "Able and ambitious, he tried for the appointment to succeed General Barnes (in 1882)."

"When General Crane died, his named forged well to the front, when General Murray retired, he was one of the most conspicuous candidates for the succession. At the time of General Moore's retirement, Baxter was the senior colonel, his personal friend, Hon. Redfield Proctor, was Secretary of War, and President Harrison was a comrade and a long-time patient."[124]

The course of Robert O'Reilly's direction toward the army surgeon generalship (1902–1909) was less tightly bound to his medical service for Grover Cleveland.[125] However, upon reelection as president, Cleveland expeditiously recalled O'Reilly to Washington from the distant post of Fort Collins, Colorado, to reassume O'Reilly's professional care. It is possible that as a result, his continued prominence in the nation's capital enhanced his chances of promotion.[126]

Earlier discussion in a previous chapter detailed Jonathan Foltz's disappointment that President James Buchanan had neglected to promote him to the navy surgeon generalship, leading to an irreparable break between the two men. Foltz had anticipated this promotion as a reward for his previous medical service to the president. However, fifteen years later, in 1871, President Ulysses Grant appointed Foltz surgeon general of the navy and chief of the Bureau of Medicine and Surgery. Foltz's promotion was more honorary than powerful, since the new appointee reached the mandatory retirement age of sixty-five only seven months later and resigned.[127] But Foltz finally got his due, however brief.

Robert Crooke Wood was twice poised to be advanced to the surgeon generalship because of his prominent postings in Washington, his excellent professional standing, and his seniority. However, despite his relationship by marriage to a former president, he was twice passed over, first in 1861 and again in 1864. In 1864, the political gadfly Joseph K. Barnes was promoted instead.[128]

Surgeon General Barnes was politically astute and viewed attendance at the treatment of prominent officials as both a requirement and a perquisite of his office. Barnes put in an appearance at the deathbed of President Lincoln and was an assistant to Bliss in the care of the assassinated President Garfield (vide supra). Barnes had been an administrator, and not a practitioner, for seventeen years, and so his professional contribution in either case is unclear.[129] Barnes's rise in 1860s Washington was due to his friendship with his superior, Secretary of War Edwin Stanton. The latter "supported Barnes in all his undertakings, even when they involved activating projects he had previously disapproved."[130] Subsequent chapters will further illuminate that the surgeon generalship became a common component of the White House physician's reward system. Future presidential doctors Presley Rixey and Ross McIntire became recipients of this patronage.[131]

To summarize, several issues involving the presidents' physicians were thrashed out during this thirty-year period (1865–1898). The first was the issue of competition for patients between civilian and military members of the profession. By the time of Grover Cleveland's operation, this had been resolved to this patient's benefit, with civilian doctors acknowledging a legitimate role for military physicians in the care of presidents and cooperating in that care when requested. A second matter was the homeopath-orthodox rivalry which subsided significantly by the end of the nineteenth century, and finally was resolved during the tenure of future presidential physician Joel Boone.[132] The full acceptance of women into medicine would not be accomplished until late in the next century.

Finally, two secondary themes also were present during this time. One was the interrelated issues of VIP medicine and physician-physician deference, that is, who controls the president's medical care at times of multiple physician involvement. The second issue was the inversion of the traditional physician-patient relationship when the patient maintains and uses the leverage of the presidency, as Grover Cleveland did during an economic panic.

Chapter 5

Admiral Presley Rixey

The First Authentic White House Physician

Captain Presley Rixey supplemented the meager pay of a navy doctor with an active moonlighting practice among the elite of the nation's capital. Among his civilian patients were Secretary of the Navy John D. Long and the members of the Long family. In the fall of 1898, the secretary, scheduled to accompany President and Mrs. McKinley on a trip to Atlanta along with his sickly daughter, self-interestedly inquired whether the president intended to designate a physician as a member of the travel party. His biographers relate: "Upon consideration, the president expressed himself as also of the opinion that it would be desirable for many reasons to identify a medical man with the party, and having no one in mind himself, asked Mr. Long to suggest some doctor."[1]

Thus, as will be discussed below, the circumstance of a substandard salary serendipitously stimulated both the initiation of continuous medical care for a sitting president and the aggrandizement of Rixey's fame and fortune.

A medical presence in the White House had been both irregular and transient, except in cases of acute emergencies caused either by a dire infectious disease or by an assassin's bullet, until the presidency of William McKinley. This changed with the arrival of Navy physician Captain Presley M. Rixey, who made regular professional appearances at the executive mansion and became a customary member of the presidential party during McKinley's travels and vacations. Other features that characterized the tenure of this first authentic White House physician were: acknowledgment that the medical care of the president and his family was his preeminent responsibility; the establishment of medical treatment space in the White House; the contemporaneous establishment of a close personal relationship with the McKinley and Theodore Roosevelt families which was social and recreational as well as professional; and the use of a close relationship with his patient to command a reward for loyal and proficient service, including the navy surgeon generalship. Previously, Dr. Jedediah Baxter likewise had parlayed his presidential connections into a desired appointment as army surgeon general.[2] Fortunately for this author, Rixey left voluminous career notes and was biographed by two friendly colleagues, all of which permit a careful analysis of his career.[3]

Rixey's White House tenure coincided with an explosive growth of American hospitals. However, neither President Cleveland nor President McKinley was treated in a traditional hospital for either their operative or postoperative care. The reasons for these seemingly contrarian decisions will be explored. Second, postgraduate physician training in the form of an internship became increasingly common as hospitals grew in numbers. Doctor Rixey did not serve a medical internship, although several presidential

Chapter 5. Admiral Presley Rixey

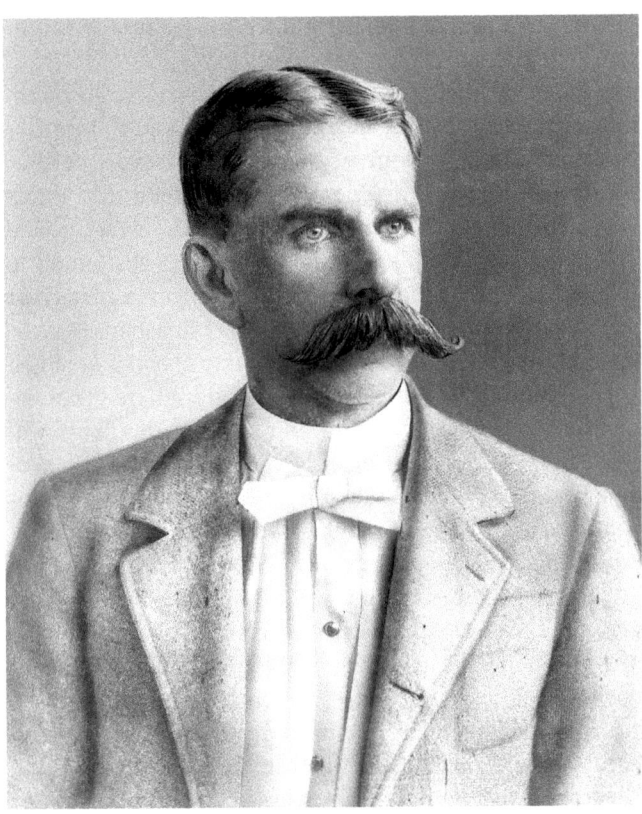

Presley Rixey. Navy physician Dr. Presley Rixey functioned as the first White House physician. President Theodore Roosevelt, as a reward, promoted him to surgeon general of the navy. (Courtesy of the Bureau of Medicine and Surgery Archives)

physicians of this era did.[4] A third major event was the 1910 publication of the Flexner report on medical education in the United States and Canada.[5] The investigation leading up to, and the widespread publicity surrounding, this report corresponded to a significant decrease in the number of American medical colleges, either through closure or consolidation. Some physicians who cared for presidents, either in a principal or subsidiary role, were alumni of schools that had disappeared.

Presley Rixey was one of nine children born into a family of Confederate sympathizers in Culpeper County, Virginia. The family farmhouse was twice expropriated during the Civil War to serve as Union headquarters. The general of the Union Armies, Ulysses Grant, who was one of many officers who used the Rixey house, signed the papers that appointed Dr. Rixey as a naval officer many years later. After receiving his secondary education in local schools, the young Rixey, a habitual user of family and social connections, apprenticed in the office of his cousin, Dr. Samuel Rixey. Apprenticeship continued to be a pathway to prepare students for medical school and often substituted for an undergraduate college education. Thereafter, Rixey was admitted to the University of Virginia School of Medicine, where he precociously completed his medical degree in a mere nine months. He burnished his skills by attending clinics at Jefferson Medical College, passed the scrutiny of the naval board of medical examiners, and was commissioned assistant surgeon in the Navy on January 28, 1874.[6]

The succeeding two decades included three lengthy sea cruises and eight years duty at the Naval Dispensary in Washington.[7] A professional détente with the District of Columbia medical society had been reached that tolerated civilian practices by military physicians. Rixey had an active civilian practice. One of his patients was Secretary of the Navy Benjamin Tracy, who retained his military doctor in Washington as long as possible.[8] During the 1898 Spanish War, Rixey was treating then Secretary of the Navy John D. Long for "an intractable condition of one of his knees." The secretary was initially very reluctant to accede to his physician's plea for warfront duty, but he finally acquiesced to the latter's importuning.[9]

Other prominent members of the naval doctor's practice at this time were Secretary of State John Hay, Senator Mark Hanna, who was the Chairman of the Naval Committee of the House of Representatives, congressmen, and members of the diplomatic corps.[10] Rixey at this time, was attending surgeon to the Washington Naval Dispensary, which included among its responsibilities the provision of medical care to the personnel at the Washington Navy Yard. During the 1860 to 1900 period, "it often was customary to order certain medical officers to Washington for special duty. These officers assisted the Surgeon General in special projects as attending physicians in the Navy Dispensary...."[11]

In the autumn of 1898, Navy Captain Presley Rixey was ordered to accompany President William McKinley and the presidential party to Atlanta, Georgia, where the president was to attend a Spanish American War victory celebration. Rixey's attendance was at the request of his patient, Navy Secretary Long. The latter's sickly daughter was scheduled to be a member of the presidential party, and the secretary intimated to McKinley that the presence of a doctor might be a useful addition to his coterie.

Shortly after the trip's conclusion, during a chance meeting, the president asked Rixey why the doctor had not accompanied him on a presidential trip to New York City the prior week. When Rixey responded that he had not received the corresponding travel orders, the president informed the physician that he wanted him "to continue to be his attending physician and also take charge of Mrs. McKinley who had been an invalid for many years."[12] Ida McKinley had been an epileptic since 1873, "subject to frequent attacks of petit mal, a brief loss of consciousness, and at irregular intervals to prolonged and violent seizures."[13] Retrospective analysis of her case concluded that Mrs. McKinley had suffered a central nervous system injury at that time, possibly involving the left frontal lobe of the brain. The pathologic sequelae were recurrent epileptic seizures and partial paralysis of her right arm.[14] Thus was initiated the ongoing practice of regular physician attendance on presidential trips away from Washington. This would not be the last time that the selection of the presidential physician resulted from the health requirements of the first lady. Dr. Rixey compassionately attended Ida McKinley even after the death of her husband. Rixey was present at her death in Canton, Ohio, in May 1907.[15]

Rixey's appointment to the White House at McKinley's request thrust the doctor into a difficult professional situation. General George M. Sternberg was then the incumbent "physician to the White House,"[16] who contemporaneously held the position of surgeon general of the army (officially, the Chief of the Medical Department of the United States Army). The demands of the latter position were significant, and the president preferred a personal physician whose primary responsibility was the ongoing health care of Mrs. McKinley and himself. Doctor Rixey adroitly solved the embarrassment of his older and more distinguished superior officer by tactfully suggesting that General Sternberg continue his visits to the White House as consulting surgeon. Sternberg accepted this arrangement and the two doctors regularly met in consultation at the White House each Sunday morning.[17]

Rixey referred to his position as "Physician to the Executive Mansion"[18] and provided a description of his duties in his autobiographical notes: "This duty was in addition to my already large practice quite a task and comprised all that was related to the health of the inmates of the Executive Mansion, in addition to my duties as Surgeon in charge of the Naval Dispensary. My special care was the President and Mrs. McKinley. By direction of the President, I made at least two visits every day, the first at 10:00 a.m., and the second at 10:00 p.m., and as many more as required."[19] In this statement, he makes clear that despite other commitments, his primary professional responsibility was to the president of the United States and his family. Margaret Leech in her biography of the president identified Rixey as the White House physician.[20] Rixey was present on all presidential journeys and attended the McKinleys during their summer vacations, including their lengthy respite in Canton, Ohio, during the summer of 1901.[21] During the White House physician's absence from Washington, his assistant, surgeon Eugene Stone, filled in at the Naval Dispensary and physician friends attended to his private patients.[22]

Ida McKinley consumed most of Rixey's attention because the president was significantly ill only once. In early 1901, McKinley came down with a severe cold that evolved into influenza. He became seriously ill, was confined to his bed for several days, and was only able to fully resume his work schedule after another week.[23] McKinley continued the practice of assigning his personal physician to the care of VIPs. At the insistence of the president, Rixey was dispatched to treat the dying vice president, Garret Hobart.[24] Previously, presidential physician O'Reilly had been dispatched to care for General Philip Sheridan.[25]

Presley Rixey accompanied the McKinleys from their Canton home to the Pan American Exposition in Buffalo, New York. It was there, on September 6, 1901, that anarchist Leon Czolgosz fatally shot the president. At the time of the assassination, the White House physician was absent, having escorted Mrs. McKinley to the presidential family's temporary Buffalo residence. Czolgosz's bullet perforated the anterior and posterior stomach walls, damaged the upper pole of the left kidney and destroyed the pancreas. The resultant pancreatitis was the probable cause of the president's death; the president expired early in the morning of September 14.[26] The catastrophic nature of McKinley's injuries convinced his attending surgeons that any surgery be immediate and that it be performed within the inadequate facilities of the temporary hospital that was constructed to attend to the urgent medical needs of the Exposition's attendees.[27]

In contrast to the professional conflict that marked Garfield's medical care after his wounding twenty years previously, deference and decorum characterized the cooperation of the many doctors who treated McKinley. Herman Mynter, a general surgeon practicing in Buffalo, was the first to arrive on the scene, but Mynter graciously deferred professional control of the case upon the arrival of Dr. Matthew Mann. Mann was well known and respected in Buffalo as the long-term chairman of obstetrics and gynecology at the university medical school, and in 1901 he was both a past and a future president of the American Gynecological Society.[28] John G. Milburn, the president's host in Buffalo and the president of the Pan American Exposition, choosing for the wounded McKinley from among the many physicians unfamiliar to the president, selected Mann as the one to take charge of the operation. After consultation with the physicians there assembled, Dr. Mann chose his operative team and asked Mynter to be his first assistant.[29] At the conclusion of the operation, Mann acknowledged the grace and skill of Dr. Mynter: "Not only was he an assistant, but he was much more, and helped me greatly by his skill and, as a consultant, with his good judgment and extensive knowledge of abdominal work. Although called first, he waived his claim, and generously placed the case in my hands, willingly assuming his share of the responsibility."[30]

Roswell Park, the medical director of the exposition and Buffalo's most renowned surgeon, was operating in Niagara Falls at the time of the assassination. He was immediately summoned to return, but arrived too late to participate in the surgery. If Park had been available, he most certainly would have been chosen to perform the abdominal operation upon McKinley.[31] Although he had reservations about the immediacy and the conduct of the surgery, Park deferred to Mann's judgment at the conclusion of the operation, upheld the professional consensus during the subsequent postoperative and postmortem interval, and kept his misgivings private.[32] After criticisms of the president's care circulated immediately after his death, Park cosigned with Mann, Mynter and others a statement, released on September 17, entitled, "No Disagreement among Those Who Attended President McKinley."[33]

Rixey arrived at the hospital as soon as he was apprised of the dire situation. The makeshift operating room contained no electric lighting, but Rixey temporarily solved the problem of inadequate illumination of the surgical wound by producing a hand mirror that reflected the setting sunlight into the operative field.[34] Ironically, the buildings of the exposition were externally illuminated by thousands of electric lights and the exposition grounds had been dubbed The City of Lights.[35]

After the operation, the president was moved to the home of his Buffalo host, John G. Milburn. From that time on, "Dr. Rixey took official charge of the case."[36] He not only directed the hour-by-hour care of his patient, but also was the official spokesman regarding the president's postoperative course and ultimate death on the seventh postoperative day. Rixey was the primary author of almost all the thirty-nine medical bulletins that were issued to the press. In a sign of professional unity, these and the official report of the case were cosigned by all the other attendants. When the president's medical course deteriorated, it was the White House physician who summoned additional consultants, doctors Charles Stockton, Charles McBurney, Edward Janeway and W.W. Johnston, from as far away as New York City.[37]

The dispensary at the Pan American Exposition had been designed by Dr. Roswell Park, who continued to serve as its medical director during the duration of the exposition. The facility included three wards, two for men and one for women, with accommodations for twenty-five beds, an operating room, and space for ambulances. The dispensary was continually staffed by physicians and nurses. Its standard operating procedure was that no patients were to be kept overnight, and indeed during its operation seventy patients were transferred to Buffalo hospitals.[38]

Adele Pillitteri explained that Mann's decision not to transport the wounded McKinley to the relatively well-equipped Buffalo General "was probably influenced by the fact that 20 years earlier when President Garfield had been shot ... his doctors had delayed so long in trying to locate the bullet ... that Garfield had developed peritonitis."[39] After the operation, the president was then cared for in a private home. Pillitteri's explanation for this choice of venue was: "Hospitals in 1901 were constructed to care for the poor, wealthy patients were cared for at home."[40]

The odd venue for President Cleveland's 1893 operation had been a medical decision that the president had wrested from his physicians by virtue of the authority of his office. The political context of the situation determined the substitution of a ship's cabin for a relatively well-equipped operating room in one of New York City's established hospitals.[41] Although New York's Bellevue Hospital had been previously "stigmatized as totally unfit to receive and house the sick in its present condition," contemporary state of the art medical facilities were available at the New York, St. Vincent's, Lenox Hill (formerly the German) and Roosevelt hospitals.[42]

Beginning in 1875, the next forty years saw a dramatic expansion of the American hospital system, as hospitals became acceptable substitutes for home care. The expansion was national in scope; as an example, twenty-two hospitals opened in Kansas City between 1874 and 1915.[43] The first American hospital survey was conducted in 1873, and it listed 178 facilities, including mental institutions, which contained a total of fewer than 50,000 beds. A subsequent census in 1909 documented 4,359 hospitals, excluding mental institutions and tuberculosis sanatoriums, with 421,065 beds.[44]

A confluence of factors was responsible for this development. Urbanization and population growth made the hospital a more convenient location for busy physicians to treat their patients. In the late 1880s, the introduction of first antisepsis, followed by anesthetic techniques, made abdominal surgery practical. As a consequence, the frequency of hospital surgeries exploded. This trend was further abetted by the availability of in-hospital X-ray and laboratory departments. Additionally, nursing schools, founded in conjunction with hospitals, served to supply the work force necessary to provide day to day patient care. Finally, internships multiplied so that young physicians could on the one hand insure continuous in-hospital treatment, and on the other acquire necessary experience before embarking on their medical careers.[45]

Theodore Roosevelt, who as the sitting vice president succeeded to the presidency upon McKinley's death, continued Rixey's duties as the White House physician. Presley, and to a lesser extent Mrs. Rixey, socialized with the McKinleys and the Roosevelts. During the Roosevelt administrations, they were frequent guests of the president and his wife, both at the White House and at the president's home in Oyster Bay, New York.[46] Moreover, the doctor became a close friend and companion to both of his presidential patients, initiating sixty years in which the military officers who fulfilled the role of White House physician became the pals of the incumbent chief executive—male buddies who shared stories, sports, and social intimacies. This intimate relationship, deviating from the usual doctor-patient professional interaction, had definite political and medical consequences in future years, but not in Rixey's case.

Rixey's relationship with McKinley was described as "More than a trusted medical advisor—he was an esteemed friend and companion, and the attachment which is widely known was not without foundation."[47] The doctor also bonded with the energetic Roosevelt. Rixey was an accomplished horseman and a dedicated hunter, and the two went on frequent rides and hunts together. The hunting trips were described as "too numerous to mention."[48] They included trips to Virginia for quail or wild turkey and a number of big game hunts in Louisiana and the far West.[49] The physician continued to accompany Roosevelt on his departures from the nation's capital. However, each of these departures from his Washington post were listed in his service records as "Special Duty," indicating that the role of the White House physician had yet to be formalized.[50]

Doctor Rixey was the first to establish a medical space in the White House, albeit an evanescent one. He equipped a "small operating or dressing room, which, among other things, included a medical case of liberal therapeutic range."[51] But it would be another thirty years before medical space became a permanent part of the White House complex.

President McKinley had been so impressed by the professional and personal talents of Dr. Rixey that he gratuitously promised the doctor that he would be appointed surgeon general of the navy upon the first vacancy in that office. This position had been an ambition of Mrs. Rixey for many years, but the president was slain before the promised appointment could be finalized.[52] Theodore Roosevelt was reminded of this promise by two cabinet secretaries who had been privy to McKinley's offer, and he, also taken by the physician's deportment and abilities, nominated Rixey for this post. On February 10, 1902, Dr. Rixey became the navy's seventeenth surgeon general, a position that automatically carried with it the rank of rear admiral. His advancement was over the heads of twenty-seven naval officers who were senior to him, but apparently was not resented, since Rixey was held in general esteem by his naval colleagues.[53]

The admiral was able to coordinate his care of the Roosevelt family with his new responsibilities. Indeed, his familiarity with and access to the president, together with the active influence of his younger brother, Representative John Franklin Rixey, a member of the House Committee on Naval Affairs, enabled the new surgeon general to be very successful in securing support for the naval medical department.[54]

The doctor was on hand to diagnose and direct the care of Archie, one of the Roosevelt's sons, when he contracted diphtheria.[55] Rixey also operated upon a soft tissue tumefaction of the president's lower leg.[56] With the assistance of an orthopedic surgeon he semi-anesthetized Roosevelt with alcohol and topical cocaine, and cut down to the tibia to remove the swelling. He was also able to monitor closely the activities of the boisterous Roosevelt who in 1905 was losing sight in his left eye, the result of a recent boxing punch.[57]

Admiral Rixey was reappointed to surgeon generalship for a second four-year term in 1906 and retired from the navy in 1910. His influence in naval matters continued with service as a member of the Naval Examining Board during the first Wilson administration. He was influential in the selection of his cousin Cary Grayson as the Wilson White House physician. In his honor, the hospital ship *Rixey* was commissioned in December 1942, and sailed with distinction in many engagements in the World War II Pacific Theater.[58]

Presley Rixey introduced a sixty-year period in which senior naval and army officers functioned as White House physicians. The medical care of the first family was their primary professional responsibility and they were constant companions of the president whenever he departed from Washington for political, diplomatic, or recreational trips. Their constant presence usually endeared them to the chief executive and usually engendered a close personal relationship. It was not unusual for these White House physicians to be rewarded for their services with promotions in rank and position.

At about the same time when Presley Rixey was defining the position of White House physician, the reach of in-hospital physician training and the character of the modern American medical college likewise were being determined. Rixey did not participate in the former since he did not spend a year after graduation as a hospital intern. Yet an internship was becoming increasingly popular among graduating American medical students during the nineteenth century. Instead, Rixey, determining that "it was absolutely necessary for him to make a decision of how he should make a living," sought a commission in the U.S. Navy instead.[59]

The seed that germinated over the course of the nineteenth century into the traditional internship year, i.e., twelve months of postgraduate hospital training that commenced immediately after graduation from medical school. The intern was also called the house physician or resident physician. In 1797 Benjamin Rush and other attending doctors on the staff of the Pennsylvania Hospital pressed for the hiring of a house surgeon to attend to outpatients, treat and admit emergencies, and carry out the orders of attending staff physicians.[60] This position became well accepted by mid-century in many hospitals as a means of providing continuous and emergency care for patients in the absence of those patients' regular physicians.[61] James C. Hall, the Pillar of the Profession, spent a year in this capacity at Philadelphia's Blockley Hospital during the 1820s.[62]

With time, a postgraduate year spent in a hospital that combined increasing patient responsibility with clinical training became desirable. It not only benefited young doctors by providing both an entrée into professional networks and clinical preparation for state licensing examinations; it also benefited hospitals whose expansion in numbers and in bed counts required continuous medical presence on-site. In urban centers the intern staff had become by 1900 the "real stuff of every hospital in the city."[63]

The first survey by the AMA Council on Medical Education in 1904 estimated that 50 percent of medical graduates were then going on to hospital training, and in 1917 it published its first comprehensive list of hospital internships.[64]

Future presidential physicians Richard Coolidge[65] and Joseph Barnes[66] served as resident physicians in New York and Philadelphia hospitals respectively in the late 1830 to early 1840 period. Coolidge's two-year service was unusual. Jedediah Baxter "after graduation ... went to New York City, where he saw some service as resident physician at Bellevue and Blackwell Island hospitals" during 1860–1861.[67]

After the Civil War, as hospitals became more numerous, the necessity for and the availability of internship positions also increased. During this period, internships were taken by Edward G. Janeway at Bellevue Hospital (1864–1866), Roswell Park at Chicago's Cook County Hospital (1876), and John Erdmann, also at Bellevue Hospital (1887–1888).[68] However, many medical school graduates continued to bypass postgraduate training in the latter part of the nineteenth century. There is no record of internship training for presidential physicians, civilian doctors D.W. Bliss and Robert Reyburn, or for military officers Robert O'Reilly and William Sternberg.[69]

Neither Dr. W.W. Keen nor Dr. Matthew Mann undertook an internship in an American Hospital. Instead, they performed their postgraduate training on the European continent. Mann studied abroad for two years before he commenced the practice of medicine in New York City in 1873. Keen did postgraduate studies in Paris and Berlin in 1861.[70] Between 1870 and 1914, approximately 15,000 American physicians departed for the European continent to study medicine at German universities.[71] Vienna, Berlin and other German and Swiss schools, rather than Edinburgh or London, were the destinations of this second wave of students of medicine from the United States. Bonner's explanation for this second medical migration was, "Nowhere in America in 1870 could a graduate physician perfect his knowledge of any branch of medicine as well as in Germany, or learn systematically the techniques of medical research and investigation. Postgraduate education in medicine did not exist even in name; modern laboratories could be found in virtually no institution of higher education [in the United States]."[72]

Significant numbers of the most prominent American physicians of this era trained in a German university, and the specialties of ophthalmology, otology, obstetrics and dermatology were the most indebted to German tutelage.[73] With the onset of the First World War in 1914, this flow of American doctors was dammed.

Contemporaneous with Rixey's reformation of the White House medical practice, a major reorganization occurred with the system of American undergraduate medical education. Medical schools witnessed increased scientific content in their courses, augmented patient and clinical exposure for their students, and saw a dramatic reduction in their numbers. A major impetus for these improvements was the 1910 publication of Abraham Flexner's historic report on "Medical Education in the United States and Canada."[74] The scrutiny upon educationally deficient, academically substandard and poorly capitalized medical colleges both during the report's preparation and after its appearance led to the dissolution of many and the consolidation of others. As a result, there were far fewer physicians in training in far fewer institutions of undergraduate medical education in 1922 than there had been in 1906.[75]

Physician Simon Flexner was influential in introducing his educator brother, Abraham, to the Carnegie Foundation's president, Henry S. Pritchett, and to several of its board members. Serendipity matched this educator, who previously had never been inside a medical school, with the headstrong Pritchett, who was determined to avoid any interference by the medical profession at a time when "swiftly moving scientific, educational, and philanthropic currents ... strongly favored reform."[76]

The indefatigable Flexner commenced his medical school examinations in 1908, and during the next eighteen months he traversed the continental United States numerous times while making 174 separate on-site inspections of medical schools. In his introductory chapter, Flexner identified the problem he was to confront: "First and last, the United States and Canada have in little more than a century produced four hundred and fifty-seven medical schools, many of course, short-lived, and perhaps fifty still-born. One hundred and fifty-seven survive today. Of these, Illinois, prolific mother of thirty-nine medical colleges, still harbors in the city of Chicago fourteen; forty-two sprang from the fertile soil of Missouri, twelve of them still 'going' concerns.... The city of Cincinnati brought forth about twenty, the city of Louisville eleven. These enterprises—for the most part they can be called schools or institutions only by courtesy—were frequently set up regardless of opportunity or need."[77]

Flexner concluded that America required fewer but better schools that would be located in population centers and attached to universities and teaching hospitals. His recommendation was draconian: that the more than 150 schools then extant be reduced to thirty-one that were strategically located and that the number of medical students be halved.[78]

However, the fate of the alma maters of presidential physicians, both those in a primary responsibility and those in a consulting capacity, reflected the above dissolution and consolidations to only a modest degree. The perquisites of the presidency probably permitted entrée to an upper class of educated medical practitioners. Cary Grayson, Woodrow Wilson's personal physician, and Robert Reyburn, who attended the moribund James Garfield, were the only graduates of schools that were already defunct by the time of Flexner's investigations.

Dr. Reyburn attended the Philadelphia College of Medicine in 1856 and 1857 and graduated with an M.D. degree in 1857. Despite a merger with the medical department of Pennsylvania College, financial difficulties and mass resignations of faculty caused the demise of the combined schools in 1861.[79] Dr. Grayson was the valedictorian of the 1903 graduating class of the University of the South (Sewanee) medical school. This school was short-lived. Founded in 1892, it closed in 1909. Sewanee was no longer able to support it despite high enrollments; moreover, it anticipated a negative evaluation by Abraham Flexner since its education was textbook, not clinical practice, based.[80]

Chapter 5. Admiral Presley Rixey

At least two consultants and one appointed presidential physician were medical graduates of schools that could survive only by consolidating with a more substantial institution: Charles Powers (Wooster Medical College, 1865), Roswell Park (Chicago Medical College, 1876), Ross McIntire (Willamette, 1912). Dr. Powers briefly attended President Garfield after the assassination attempt.

The Flexner report on Willamette was devastating. After taking into account that the requirement for entrance was less than a high school education, that the chemistry laboratory had little material and no running water, and that the clinical facilities were little more than nominal, he concluded that it "…is an utterly hopeless affair, for which no word can be said."[81]

Rixey's tenure occurred during a period of significant change in American medicine. Medical school education was significantly tightened and strengthened; the beginnings of postgraduate training appeared; and hospitals began to assume an increasingly important role for the medical profession. Presley Rixey expanded the medical presence in the White House to a degree that he rightly qualifies as the first White House physician. Twenty years later another navy physician, Joel Boone, would institutionalize this office.

Chapter 6

Captain Joel Boone and the Institutionalization of the Office of the White House Physician

On his inauguration day, March 4, 1929, President Herbert Hoover directed his newly appointed presidential physician, Joel Boone, to take him to the doctor's White House office to treat a sore finger. Boone dutifully "…led the president to a linen closet in the center of the long hall on the second floor. After he had opened the double doors, revealing shelves lined with bottles, dressings, and medical instruments," Hoover repeated, "…with a note of annoyance, 'But I want to go to your office.' 'This is our office,' was the reply."[1]

The tenure of navy doctor Joel T. Boone, first as the assistant White House physician to presidents Warren G. Harding and Calvin Coolidge (1922–1929), and then as the White House physician to President Herbert Hoover (1929–1933), coincided with significant enhancements of the duties, physical space and official recognition of this position. Acts of Congress in 1928 and 1930 that codified the rank and perquisites of military physicians assigned to the White House provided its first official acknowledgment.

Joel Boone was a prolific chronicler of his White House experience, leaving a diary, oral histories, and copious notes and papers that are available in several presidential museums and the Library of Congress. Additionally, he was the beneficiary of an admiring biography by his son-in-law.[2] With rich detail Boone elaborated on several aspects of the White House physician's unique position: an expansion of his responsibilities to include not only the health care for the presidential extended family but also for political associates, and the assumption of additional ceremonial and social responsibilities peculiar to the office. Joel Boone also was an interesting example of a physician to the president; he was both a homeopath[3] by training and the only Congressional Medal of Honor recipient to serve in this capacity.[4]

When Boone was first assigned as assistant White House physician in 1922, he was stunned by the primitive facilities then dedicated to medical care in the White House. Brigadier General Charles Sawyer, White House physician to President Warren G. Harding (1921–1923) and Boone's superior, had been able to secure a linen closet on its second floor, which he had converted into a medical facility with shelves, a folding table and an overhead light. The closet also provided space to store his doctor's bag containing medical equipment and assorted medicines. Despite the prior efforts of Presley Rixey, for most of its history a doctor's bag toted around by the presidential physician as he made his patient rounds had been his sole medical venue in the White House.[5]

Chapter 6. Joel Boone and Institutionalization of the Office

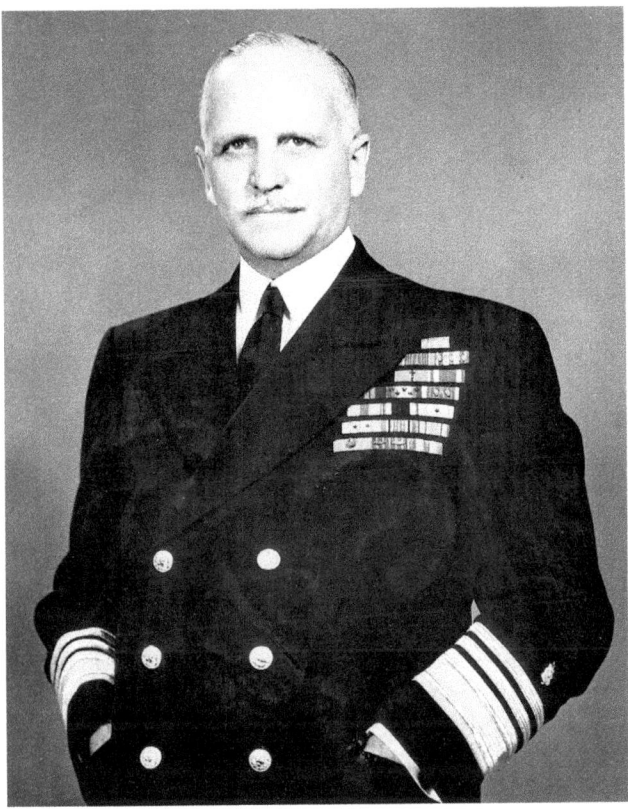

Joel Boone. Navy physician and homeopathically trained, Dr. Joel Boone served as a White House physician under Presidents Harding, Coolidge and Hoover. After his appointment as Herbert Hoover's presidential physician, he institutionalized White House medicine. (Courtesy of the Bureau of Medicine and Surgery Archives)

As described earlier, shortly after his inauguration as president in 1929, Herbert Hoover, while being treated for a sore finger by Boone, was amazed to discover that the location for treating a president in the White House was a closet! He subsequently charged Boone to locate more appropriate space in the executive mansion. The latter identified rooms in the basement for an office and a treatment clinic which previously had served as a poolroom and valet's quarters respectively. Hoover, trained as a mining engineer, saw no difficulty in drilling a doorway through the four-foot wall that separated these two rooms in order to establish a functional work area.[6]

Boone also increased the size of the permanent White House medical staff from one to two. He requested the reassignment to the executive mansion of navy corpsman George A. Fox to assist the presidential physician in his duties. Although nurses and ancillary health personnel including Fox had been assigned to presidential care on previous occasions, the assignments had been temporary. Fox was the first to fill a permanent slot on the White House personnel roll.[7]

Additionally, Boone may have been the one to inaugurate regular and comprehensive physical examinations of the president, a practice that has become institutionalized. This doctor initiated periodic examinations on the sixth day after Hoover's inauguration,[8] and thus presaged a commitment to health maintenance and disease prophylaxis that went beyond the prompt diagnosis and treatment of acute medical problems that had risen episodically.

At Hoover's insistence[9] the Seventy-first Congress of the United States codified the rank of those military physicians who were assigned to duty as physician to the White House. On April 4, 1930, both houses of Congress approved the following: "That the officer of the Medical Corps, United States Army, or of the Medical Corps, United States Navy, below the rank of colonel or captain, respectively, who is now, or hereafter may be, assigned to duty as physician to the White House, shall have the temporary rank and the pay and allowances of a Colonel, Medical Corps, United States Army, or of Captain, Medical Corps, United States Navy, while so serving: Provided that the officer now assigned to that duty shall have the rank, pay and allowances herein provided from March 6, 1929, the date of assignment as such."[10]

This statute retroactively applied to Boone, since a previous act of the Seventieth Congress, approved May 16, 1928, had applied only to army medical officers.[11] Boone complained to Coolidge about the initial act's oversight of naval officers, namely himself, then a navy commander. He also requested that the travel and related expenses that he incurred related to his duties be compensated. Coolidge, angered by Boone's request, insisted that the temporary promotion of his personal White House physician, Dr. James Coupal, was only fair since the latter had incurred significant expenses while spending summer vacations with the Coolidge family.[12] President Hoover satisfied Boone's ambition when he promoted the doctor to navy captain retroactive to the date of Hoover's inauguration.[13] An act of Congress, August 10, 1956, simplified the wording of the 1930 law by declaring the "temporary" as surplusage.[14]

Joel T. Boone was a native of Pennsylvania. His choice of a medical career was heavily influenced by his admiration of his uncle, Dr. George Boone.[15] Upon graduation from Mercersburg Academy, Boone was admitted directly to medical school; a college education still was not a prerequisite for admission in the late nineteenth century. Boone selected the homeopathic medical school Hahnemann Medical College in Pennsylvania, graduated in 1913, and continued at Hahnemann for his internship year.[16] Boone later joined doctors Susan A. Edson, Silas Boynton, and Charles Sawyer as the only homeopathically trained physicians to serve as medical caregivers for a United States president. Doctors Edson and Boynton participated in the nursing care of the moribund James Garfield. However, in contrast to both Edson and Sawyer, Boone was trained at a time when the treatment and diagnostic practices of homeopathic and allopathic medicine had converged.[17]

At the turn of the century, homeopathy in America was at the peak of its influence, just before it began its slide into the valley of medical irrelevance. It was not until the last decades of the twentieth century that it began a slow climb back toward significance as a part of the growing popularity of alternative medicine.

In 1900 between 8 and 10 percent of doctors were homeopaths and the percentage was even higher in the urban states of the East and Midwest. Twenty-two homeopathic medical schools were extant in 1900, and in 1898 American homeopathy hosted nine national medical societies, thirty-three state medical societies, eighty-five local societies, sixty-six general homeopathic hospitals, seventy-four specialty homeopathic hospitals, fifty-seven homeopathic dispensaries, and thirty-one medical journals.[18]

Toward the end of the nineteenth century, regular physicians found a need to cooperate with homeopathic doctors in order to effect meaningful state licensure laws. Both sets of physicians realized that a common front was necessary to ensure a system of quality health care. The coalition's goals were twofold: to drive incompetent physicians from the practice of medicine and to limit the prerogatives of newer medical sects, e.g., chiropractors, osteopaths and Christian Scientists.[19]

The Flexner report on American medical education in 1910 savaged the homeopathic medical colleges. Already by the date of its publication the number of medical colleges of this sect had declined from twenty-two in 1900 to fifteen. Flexner criticized the educational position of these schools as self-contradictory, "...when, having pursued ... the normal scientific curriculum with his student for two years, he is at the

Chapter 6. Joel Boone and Institutionalization of the Office

beginning of the third year produces a novel principle and requires that thenceforth the student effect a compromise between science and revelation."[20] His criticisms included the admission standards,[21] laboratory investigation, and financial underpinnings of homeopathic education.[22] Flexner successfully accomplished his mission to reduce the number of American medical colleges; only two homeopathic medical schools existed in 1930 and none in 1950.[23]

The rapid progress of scientific medicine in the 1890s and beyond persuaded many homeopathically trained doctors to dispense allopathic remedies in conjunction with their traditional homeopathic treatments. The great majority of sectarian doctors began to disbelieve in infinitesimal doses, to reject the universality of the law of similars, and thus to prescribe according to the principles of orthodox medicine. As the differences between orthodoxy and homeopathy blurred, there was a decreasing interest on the part of practitioners to select the latter as a method of education or practice. Finally, the desire of homeopathic physicians to benefit from scientific progress, to consult with their orthodox colleagues, and to specialize in the new branches of medicine combined to affect the near demise of homeopathy in the early decades of the 1900s.[24]

Boone enlisted in the United States Navy in 1914; shortly thereafter Lieutenant Boone was dispatched to Haiti to join the marines then engaged in a lengthy peacemaking mission.[25] With the United States entry into World War I, Boone was assigned as assistant regimental surgeon to the Sixth Marine Regiment in France. It was there that his heroic behavior was recognized with the Congressional Medal of Honor. In an accompanying citation, President Woodrow Wilson stated in part: "For extraordinary heroism, conspicuous gallantry, and intrepidity while serving with the Sixth regiment, United States Marines, in actual conflict with the enemy at and in the vicinity of Vierzy, France, 19 July 1918. With absolute disregard for personal safety, ever conscious and mindful of the suffering fallen, Surgeon Boone, leaving the shelter of a ravine, went forward onto the open field where there was no protection and, despite the extreme enemy fire of all calibers, through a heavy mist of gas, applied dressings and first aid to the wounded Marines."[26]

Boone's journey to the White House was serendipitous. At the conclusion of the war, he was assigned to the Navy's Bureau of Medicine and Surgery (surgeon general's office) in Washington, D.C. (1919–1922).[27] However, the medical needs of a first lady again intervened and dramatically altered a physician's professional career. In March 1922 Boone and his wife, Helen, were invited to the White House for an interview by Florence Harding, the wife of the president. Mrs. Harding took a liking to the couple, and her favorable evaluation, together with Boone's heroic war record and his friendship with navy surgeon general Edward Stitt, led to his new assignment—the medical officer of the presidential yacht, *Mayflower*.[28] The major responsibility of this post was the health of its crew of seven officers and 315 men. However, this medical officer also was responsible for the care of President and Mrs. Harding whenever they stayed on the *Mayflower* and the incumbent White House physician, Dr. Charles Sawyer, was absent.[29] Boone's position as medical officer of the *Mayflower* also entailed many social and ceremonial duties.[30]

Subsequently Florence Harding began to rely upon Dr. Boone's care for her chronic kidney problems and insisted that he make consultation visits to the White House.[31] As a result, he was appointed assistant White House physician, a position that was reaffirmed when Calvin Coolidge became president upon Harding's death in 1923.[32]

Boone's eleven years at the White House involved him in the medical emergencies that afflicted the nation's first families during this period—the periodic flare-ups of Florence Harding's kidney, the death of Warren Harding in San Francisco, and the sudden illness and death from bacterial sepsis of the Coolidges' younger son, Calvin.

It was Boone's practice to check President Coolidge's pulse every morning at precisely 8:00 a.m. and again in the evening at 6:30 p.m.[33] He defined his responsibility toward the Coolidges as keeping them "as healthy as possible, support them in their performance, and be a reassuring influence. He recognized a responsibility to care for his charges without disclosing to the public every detail of an indisposition and nonetheless keep the public informed."[34]

The White House physician's medical responsibilities included the members of the president's immediate family.[35] It occasionally expanded to include members of their extended families, e.g., Dr. Boone accompanied Grace Coolidge, the President's wife, on three separate occasions to Northampton, Massachusetts, to treat her mother, Lemira Goodhue. Consequently, Boone did not accompany the presidential party to their 1928 summer vacation in Wisconsin, in order to be more available to take care of Mrs. Goodhue.[36] Doctor Coupal, Coolidge's White House physician, was dispatched to treat Colonel John Coolidge, the president's father at his Vermont home for extended periods of time when the senior Coolidge was recovering from a prostate operation. Subsequently, Coupal remained at the colonel's side during his final illness and was ordered to telephone the President when his father's death was imminent.[37] Yet another example of this new duty was Boone's mission to the Harvard Business School at the request of Hoover to check on son Allan's health and to confer with one of Allan's teachers[38] when the younger Hoover was experiencing adjustment problems at the college.

Harding requested that Boone treat his closest political associate and friend, attorney general Harry M. Daugherty, who suffered from hypertension and a minor stroke. As a consequence, the doctor absented himself from the presidential party to treat Daugherty for an extended period of time. While in attendance the doctor also performed secretarial chores for the ill Attorney General.[39] Daugherty also asked that Boone take care of his political crony, Jess Smith, who was a diabetic.[40] President Hoover continued the practice of providing uncompensated medical treatment to visitors when it may have been politically opportune—Boone was requested to care for presidential guests Madam Curie and Thomas Edison.[41] During this period the presidential physician attended not only the president and his family but also assumed the care of other individuals in the executive branch of the government. Boone's medical practice included the White House staff and cabinet members and their families. He was subject to call at any time.[42]

Social and ceremonial duties often occupied Boone during the Harding and Coolidge administrations.[43] He taught Florence Harding how to dance, swam with Grace Coolidge,[44] and played tennis with the Coolidge sons.[45] First lady Grace Coolidge developed a lifelong friendship with Joel Boone, which extended to the entire Boone family, including daughter Suzanne. Suzanne spent many nights in the White House as the guest of Mrs. Coolidge and was a guest of the Coolidges at Washington Senators baseball games.[46] Grace Coolidge discussed many personal family issues with Dr. Boone, and continued a correspondence with the Boones for many years after she had departed the White House. Boone attended her funeral in 1957.[47] When Grace Coolidge sought out Boone's counsel for a proper school for her sons, the doctor convinced her

Chapter 6. Joel Boone and Institutionalization of the Office

to select his alma mater, Mercersburg Academy, in Pennsylvania.[48] Boone became close friends with the two Coolidge sons and frequently played tennis and went horseback riding with them.[49]

Doctor Boone saw President Hoover daily and organized the daily dawn Hooverball games on the White House lawn.[50] This was a concoction by Boone to provide scheduled exercise for the portly president. Hooverball consisted of tossing about a weighted medicine ball in a volleyball format. When the diagnosis of tuberculosis was made on son Herbert Jr., the Hoovers exhibited their confidence in their White House physician by recalling their son to the White House for Boone to confirm the diagnosis.[51] In November 1936, Lou Hoover, the ex-president's wife, saw to it that her favorite uncle, Will Henry, age 89, when he became ill, was transported to the San Diego naval hospital, where Dr. Boone was then stationed, in order to keep Mrs. Hoover abreast of uncle Will's diagnosis and treatment.[52]

During the eras of Presley Rixey and Joel Boone the routine medical responsibilities of the White House physician were modest, permitting these doctors to become the friends, and even the confidantes, of members of the first family. The development of a personal intimacy with the patients of a physician, however, may introduce unnecessary conflicts into a medical relationship; such a personal relationship might prove problematical in the delivery of objective medical care. Political psychologists Jerrold Post and Robert Robins analyzed the special conditions of the relationship between a national leader and his physician.[53] They emphasized that when the "contact, physical and emotional, is very close, an unusual degree of intimacy results that has important consequences for the physician's judgment and for the health management of the physician's special charge."[54] Chapter 7 will document examples of personal attachments influencing and trumping professional decisions.

Issues of authority and control may arise whenever a medical team involves more than a single physician. Conflict is especially prevalent during medical emergencies, such as the terminal illness of Warren G. Harding in San Francisco in 1923 when as many as five physicians composed the medical team. In his writings, Boone describes in detail his problems with deference to his nominal medical superiors in the White House. Boone bridled at the chain of command that subordinated his medical opinion to those of physicians whose professional competence he considered to be inferior: Brigadier General Charles Sawyer and Colonel James F. Coupal, the ranking White House physicians to presidents Harding and Coolidge respectively.[55] Sawyer, the civilian homeopathic proprietor of the White Oaks Clinic in the Hardings' hometown of Marion, Ohio, was brought to the White House at the request of Mrs. Harding only through the dual inducement of a commission as brigadier general in the U.S.A. Medical Reserve Corps and chairmanship of the Federal Hospitalization Board.[56] Sawyer thereby became "the suddenest Brigadier General in U.S. History."[57] This doctor had a long social relationship with the Hardings; moreover, Florence Harding became very dependent upon his treatment for her chronic kidney condition.[58]

A digression into the complex long-standing Sawyer/Harding relationship may serve to illuminate the peculiarities of the selection and reward system of White House physicians. Both of Warren G. Harding's parents were practicing homeopathic physicians in central Ohio. Doctor Charles Sawyer made his debut in the Harding saga in July 1897 as a consultant to Phoebe Harding, the future president's mother. She had diagnosed "cholera infantum" in an eighteen-month-old child and had provided a bottle of "lacto-pepsin and carbo vegetables" as treatment. The child became comatose and died suddenly. The decedent's father brought the prescribed powder to a pharmacist, who upon testing concluded that it contained morphine. The father then accused Phoebe Harding of negligently killing his child.[59]

According to Harding biographer Francis Russell, "For a few days it seemed that the Hardings' medical practice was in ruins and Warren's career indirectly marred. But Dr. Sawyer, from the respectable background of his sanitarium, pronounced the death as owing to a brain fever 'that often develops from cholera infantum.' He ... assured the public that the baby had not died from the effects of the drug [morphine]." The local newspaper commented, "This statement, from a man of Dr. Sawyer's ability and standing in the community relieves Mrs. Harding from all responsibilities in the affair."[60]

Charles Sawyer, an 1881 graduate of the Homeopathic Hospital College of Cleveland, was a prominent homeopathic physician who continued to provide significant services to the Harding family. He was chairman of the American Surgical and Gynecological Association, president of the American Institute of Homeopathy, and president of the Ohio State Homeopathic Medical Society.[61] Additionally, he occasionally authored articles published in the *Journal of the American Institute of Homeopathy*.

The Sawyers and the younger Hardings became very friendly and often traveled together after 1904.[62] Florence Harding had a kidney removed at Grant Hospital in Columbus in February 1905. In early 1913 Sawyer assumed responsibility for her medical care, and Mrs. Harding, known not too affectionately as "The Duchess," became very dependent upon Sawyer. Sawyer's personal correspondence documents at least one emergency trip from Ohio to Washington, D.C., to attend to Mrs. Harding's acute illness.[63]

Since Mrs. Harding was convinced that only Sawyer could keep her alive, Warren Harding insisted that the doctor become his White House physician. It was only the inducements of a brigadier generalship and an additional bureaucratic sinecure that secured Sawyer's acceptance.[64] Sawyer rendered one significant service to The Duchess as first lady. In November 1922 she developed a critical urinary tract illness of her remaining kidney. Two famous consultants, Charles Mayo and John Finney, wanted to operate. Sawyer refused and Mrs. Harding recovered without surgery.[65]

As a *quid pro quo* of sorts, Harding reciprocated by presenting various considerations to his physician. Harding, as a United States senator, was instrumental in Sawyer's somewhat controversial appointment to the Ohio State medical board.[66] Moreover, Harding was induced to speak at the homeopathic Hahnemann Medical College in Philadelphia, and referred in correspondence with Sawyer to a "very acceptable honorarium" for his presentation.[67] At Sawyer's urging, President Harding issued a proclamation "cordially sympathizing with the work of homeopathic physicians,"[68] and wrote a dedication for *The War History of Homeopathic Doctors*.[69]

Sawyer jealously guarded his favored position. Irate that Boone had treated the president for a minor problem, Sawyer ordered Boone never again to treat Harding without his knowledge. Thereafter Boone always visited the president in Sawyer's company.[70] Later Sawyer was resentful that his subordinate had treated President or Mrs. Coolidge during Sawyer's absence.[71] After Harding had taken ill during his ill-fated trip to Alaska in 1923, Boone and Secretary of the Interior Hubert Work, also a physician, disagreed with Sawyer's diagnosis that Harding's intestinal symptoms were due to tainted crabmeat. They circumvented Sawyer by directly appealing to Secretary of

Chapter 6. Joel Boone and Institutionalization of the Office

Commerce Herbert Hoover to wire Dr. Ray Lyman Wilbur, then president of Stanford University and former dean of its medical school, to meet the presidential train in San Francisco, together with the best cardiologist in the area.[72] It was all to no avail, as the president died shortly thereafter in San Francisco from heart disease.

President Coolidge, much to Boone's frustration, selected as his White House physician Major James Coupal after Sawyer resigned. Coupal previously had served as Coolidge's doctor when the latter was vice president.[73] Coupal, a Massachusetts native, obtained both his bachelors and his medical degrees from Tufts University. He entered the army in 1915 and saw service both on the Mexican border and in France. Coupal, then a curator of the Army Medical Museum in Washington, D.C., was recommended to the incoming vice president by Coolidge's Boston physician.[74]

Boone considered Coupal's ability to be that of a family physician of the sort that one might have discovered at that time in towns and small cities in the United States, and he resented the quality of Coupal's medical treatment of Grace Coolidge.[75] However, these two physicians closely cooperated in the care of Calvin Coolidge Junior's fatal illness and jointly selected outside specialists for consultation during that medical emergency.[76] Appropriate deference between physicians is difficult even today among doctors practicing under far less duress.

Calvin Coolidge understandingly believed that James Coupal, then a major and his White House and personal physician, should hold a rank comparable to those held by his immediate two predecessors, Cary Grayson and Charles Sawyer. The two physicians had been promoted to the ranks of rear admiral and brigadier general respectively. On August 5, 1926, President Coolidge fired off a telegram to Secretary of War Dwight Davis that read, "I want specific information whether I have any authority in law to make Coupal a Brigadier temporary or permanent." Bureaucratic maneuvers continued to frustrate the president in his repeated attempts to obtain a promotion for his physician until Dr. Coupal was promoted to the temporary rank of colonel as a result of the congressional statutes

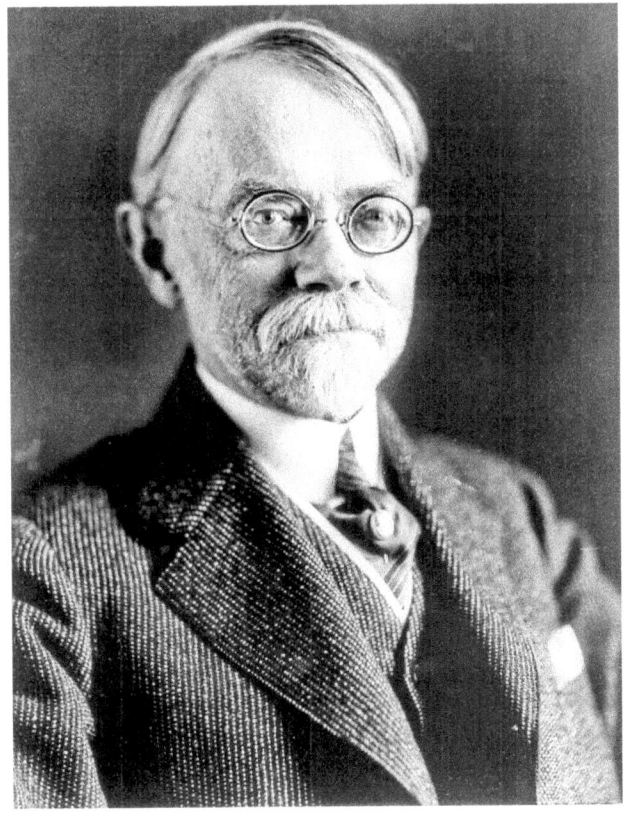

Charles Sawyer. Homeopath Dr. Charles Sawyer was lured from his prosperous Ohio sanitarium to serve as Harding's presidential physician by a brigadier generalship, a horse, and a prestigious governmental appointment. (National Library of Medicine)

discussed previously.[77] Coolidge quickly rewarded this White House physician by assuring that Coupal's colonelcy be retroactive to the date of his appointment as his personal physician. As a result, a special order of the War Department, dated May 17, 1928, read, "The assignment of Major James P. Coupal, as personal physician to the President, with the rank, pay, and allowances of a colonel, Medical Corps, to date from July 1, 1924, under the provisions of an Act of Congress approved May 16, 1928, is announced."[78]

However, President Coolidge was unsuccessful in his attempts to secure for Coupal a permanent promotion to the rank of colonel. As a result, Coupal was reduced to his prior rank of major when Coolidge's successor, Herbert Hoover, failed to reappoint him as presidential physician.[79] Perhaps as a consequence, the doctor resigned from the army on July 12, 1929. He had a private medical practice in Washington until his death in January 1935.[80]

Joel Boone was not reappointed as White House physician by Hoover's successor, Franklin Roosevelt. He likewise was reduced in rank to that of a navy commander with a corresponding reduction in pay. His prior rank of captain had been linked by statute to his position rather than to his person.[81] Boone's subsequent military career was spent first on the West Coast, and then as a member of Admiral William Halsey's staff during the war in the Pacific. He witnessed the formal surrender of the Japanese on Halsey's flagship, the battleship USS *Missouri* on September 2, 1945.[82] Boone retired with the rank of vice admiral in 1950 and served afterward as medical director of the nation's network of Veterans' hospitals.[83] Admiral Boone similarly was honored as his predecessor, Admiral Rixey, by the naming of a United States naval vessel in his honor. The guided missile frigate USS *Boone* was commissioned on January 16, 1980, and remained in active service until decommissioned on February 23, 2012. She was the last active warship to be named after a Navy physician.[84]

In a February 4, 1961, letter to Dr. Janet Travell, one of his successors, Admiral Boone claimed for himself historical notice as the first official White House physician. He wrote: "…and [I was] the first physician to be benefited by Public Law No. 89–71 Congress (S. 2515), as approved April 4, 1930, which, by statute for the first time, established the position and provided the title of Physician to the White House.…" His letter also noted that he and all subsequent White House physicians were the recipients of President Hoover's determination to make suitable space in the White House available for presidential physicians.[85] More recently, Dr. Connie Mariano, the White House physician to President Bill Clinton, acknowledged Boone's significance in the institutionalization of the office by writing that by enacting the above referenced statute, "Congress recognized the title 'White House Physician' as that of the doctor responsible for the medical care of the president. This physician would also serve as the director of the WHMU (White House Medical Unit)." She further noted Boone's and Hoover's roles in establishing a physician's office on the ground floor of the White House, which, in her words, "…remains to this day as the Doctor's Office and serves as the medical office for the president's physician."[86]

CHAPTER 7

The Military Keepers of the Stethoscope

Doctors Cary Grayson,
Ross McIntire and Howard Snyder

In April 1944, the third year of America's involvement in the Second World War and six months before Franklin Roosevelt would be elected president for an unprecedented fourth term, a thorough physical examination at Bethesda Naval Hospital disclosed that the 62-year-old president was severely ill with accelerated hypertension and congestive heart failure. Newspaper and magazine reporters, alerted by rumors that Roosevelt's health was in decline, clamored for a clarification from the president's White House physician, Vice Admiral Ross McIntire.

The Admiral appeared before the press wearing "...the smile of a physician relieved of worry." "When we got through," he said, "we decided that for a man of sixty-two-plus we had little to argue about, with the exception that we had to combat the influenza plus the respiratory complications that came along after.... The greatest criticism we can have is that we haven't provided him with enough rest and exercise."[1]

Three of the most controversial White House physicians were military officers: Cary Grayson, Ross McIntire and Howard Snyder. Their lengthy tenures were a result of their devoted attachment to their patient sponsors, the successful presidents Woodrow Wilson (1913–21), Franklin Delano Roosevelt (1933–45), and Dwight Eisenhower (1953–61). Grayson, McIntire and Snyder were in charge of the medical care of presidents Wilson, Roosevelt, and Eisenhower for eight, twelve, and eight years respectively.

All three military physicians managed critical medical emergencies during their tenures. Woodrow Wilson experienced a series of incapacitating strokes; Franklin Roosevelt developed severe hypertension which resulted in congestive heart failure and then in a fatal cerebrovascular accident; Dwight Eisenhower suffered a major heart attack that was followed first by a recurrence of his chronic Crohn's disease that required emergency intestinal surgery, and later by a mild stroke known medically as a transient ischemic attack.

In the period before the massive expansion of the modern presidential staff, Grayson, McIntire and Snyder were able to develop close friendships with their respective presidential patients. Indeed, the relationships became both personal and intimate. This was particularly exemplified by Cary Grayson, who not only introduced the recently widowed Woodrow Wilson to Edith Bolling Galt, his second wife, but also was essential in preserving their engagement when political opportunism threatened to scuttle the marriage.[2]

This chapter examines the unusual confluence of dramatic historical events, serious personal illnesses, and fiercely loyal friendships upon the professional deportment and clinical judgment of the presidential physician. Although other military White House physicians, for example admirals Rixey and Boone, had developed close attachments to their president-patients, the appearance of debilitating chronic illness during times of foreign policy crises or domestic political disputes presented unique challenges to the occupants of the White House physician's office. The responses of this physician trio to their challenges affected the subsequent evolution of the role of the presidential physician.

Grayson, McIntire and Snyder all misled the press and the public over the nature and the seriousness of their patrons' medical illnesses. Cary Grayson downplayed the extent of Wilson's incapacity after the president's major stroke in 1919.[3] Ross McIntire repeatedly denied that his patient had significant heart disease throughout FDR's entire life. He continued his denials in his memoir, *White House Physician*,[4] published one year after his patient's death. Howard Snyder became increasingly adept in the political and media management of Eisenhower's illnesses.[5]

Additionally, each may on occasion have misled their illustrious patient. Cary Grayson deliberately minimized the seriousness of the chronic renal failure of Ellen, Wilson's first wife. The kidney malfunction most likely was a result of the toxemia that had occurred during her 1889 pregnancy.[6] When Ellen Wilson's renal failure became critical in 1914, Dr. Grayson, also serving as her physician, procrastinated for some time before he requested the assistance of kidney specialists. He had decided not to alert Wilson to his wife's dismal prognosis out of concern for the president's neurotic temperament.[7] Edwin Weinstein succinctly portrayed the doctor's dilemma, pointing out that as a virtual member of the Wilson family, Grayson lacked professional detachment: "As a military officer, serving under, and primarily responsible for, the health of the President … he could not risk upsetting Wilson by trying to penetrate his denial system and possibly precipitate another stroke."[8]

Navy Commander doctor Howard Bruenn was tasked by his superior officer, Vice Admiral Ross McIntire, to assume the cardiac care of President Franklin Roosevelt during the last year of the president's life. Bruenn was astonished that FDR appeared completely disinterested in his own daily medical examination.[9] When the diagnosis of severe hypertension and consequent congestive heart failure was established in April 1944, McIntire insisted that the consulting physicians agree to avoid any mention of arteriosclerosis or heart disease in order not to worry the presidential patient.[10] Bruenn was commanded not to discuss Roosevelt's health with anyone except McIntire. The admiral was the only person with the self-designated authority to discuss these matters either with the family or anyone outside the family.[11] The extent to which the admiral discussed his diagnosis and prognosis with his patient will be forever undetermined.

White House physician Howard Snyder gave his presidential patient, Dwight Eisenhower, "plausible deniability" in May 1956, when he announced to the press that the X-ray examination of the president's intestine showed normal function, despite the presence of radiologically diagnosed Crohn's disease.[12] This intestinal ailment is a persistent chronic inflammation that eventually results in small bowel obstruction. Significantly,

Snyder also withheld this radiographic diagnosis from his patient. At the time, Eisenhower's health was the object of intense national scrutiny as he recovered from a significant heart attack on his way toward a second campaign for the presidency. Ironically, Eisenhower's Crohn's disease required emergency intestinal surgery two months later, a few short months before the onset of his successful campaign for reelection.

Grayson, McIntire and Snyder benefited from their loyal service, not only by the expected perquisites inherent in the proximity to power, but also by dramatic military promotion. In 1916, after four years of faithful service to Wilson, Cary Grayson was promoted from the rank of a navy lieutenant to rear admiral. According to Braisted and Bell, "The rapid promotion of Dr. Grayson from Passed Assistant Surgeon with the rank of Lieutenant to Medical Director with the rank of Rear Admiral was unprecedented and was due to his position as White House Physician."[13] Ross McIntire assumed his new position as White House physician in 1933 as a lieutenant commander[14] and retired in 1945 as a vice admiral. In addition, in 1938 FDR appointed him surgeon general of the navy, a reward not unfamiliar to presidential physicians.[15] Doctor Howard Snyder was already a major general at the conclusion of World War II. When Eisenhower subsequently appointed Snyder his personal physician, the doctor twice was recalled from retirement to active duty status[16] and was continued with the rank of major general. Upon his final retirement from the army in 1961, Snyder received an office near Walter Reed National Military Medical Center so he could work on a proposed medical history of Eisenhower.[17]

The authorship in book form of one's White House experience has been a perquisite of former presidential physicians. This is not a recent phenomenon, since both Grayson and McIntire published their memoirs as apologias after their controversial tenures. Grayson's *An Intimate Memoir* was published in 1960 and reissued in 1977.[18] McIntire's *White House Physician* reached bookstores in 1946.[19] Howard Snyder accumulated Eisenhower's abundant medical records with an eye toward publication. He was forced to abandon his book project due to a lung tumor and a series of strokes that left him in a "vegetative state."[20]

In which ways, if any, did the professional behavior of these three physicians affect the evolution of the office of the White House physician? The answer may be alliterated as permanence, prominence, and public perception. FDR discharged Dr. Joel Boone from his duties at the White House shortly after his inauguration. The president, either because of political guile or a philosophical principle, voiced the opinion that he did not require a presidential physician.[21] However, shortly thereafter he appointed the aforementioned McIntire to fill this post, and ever since then an appointed White House physician has been an unchallenged permanent fixture of the presidential staff. The public illness of their presidential patients illuminated the personality and professional competence of these three physicians, and henceforth the identity of the White House physician would be far from anonymous. The handling, perhaps more appropriately the mishandling, of the presidents' illnesses became a factor leading to the discussions that eventuated in the passage of the Twenty-fifth Amendment to the U.S. Constitution in 1967. A political consensus formed that a presidential disability ought to be a public and not only a private matter determined by the president's physician.

Cary Grayson, like his patron Wilson, was born into an educated Virginia family; both his father and grandfather were physicians. The young Grayson attended William and Mary College in Williamsburg and afterward took his medical degree from the now defunct medical school at University of the South in Sewanee, Tennessee, in 1902. His internship training was at the Columbia Hospital for Women in Washington, D.C.[22]

In 1903 Grayson was commissioned as Acting Assistant Surgeon in the United States Navy[23] and subsequently assigned to the presidential yacht, *Mayflower,* as its medical officer, where he got to know both presidents Theodore Roosevelt and William Howard Taft.[24] Future White House physician Joel Boone also turned this billet into a precursor for the more prestigious tour of duty as White House physician.

Grayson's career was immeasurably abetted by the interest and friendship of Presley Rixey, who was William McKinley's and Theodore Roosevelt's White House physician. Rixey was a Virginian like Grayson and was related to him by marriage: Grayson's half-sister was the wife of Rixey's youngest brother.[25] Rixey wrote: "I had known Dr. Grayson for many years prior to his entry in the Navy and advised him how to proceed with his entry into the Navy and advised him how to proceed with his medical education so as to become a naval surgeon, and in the service he made good in every assignment I gave him."[26] Rixey's interest in the younger man's career occurred after the death of Grayson's parents when he was a boy.[27] Grayson, like Rixey an experienced horseman, accompanied Theodore Roosevelt and an army aide on a one-day 104-mile ride to and from Warrenton, Virginia. Rixey previously had suggested to the president that a fitting qualification of naval officers' physical competence would be a 100-mile horse ride in one day, as compared with Army officers' march of fifty miles or ride of 100 miles in three days. Roosevelt, always eager for adventure, insisted that he accompany Rixey on this qualifying exercise.[28]

Grayson served on *The Maryland* during the 1907–1909 tour of the Great White Fleet, and upon its return he joined the medical staff of the White House as medical officer of the presidential yacht. Grayson's appointment as White House physician may have resulted from the recommendation of the outgoing president, William Howard Taft.[29] A second reason may have been his capable attendance to

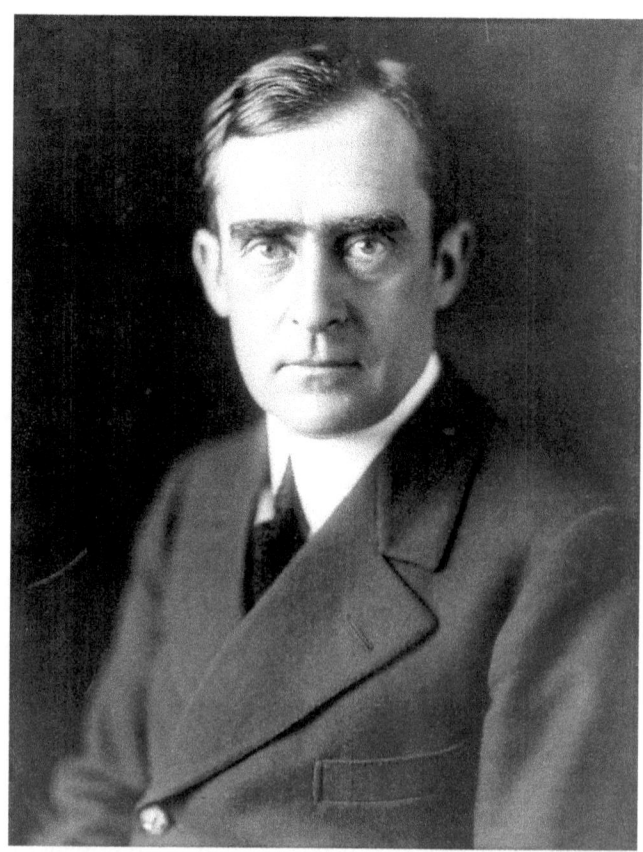

Cary Grayson. Admiral Cary Grayson had an extremely close personal relationship with his patient, President Woodrow Wilson. (National Library of Medicine)

Woodrow Wilson's sister, Mrs. Annie Howe, who had injured herself in a fall on Wilson's inauguration day in March 1913.[30]

The well-being of the president was Grayson's overriding, and usually his sole, responsibility during Wilson's two-term presidency (1913–1921). Grayson did take care of the president's first wife, Ellen, and most probably also treated Edith, his second wife.[31] There is also a record of a single consultation on the health of the president's principal adviser, Colonel Edward House.[32]

Bernard Baruch, in a foreword to Grayson's memoir, wrote, "Grayson was more than a doctor.... He was also a discreet and able aide who could be entrusted with difficult and delicate tasks. Above all, Grayson was the loyal and understanding friend."[33] Grayson explained this relationship in a similar fashion: "The official relationship grew rapidly into a very close personal relationship. Not in boastfulness, but as a statement of fact, I can say that I saw him more intimately than any other man during those eleven years."[34] The doctor resided in the White House much of the time prior to his marriage and lived with Wilson during the Paris Peace Conference in 1919.[35] The doctor frequently played golf with the president, was a companion to the Washington theater,[36] and accompanied him on afternoon automobile excursions. Edmund Starling, the secret service agent assigned to Wilson, described these golfing outings: "He is terrible. So is Grayson. [It is] a melancholy prospect—following two poor golfers over a wind-swept course on a winter's morning."[37]

The most striking personal aspect of this physician-patient relationship was the role played in the courtship of the widowed president's second wife, Edith Bolling Galt. In an attempt to dispel the president's depression after Ellen Wilson's death, Grayson intrigued to arrange an encounter with the wealthy Washington widow, Edith Galt. Mrs. Galt's "time tried traveling companion" was Alice Gertrude Gordan, who happened to be the doctor's fiancé and later his wife.[38] On April 30, 1915, Dr. Grayson escorted both Edith and Alice to dinner at the White House, and after this introduction the presidential romance blossomed.[39] When Colonel House crudely attempted to discourage Wilson's remarriage for political reasons, Grayson was the intermediary who successfully resolved the problem.[40] According to the leading Wilson scholar, Arthur Link, "Grayson was like a son to Wilson and Grayson worshipped Wilson and Wilson thought Grayson was one of the finest people he'd ever known."[41] The doctor felt an obligation to honor Ellen Wilson's dying words: "Doctor, I realize that I am going. You know him and he is devoted to you. Take good care of Woodrow."[42] And he did.

Cary Grayson served as a trusted aide in matters both personal and political. Presley Rixey, in his defense of his protégé's promotion to rear admiral, wrote that Grayson "had made himself personally and professionally indispensable to the President."[43] A long letter from Grayson to Rixey described the former's activities at the Paris Peace Conference at the conclusion of World War I: "In addition to my professional duties, the President gives me a lot of things of a personal nature to attend to, and as a personal aide, I have to be on hand all the time."[44] Edmund Starling related two instances in which this White House physician was the intermediary in political and personnel matters: Notification of Colonel House's unauthorized press conferences in Paris,[45] and a recommendation to the chief of the Secret Service, Moran, that Starling should be promoted with a raise in pay.[46]

The staffing of the White House physician's office was a one-man show during most of Grayson's tenure; apparently there was no military medical backup. When the doctor was away on a Liberty bond trip during World War I, Edith Wilson was required to call in Sterling Ruffin, her former personal physician and an old friend, to treat her "grippe."[47] A visit by the prominent Philadelphia ophthalmologist, George Schweinitz, was one of the rare physician consultations at the White House prior to the president's massive stroke in October 1919.[48]

The chronology of President Wilson's massive stroke and resultant disability has been extensively documented.[49] After a premonitory episode in Pueblo, Colorado, Wilson suffered a complete paralysis of his left arm and leg, the loss of vision in the left half of the visual fields of both eyes, difficulty in swallowing and impairment of his speech, and changes in both his cognitive behavior and emotional stability. Wilson's condition slowly improved after several months, but he left the White House in March 1921 as a semi-invalid.

Crispell and Gomez harshly criticized Grayson's conspiracy with Edith Wilson and presidential political aide Joseph Tumulty in masking the president's disability: "Grayson's behavior during these days exceeded the bounds of physician responsibility. Grayson was using the office of the president of the United States as therapy for his patient."[50]

When the seriousness of Wilson's neurological disability became apparent, Dr. Grayson, as the president's physician, exercised his prerogative in summoning consultants. However, Grayson remained in charge of the case and was the sole designated conduit for information regarding the president's condition. He called into consultation Philadelphia neurologist Francis X. Dercum, Admiral E.R. Stitt, and Mrs. Wilson's physician, Sterling Ruffin. Later, when the president developed urinary tract obstruction, Baltimore urologist Hugh Young, Washington, urologist H. Fowler, Rochester, Minnesota, surgeon Charles Mayo, and Philadelphia ophthalmologist George Schweinitz were called to the White House.[51]

United States presidents have always possessed an advantage that is not shared with members of the American electorate, namely, the availability of the most prestigious medical talent as the need arises. This was exemplified by the prominence of the physicians who responded to Dr. Grayson's request for urgent consultation in 1919. Doctor Francis X. Dercum was a renowned neurologist who served as clinical professor of mental and nervous diseases at Jefferson Medical College and had authored several books in this field.[52] George Schweinitz was professor of ophthalmology at the University of Pennsylvania and served as president of the International Congress of Ophthalmology.[53] Doctor Charles Mayo, described as a "surgical genius," together with his older brother founded the world famous Mayo Clinic.[54] Hugh D. Young was professor of urology at the Johns Hopkins School of Medicine and was "universally acknowledged ... the father of modern urology."[55]

In 1916 Colonel and Mrs. House persuaded Woodrow Wilson to promote his devoted physician to the rank of rear admiral over 100 more senior officers.[56] Subsequently, Secretary of the Navy Josephus Daniels ordered the retired surgeon general of the navy, Admiral Presley Rixey, as president of the Naval Board of Examiners, to examine Lieutenant Cary Grayson for promotion to the rank of medical director, which carried with it the rank of rear admiral. As a result of the board's positive report, Grayson skipped the grades of surgeon and medical inspector. Rixey defended "the rapid promotion of Dr. Grayson from Passed Assistant Surgeon with the rank of Lieutenant to Medical Director with the rank of Rear Admiral ... [It was] unprecedented

Chapter 7. The Military Keepers of the Stethoscope

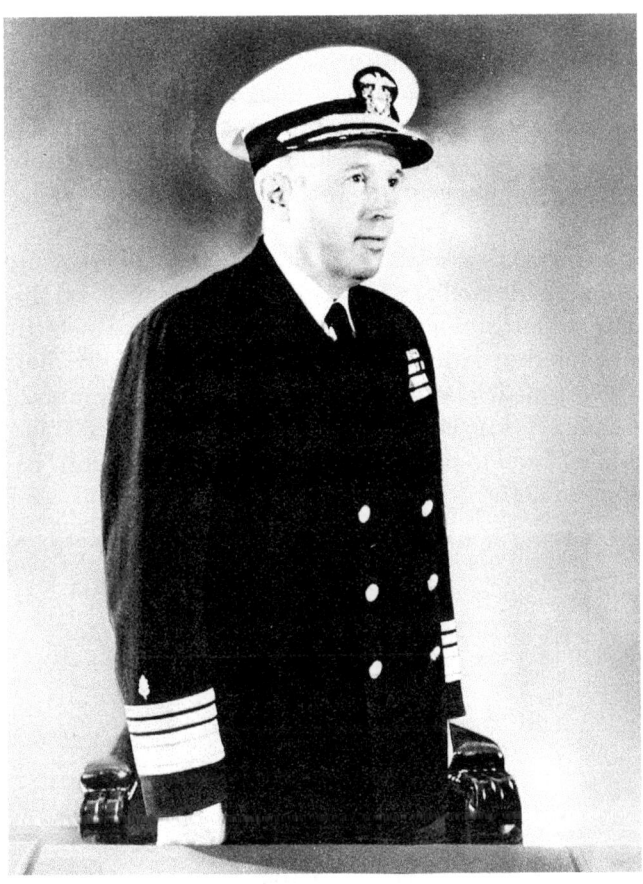

Ross McIntire. Navy physician Dr. Ross McIntire was President Franklin Roosevelt's personal physician for the twelve years of Roosevelt's presidency. An otolaryngologist, McIntire was ill-prepared to handle the president's worsening hypertension in 1944. (Courtesy of the Bureau of Medicine and Surgery Library and Archives)

and was due to his position as White House Physician."[57] Not surprisingly the unprecedented promotion produced great controversy among the navy officers' corps.

Grayson's prestige outlived his service to Wilson. He was twice (1933, 1937) inaugural committee chairman for Franklin Delano Roosevelt and was chosen (1935) chairman of the American Red Cross.[58] He was able to recommend a protégé, Lieutenant Commander Ross McIntire, to newly inaugurated Franklin Delano Roosevelt as his White House physician.[59] Decades later Wilson's disability and Grayson's connivance in masking it became oft-used arguments for the passage of the Twenty-fifth Amendment to the Constitution of the United States.[60]

Ross McIntire was born in Salem, Oregon, and graduated from Willamette (now the University of Oregon) Medical School in 1907. He was commissioned assistant surgeon with the rank of lieutenant (j.g.) in the navy medical corps when the United States entered World War I. McIntire remained in the Navy after the war, and during the following ten years he took advanced training in otolaryngology, practiced at navy hospitals in San Diego and Washington, D.C., and served three tours on the hospital ship *Relief*.[61]

Cary Grayson recommended McIntire to Roosevelt as his White House physician when McIntire was stationed at Washington Naval Hospital in 1933. McIntire first met Grayson in 1917 when the young lieutenant was assigned to the Washington Naval Hospital. The acquaintance was renewed in 1925 when McIntire was again billeted in Washington, this time to the Naval Dispensary where Admiral Grayson was his commanding officer. When McIntire commenced a third tour of duty in the nation's capital, this association was renewed once again. McIntire recounted, "As one of Franklin Roosevelt's oldest and dearest friends, the Admiral became a White House intimate after the 1932 election, and thought of me when the President asked him about a physician."[62] Grayson reassured McIntire of the propriety of his selection as White House physician by noting that McIntire had been trained as an ear, nose and throat (ENT) specialist: "The President is as strong as a horse with the exception of a chronic sinus condition that makes him susceptible to colds. That's where you come in."[63] McIntire was indeed qualified to practice the specialty of otolaryngology; he was later (1942) certified as a specialist by the American Board of Otolaryngology, thus becoming the first presidential physician with specialty certification.[64]

McIntire, in agreement with Grayson's assessment of the role of the physician to the president, wrote: "The job is to keep him well, to guard him against illness, and that entails daily observation and constant watchfulness."[65] For more than a decade McIntire diligently irrigated FDR's sinuses and dosed him with nose drops and sprays.[66] There is little evidence that he provided any medical care to other members of the Roosevelt family or to presidential advisers and service personnel, aside from visits to FDR's closest adviser, Harry Hopkins, at Malta,[67] and to the comatose military aide General "Pa" Watson onboard the cruiser *Quincy* in 1945.[68]

McIntire made twice daily inspections to assess FDR's well-being, one at 9:30 a.m. over breakfast, and a more thorough once over in the evening. McIntire, in a self-congratulatory vein, smugly related that the intervening rest of the day was devoted "to my own affairs." These consisted of the chairmanship of the ear, nose and throat department at the Washington Naval Hospital and teaching at the Naval Medical Center. In 1938 McIntire was appointed Rear Admiral and Surgeon General of the Navy. It was an important job: During World War II the medical department of the navy expanded to 175,000 personnel and over 300 fixed and mobile hospitals.[69]

FDR, who had a penchant for affectionate nicknames, addressed McIntire as "The Doc."[70] "The Doc" accompanied the president on most of his trips outside

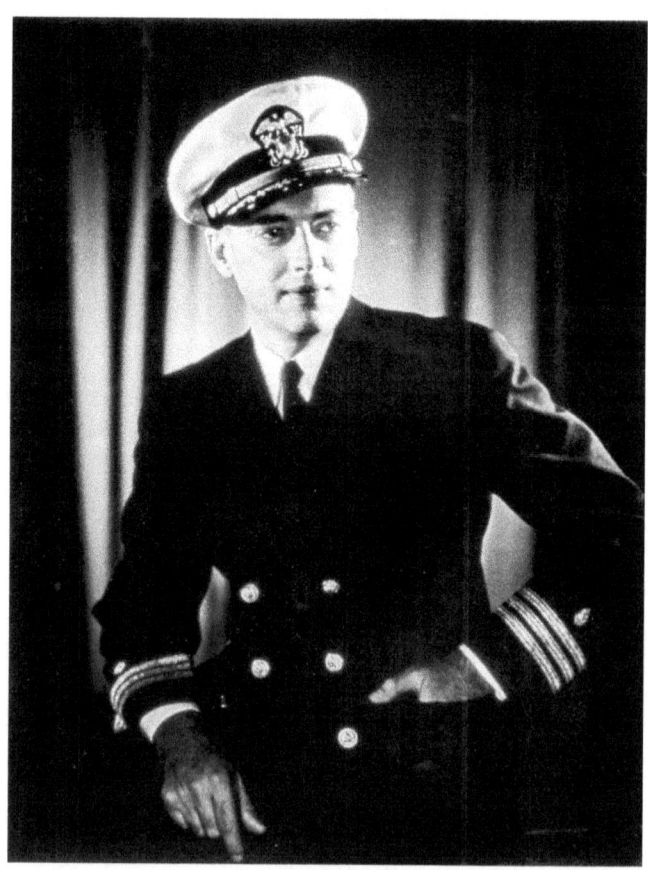

Howard Bruenn. Navy cardiologist Dr. Howard Bruenn correctly diagnosed and treated Roosevelt's hypertensive heart disease and congestive heart failure in early 1944. He was commanded to communicate his medical findings only to his commanding officer, Admiral Ross McIntire. (National Library of Medicine)

Washington, including all foreign journeys and FDR's frequent vacations.[71] He was an enthusiastic companion on the president's frequent fishing excursions[72] and accompanied FDR on a 1940 overnight cruise of the presidential yacht *Potomac*.[73] He also was a frequent guest at the intimate dinners hosted by Roosevelt.[74]

McIntire relied upon medical consultants who were almost exclusively navy officers. He justified this decision: "Not only did I consider them to be as good as the best, but there was an advantage that journeys to [Bethesda] Medical Center could be made without exciting comment."[75] It also suited his purposes that the secrecy of medical records could be maintained with the expected results, as commented upon by Dr. Howard Bruenn: "The original hospital chart in which all of the clinical progress notes as well as the results of the various laboratory tests were incorporated was kept in the safe at the U.S. Naval hospital, Bethesda. After the President's death this chart could not be found."[76]

In early 1944 the Roosevelt family noticed that FDR, after a grueling overseas trip, did not bounce back with his usual vigor from an attack of his recurrent sinobronchitis. Anna Roosevelt, the oldest of the Roosevelt's five children, was the most determined to seek a second medical opinion. McIntire's reassuring blandishments were not accepted and, forced to seek a second opinion, he scheduled an outpatient cardiac examination at Bethesda Naval Hospital by Commander Howard Bruenn, a cardiologist.[77] Doctor Bruenn's examination diagnosed marked hypertension, cardiac enlargement, and congestive heart failure.[78] However, his diagnoses and recommended therapy initially were rejected on March 30, 1944, by a medical board that had been hastily convened by McIntire.[79] Its membership consisted of McIntire, Bruenn, Navy Captain John Harper, commandant of Bethesda Naval Hospital; Captain Robert Duncan, Harper's executive officer; Captain Charles Behrens, chief of radiology at Bethesda, and a token civilian physician, Paul Dickins, clinical professor of medicine at George Washington School of Medicine. The following day the board was enlarged by the arrival of honorary medical Consultants to the navy, the prestigious civilian physicians, surgeon Frank Lahey, of Boston, and Atlanta internist James E. Paullin.[80] At this second meeting, Bruenn, secure in his professional judgment, persuaded his colleagues to accept the correctness of his diagnoses and treatment regime.[81]

Parts of this consultative board met periodically over the next year to review FDR's medical situation.[82] The convening of this medical committee may have presaged the routine practice of consultation by medical committees both in the management of a president's chronic illness and in the annual review of his health status.

McIntire was extremely secretive and uniformly deceptive regarding the status of FDR's health during the twelve months that preceded the president's fatal stroke in April 1945. The White House physician's rationale for his behavior may have been complicated and was probably due to a conflation of reasons: wartime security, the doctor's investment in the personal and political success of his patron, and compassion for the well-being of his patient. Historian Robert Ferrell painted McIntire's support for a fourth Roosevelt term in 1944 with this cynical brush: "McIntire was beholden to Roosevelt for rapid advance, from lieutenant commander to vice admiral. If he had opposed the president he would have had to resign, unthinkable in the midst of a great war, or risk reassignment. The latter would have involved demotion, for there was no other vice admiral's billet in the bureau of Medicine and Surgery."[83] Popular historian Jim Bishop characterized McIntire's mission after Roosevelt's March 1944 examination as one to disarm the correspondents and, through them, the U.S. electorate.[84] He wrote that on April 4, 1944, "McIntire blithely assured the press that nothing was wrong, that the president was simply suffering from a case of bronchitis. The results of the checkup were excellent."[85] When Winston Churchill, visiting at Hyde Park, asked the doctor about FDR's health, he responded to Roosevelt's most important foreign ally that everything was fine.[86] The deception over the president's condition continued in McIntire's memoir, *White House Physician*.

Professional deference had been replaced by military command. Bruenn was ordered to limit any discussion of the president's health to McIntire alone. The admiral thereby assumed control of the flow of medical information; he became the only agent to discuss FDR's medical condition.[87] The control was so tight that Eleanor Roosevelt found that Dr. Bruenn was practically inaccessible to her due to McIntire's orders.[88] At Yalta, FDR's daughter Anna was only able to breach the chain of medical command after Bruenn extracted from her the promise that she not "tell Ross that this ticker situation is more serious than I ever knew."[89] Anna, FDR's daughter, not his wife Eleanor, accompanied the president to the fateful Yalta Conference in early February 1945. Anna, together with cardiologist Bruenn, attempted, with only occasional success, to shield FDR from the incessant turmoil of the conference. FDR's cardiac health declined; the cardiologist was frightened when his patient developed an episode of pulsus alternans.

FDR risked his life by agreeing to meet with Stalin and Churchill in the Crimea in the winter. Yalta could only be accessed by air. A plane flew the president from Malta to Yalta. "The President's bed was perpendicular to the plane's axis. It was a big, wide bed. But he refused to have a safety belt. We were afraid that if there was a sudden stop of something he would be tossed right out of the bed. Michael Reilly, Chief of the White House secret service detail ... decided that when all the lights were out, I would creep in and position myself on one side of the bed so that if he fell out of bed, he'd fall on me."[90]

McIntire did not accompany the president on his final trip to Warm Springs, Georgia, but he ordered Bruenn to communicate with him by telephone only and not to consult with any other doctor during this stay.[91]

Admiral McIntire's reputation remained unscathed after FDR's unexpected death. He retired from the navy at the end of 1946. He organized the Red Cross regional blood program the following year and resigned as its national administrator in 1951. McIntire also served as the first chairman of the President's Committee for Employment of the Physically Handicapped and as executive director of the International College of Surgeons before his death in 1959 at the age of seventy.[92]

Howard Snyder became President Dwight Eisenhower's White House physician in 1953 at age seventy-one, and served his patient with great loyalty for the next eight years. Doctor Snyder already was a major general when he first met Eisenhower (Ike) during World War II.[93]

Snyder was born in Cheyenne, Wyoming, in 1881, attended the University of Wyoming, and graduated from Thomas Jefferson Medical College in 1905. He worked as a contract physician for the army for several years before enlisting in 1908. Snyder, a surgeon, had a distinguished medical career in the military, and was asked by Army Chief of Staff George Marshall to treat Mamie Eisenhower, which he did on numerous occasions during the prolonged separation from her husband during the war.[94] General Eisenhower then met Snyder during the war as the doctor had traveled widely as assistant inspector general for the War Department.[95]

In mid–1945 the doctor rushed to Boone, Iowa, where Mamie had contracted bronchopneumonia. After her condition was stabilized, Snyder accompanied Ike to Chicago for a speaking engagement and treated him there for "speaker's throat." Subsequently, he traveled to Washington, D.C., where he first treated the future president for sinusitis and then had him hospitalized at Ashford General Hospital in West Virginia with severe bronchitis.[96] Mamie Eisenhower's positive rapport with Dr. Snyder was a third example of a first lady's influence in identifying her husband's White House physician. Ida McKinley and Florence Harding were the patients of Presley Rixey and Charles Sawyer prior to their husbands' appointment of these physicians.

Eisenhower saved Snyder from a military retirement by assigning him as the Eisenhowers' personal physician while Ike served as army chief of staff. When Ike became president of Columbia University in New York City, he requested that the doctor retire, move to New York City to become senior adviser to the university's Conservation of Human Resources Project, and thereby continue as the Eisenhowers' personal physician. Snyder agreed, but was restored to active-duty status when Ike was appointed the first military commander of NATO. He continued on active-duty status during the two-term Eisenhower presidency.[97]

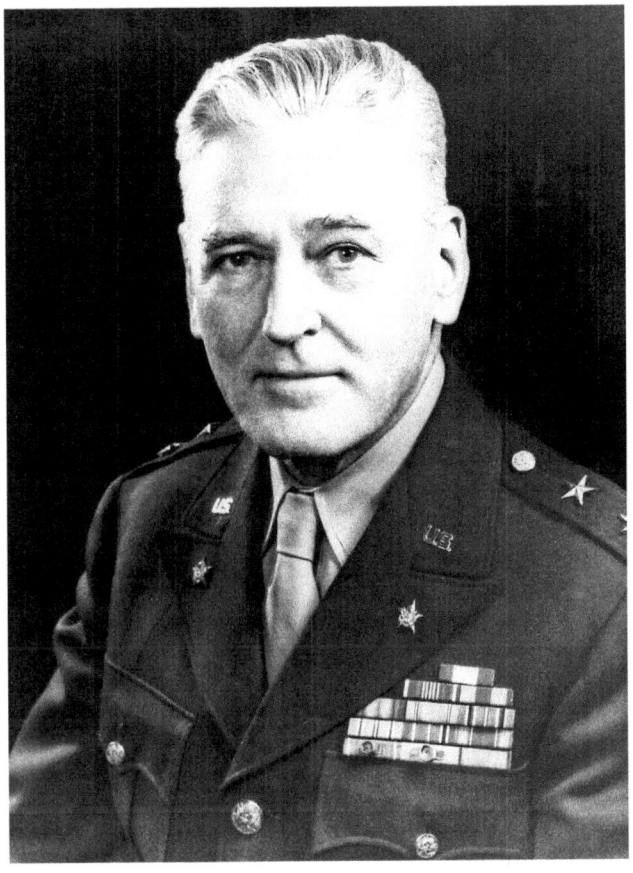

Howard Snyder. Major General Howard Snyder, Eisenhower's presidential physician, adroitly managed the political implications of his patient's three serious illnesses during Eisenhower's presidency. (National Library of Medicine)

As White House physician, the Snyders lived in a luxurious Connecticut Avenue apartment and were often at the White House in the evening playing cards or watching movies. Clarence Lasby states that "They were more than friends of the Eisenhowers; they were part of the family."[98] Robert Ferrell portrayed Snyder as shrewd, intelligent, and sociable: "He was a good conversationalist and just the man to have around for a card game. Like all old army officers, he had learned how to stow the liquor away and could do whatever drinking was necessary."[99] Decades later, Ronald Reagan's White House physician, Burton Smith, referred to this military camaraderie by commenting, "In the old days I think Dwight Eisenhower and his doctor used to have a scotch together before bed.... I think FDR and his doctor used to sit around and drink together."[100] Doctor Snyder accompanied Eisenhower on almost all (and after 1955, at the demand of press secretary James Haggerty, all) of the president's trips; he often remained at the Eisenhowers' Gettysburg farm during Ike's frequent visits there.[101] In May 1959, when Eisenhower took an afternoon off to take grandson David to a Washington Senators–New York Yankees baseball game, Snyder went along.[102]

Ike reciprocated Snyder's loyalty and affection. In November 1954 Lucius Clay, a leading Eisenhower supporter, advised the president "...that there was a feeling among his friends that Dr. Snyder, being seventy-three years of age, was really not capable of providing the medical care and advice that the President ought to have."[103] Eisenhower strongly disagreed with this advice and gave his doctor a superior rating on Snyder's 1955 efficiency report.[104]

Snyder made the health of the President his full-time job. After Ike's severe heart attack in August 1955, his professional care was depicted by Clarence Lasby: "He waits each night to check over the patient before he goes to bed—and then is around in the morning before he gets up. There is no more devoted a man."[105] Snyder's professional responsibility became exclusively and obsessively focused upon the President.

However, when a medical emergency occurred, as it did three times during Ike's eight-year presidency, Snyder convened consultative groups that consisted of both military and nonmilitary physicians. The most important of these was organized at the time of Ike's 1955 heart attack in Denver, which necessitated a seven-week convalescence at Denver's Fitzsimmons Army Hospital. The group's members were cardiologist Colonel Byron Pollock and internists Colonel George M. Powell and Lieutenant Colonel John A. Sheedy. Ike's cardiologist from Walter Reed, Colonel Thomas Mattingly, was flown in from Washington, but the most significant addition was the world-renowned Boston cardiologist Paul Dudley White.[106] The

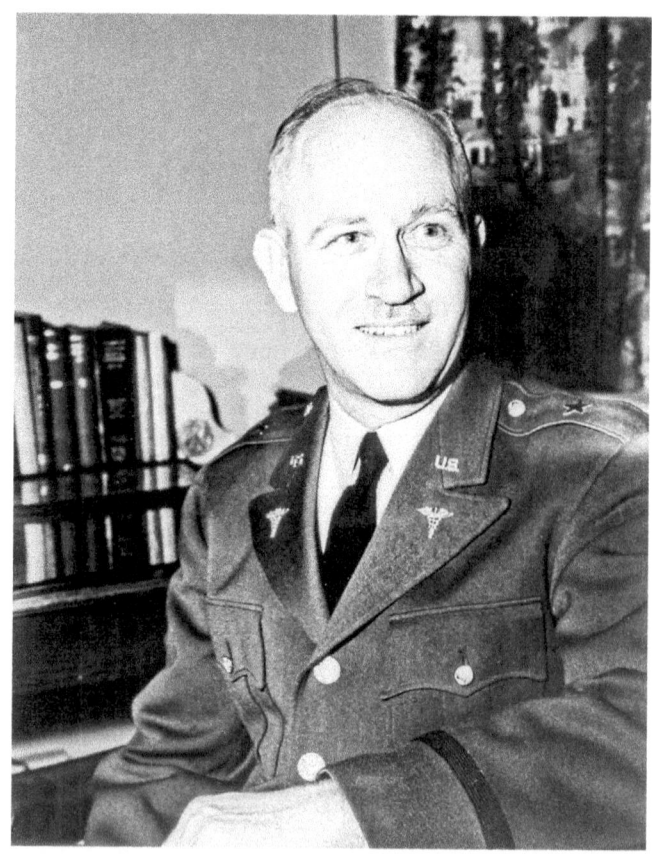

Thomas Mattingly. Cardiologist Thomas Mattingly monitored Dwight Eisenhower's heart disease during his presidency. Mattingly's military superiors, Generals Snyder and Heaton, tightly controlled his remarks to the press. (National Library of Medicine)

Eisenhower administration, very cognizant of the skepticism that had accompanied the coverage of the presidential disabilities of Wilson and Roosevelt, was insistent that a respected nonmilitary physician serve in a prominent role for the president's treatment.[107] In the selection of Dr. White, Howard Snyder apparently adhered to the army chain of command, first consulting with Major General Martin E. Griffin, the Fitzsimmons Hospital commander, and then discussing the decision with the army surgeon general in Washington, D.C. It was the latter, Major General Silas B. Hays, who extended the invitation to White to fly to Denver in consultation.[108]

Segments of the consultant group continued to monitor Ike's recovery over the next year. On February 14, 1956, White was maneuvered, mainly by Snyder, to declare that Eisenhower was fit to serve a second term as president.[109] Colonel Mattingly, a very talented cardiologist, disagreed with the public prognoses of his military superiors and was reluctant to clear the president for a second campaign for the presidency. Snyder managed to silence any public opposition by his military subordinate.[110] When the army cardiologist attempted to secure his integrity by begging off attending a December 1955 press conference intended to bolster the image that candidate Eisenhower was fit to run for reelection, "The generals [Snyder and Heaton] insisted he attend because … the press would expect a cardiologist to be present."[111] He attended. Whether related to this incident or not, in the spring of 1957 the president-patient sent a personal letter to the secretary of the army suggesting that Colonel Mattingly be promoted to brigadier general.[112]

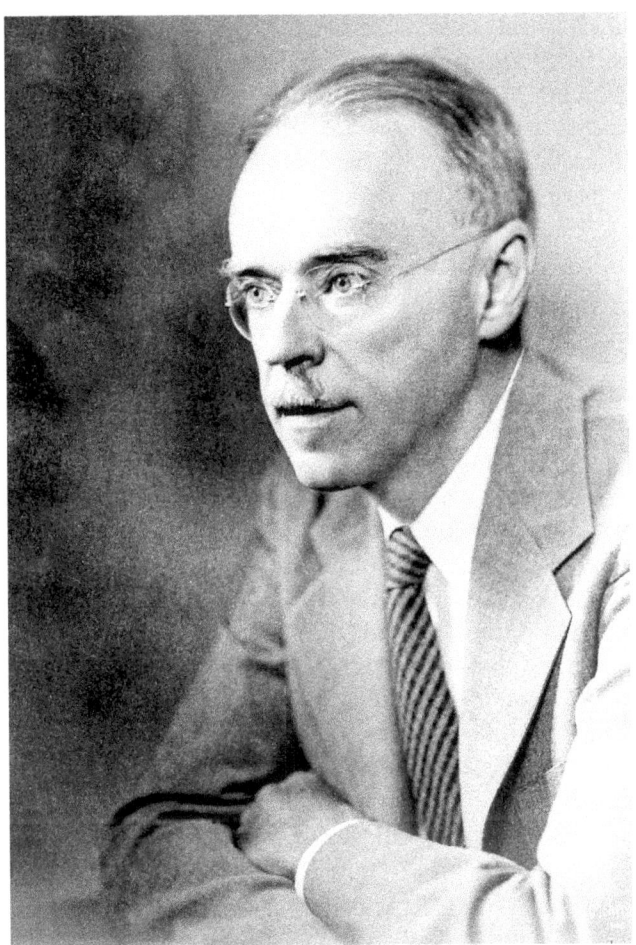

Paul D. White. Prominent cardiologist Paul Dudley White was recruited as consulting cardiologist after President Eisenhower had a heart attack in 1955. White's presence dispelled any notion of a medical cover-up by the military physicians who surrounded the ailing president. (National Library of Medicine)

It is remarkable that when President Eisenhower was admitted to Fitzsimmons Army Hospital in September 1955, he became only the second president of the United States to be hospitalized while in office. His predecessor, Harry Truman, was briefly hospitalized in Washington in 1952 with viral pneumonia.[113] Previous chapters have recounted the operations that had been performed upon sitting presidents in 1893 and 1901, but in neither the case of Cleveland nor that of McKinley did the surgery occur within a standard hospital setting. However, future presidents Lyndon Johnson and Ronald Reagan would undergo in-hospital surgery, and presidents Richard Nixon, George H. Bush, and Donald Trump would be hospitalized for medical conditions.[114]

Franklin Roosevelt had a habit of visiting Bethesda Naval Hospital as an outpatient but was never admitted for treatment for either his hypertension or congestive heart failure. Roosevelt became the seventh president of the United States to die in office. Two (William Henry Harrison and Zachary Taylor) died in the White House, Abraham Lincoln in a private home across the street from Ford's Theater in Washington, William McKinley in a private home in Buffalo, New York, James Garfield in a private home in Elberton, New Jersey, and Warren G. Harding in a hotel room in San Francisco.

Why would this be? Why did the presidential physicians avoid hospitalizing their sick patients? An appropriate answer consists of equal parts of subterfuge, safety, and skill. Franklin Roosevelt, a skilled practitioner of secrecy and deceit,[115] certainly considered any publicity of his health concerns to be impolitic. Moreover, there was little more that a physician could accomplish in a hospital in 1875 than could be performed with safety and skill in 1830.[116]

However, in the succeeding decades, hospitals grew rapidly to number more than 5,000 institutions by 1915.[117] Physicians increasingly oriented their practices around hospitals. In New York City, the percentage of hospital-affiliated doctors increased from 36.8 percent to 52 percent between 1921 and 1927. By 1933 five-sixths of American physicians held a hospital appointment.[118]

The major impetus for hospital growth was a significant increase in surgery. In-hospital abdominal surgery became both practical and safe with the combination of anesthesia, aseptic operating room technique,

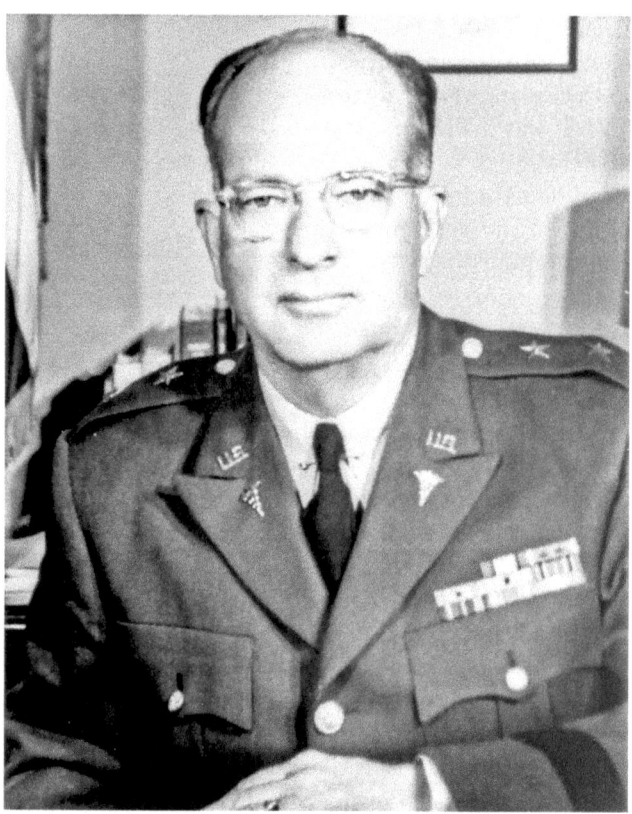

Leonard Heaton. General Leonard Heaton was the principal surgeon during President Eisenhower's intestinal surgery during the 1956 presidential election campaign. Heaton later was promoted to the rank of lieutenant general and to the position of surgeon general of the army. (National Library of Medicine)

Chapter 7. The Military Keepers of the Stethoscope

and the easy availability of X-rays and the clinical laboratory. Hospital expansion generated both the professionalization and increased numbers of nurses; the requirement of round-the-clock house staff, both interns and residents in post-graduate training, added to a medically safe environment. However, it was the growth in surgical volume, pioneered by the Brothers Mayo, that was pivotal for hospital growth in the twentieth century.

An ileocolic bypass was performed at Walter Reed in June 1956 by Major General Leonard Heaton, who contemporaneously was the commander of the hospital. Assisting him was Isidor S. Ravdin, professor of surgery at the University of Pennsylvania School of Medicine. Ike's chronic Crohn's disease of the small intestine had produced an intestinal obstruction that could not be repaired by nonsurgical measures.[119] After an uncomplicated recovery, one month later a grateful Eisenhower officially designated Heaton as his surgeon.[120] Reelected easily in 1956, Ike suffered a minor stroke in November 1957. Snyder and Heaton called in famed civilian neurologists Francis M. Forster of Georgetown and H. Houston Merritt and James Hammill, both of Columbia.[121]

Howard Snyder skillfully maneuvered to limit any political damage to Eisenhower from his medical difficulties. He delayed for at least ten hours the announcement of Eisenhower's heart attack and then tried to stage manage the event by having the stricken president walk down a flight of stairs, transporting him to the hospital by private car rather than an ambulance, and directing that the automobile take a somewhat circuitous route to allow the patient to enter the hospital by a side entrance.[122] Snyder, more subtly than McIntire and with some assistance from Heaton, was successful in controlling Mattingly's public comments regarding Eisenhower's cardiac status. Mattingly's medical opinions were consistently less sanguine than Snyder's.[123]

Snyder deliberately issued a misleading statement after a crucial pre-election comprehensive examination which included an intestinal X-ray showing Crohn's ileitis as the cause of Ike's chronic intestinal problems. Snyder deviously authorized a statement that the X-rays "showed a normally functioning digestive tract," and slyly withheld this information from his patient.[124] Later, in 1957, Snyder and Heaton, with the assistance of press secretary James Haggerty, were able to obscure and obfuscate the nature of Eisenhower's minor stroke.[125]

After the ileitis operation, White House physician Howard Snyder slipped into a joint management arrangement for maintaining the president's health with Leonard Heaton.[126] There had been significant deference issues between General Snyder and the civilian physician, Dr. White. Eisenhower, comfortable with a military chain of command, was angered by White's reporting to Mattingly or directly to the president, and not through the nominal chief of medical care, Snyder.[127] As previously stated, Mattingly also had significant disagreements with both Snyder and Heaton.[128] Howard Snyder died in 1970, one year after the demise of his famous patient.[129]

Leonard Heaton was an accomplished surgeon. He underwent training in this specialty by completing both a surgical internship and a surgical residency in military teaching hospitals. Heaton was one of the first presidential physicians to be board certified in a medical specialty. At age forty-six, he passed the American Board of Surgery examination in 1948.[130] The American Board of Surgery had been established in 1937.[131] The practical experiences of World War II had accelerated the growth of specialization within American medicine. The diversity of war related illness and injury encouraged the rise of specialization and enhanced the attractiveness of board certification. Between 1940 and 1949 the number of American medical specialists rose from 36,880 to 62,888 and the number of part time specialists and generalists declined from 120,090 to 110,441.[132]

Heaton commenced a lifelong friendship with Howard Snyder when both were serving as military physicians in England during the war. As career army men they had a compatible worldview and a deep respect for military medicine. It was not surprising that Heaton subsequently fulfilled a major role on Eisenhower's medical team "…as an 'old army' man whom the president liked and trusted."[133]

Heaton's successful care of Eisenhower evolved into a "warm friendship between the two families that continued until Mrs. Eisenhower's death. Both couples, their wedding anniversaries within days of each other, subsequently spent these times together when they could, either directly or by phone."[134] The friendship endured as Heaton accompanied the then ex-president to Great Britain for Winston Churchill's funeral in 1965.[135] President Eisenhower nominated his surgeon to be Surgeon General of the Army when this post became vacant on May 1, 1959. Heaton served in this post for ten years until he retired in September 1969.[136] The president further honored Dr. Heaton in August 1959, when he asked the Senate to approve an additional star, which would elevate his doctor to the rank of lieutenant general.[137] At the time of this promotion, Heaton became the first physician to achieve this rank.[138] The surgeon was not a mere passive recipient of his third star. Instead, when it appeared that his promotion might be blocked by Pentagon bureaucrats, Heaton actively lobbied Jerry Parsons, assistant to President Eisenhower, for his promotion. Congressman Mendel Rivers, the very powerful chairman of the House Armed Services Committee, expedited Heaton's elevation to lieutenant general. Rivers was a patient of Dr. Heaton.[139]

Medical consultants also have benefited from their association with a president's care. In his autobiography, Dr. White commented: "The public prestige that came my way increased my usefulness as a speaker at meetings, both medical and lay, and I know that frequently my name has helped in fund-raising or even the passage of useful legislation. Also, my contacts abroad have been enhanced. Happily. some of the affection that most people of the world held for Ike passed down to me." He continued by mentioning a few troublesome effects of his publicity; these included the swamping of his mailbox and home telephone lines by the press and public, and the unauthorized use of his name and photograph in newspaper and journal advertisements.[140]

There is no record of any bill that was presented by White to the government or to the president for professional services rendered.[141] If Dr. White had submitted a bill, he would have been reimbursed by the Department of Defense as a consultant to the surgeon general at the 1956 rate of $50 a day. Eisenhower's 1956 hospitalization of ileitis lasted for twenty-two days. "As Commander in Chief of the Armed Forces, he was not charged for his four-room suite at Walter Reed. The services of all the military personnel at the hospital—from the commanding officer, Maj. Gen. Leonard D. Heaton, who performed the operation, to technicians and nurse—also were free."[142] However, Eisenhower did reimburse the government for meals at $1.05 per diem for himself and $1.55 per diem for Mrs. Eisenhower, who had remained with him at Walter Reed.

Military physicians protected three presidents from full public disclosure of their significant medical diseases. Personal commitment by their loyal doctors shielded these leaders from a scrutiny that would be impossible today. These White House doctors probably justified their deceptions on the basis of security and policy exigencies. Roosevelt was contemporaneously the leader of the Allies in the midst of fighting the Second World War, and Woodrow Wilson was unsuccessfully engaged in securing congressional approval of the treaty that ended the First World War. The Treaty of Versailles optimistically proposed a formula for obviating all future wars by the organization of the League of Nations. Dwight Eisenhower was engaged in a contest to be reelected to the White House when he suffered first a heart attack, and second an intestinal obstruction. Their physician's secrecy and obfuscation elevated political considerations over any medical concerns. The intimate "pal ship" that characterized the relationship that these three doctors enjoyed with their respective presidents undoubtedly influenced their secretive and protective behavior in matters medical. Such conduct became less likely after Snyder; the increasing bureaucratization and transparency of the White House physician's responsibilities made such a close relationship increasingly difficult, albeit not impossible, for succeeding White House physicians.

Wallace Harry Graham was yet another military physician who served a long tenure as the White House physician. Graham was President Harry Truman's doctor from September 1945 until Truman departed the White House in January 1953.[143] Graham's patient remained in excellent health and battled no significant illnesses during his presidency,[144] and, as a result, controversies over professional deference and public disclosure, so prominent during the Grayson, McIntire and Snyder tenures, did not arise. As a consequence, Graham's prominence in this narrative is a diminished one.

In many ways, Graham's White House incumbency mirrored those of other White House physicians in the first half of the twentieth century. He was the recipient of rapid promotion. In September 1946 the president made him a brigadier general at the young age of thirty-six years.[145] In March 1951 Truman recommended that Graham be advanced to the temporary rank of major general in the Air Force Reserves.[146]

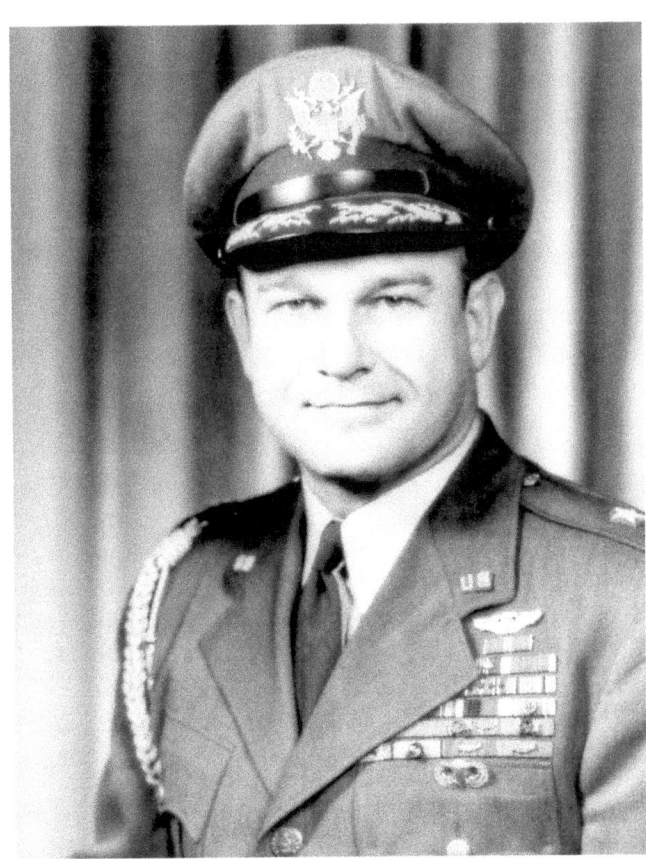

Wallace Graham. General Wallace Graham, President Truman's personal physician, became embroiled in politics, and suffered professionally as a consequence. (National Library of Medicine)

Doctor Graham's age differential of thirty years with his patient may have lessened his camaraderie with the president, but he was a regular player in Truman's frequent poker games,[147] often swam with the president in the White House pool,[148] and was occasionally invited to dinner with the first family.[149]

Harry Truman was profligate in his use of the White House physician's office for the treatment of family, administration officials, and foreign dignitaries. On March 15, 1947, the president's mother fractured her hip in her Missouri home; Graham was immediately dispatched to attend to her.[150] Graham also treated Truman's sister Mary Jane for an upper respiratory problem. "I treated her mother also. I was flown out to Kansas City-Independence a few times to treat them."[151] When cousin Ralph Truman was hospitalized in the Hot Springs, Arkansas, Army and Navy Hospital, Truman wrote, "I sent my Brig. General Doctor down to see him...."[152]

Administration officials also benefited from Graham's medical care. He would see "Generally, anybody who wanted treatment, yes. That's how it ran. Jimmy Byrnes would come in occasionally. The Secretary of Agriculture, Clinton Anderson, would come in occasionally, and Lord Halifax, when in the city."[153] Dr. Graham was not the first presidential physician to treat foreign VIPs, but this practice became commonplace during his tenure. Additionally, Graham traveled to Saudi Arabia where he removed an esophageal tumor that was choking King Ibn Saud,[154] and to Lima, Peru, to surgically correct a Dupuytren's contracture of the hand of President Manuel Odria.[155]

Harry Truman had not met Dr. Graham prior to selecting him as White House physician. Truman, shortly after succeeding to the presidency upon the death of Franklin Roosevelt, attended the 1945 end of the war conference in Potsdam, Germany. While there he arranged a meeting with the available serving medical officers from the state of Missouri, the president's home state. Among the gathering was Colonel Graham, the son of Dr. James Walter Graham, a long-time colleague of Truman when both were active in the Reserve Officers Association in Missouri. The president's close aide Harry Vaughn took an immediate liking to military doctor Wallace Graham and asked him to return to Washington as President Truman's White House physician. The surprised and bewildered Graham's response was unexpected, saying in part, "If you ask me how I would like it, I don't think I would like it." A second interview a few days later secured Graham's acceptance with reservations. The president finally responded, "Do you realize who you're talking to?" Graham answered, "Yes, sir. I'll obey orders, sir."[156] However, the president did allow Graham to serve contemporaneously as chief of surgery at Walter Reed National Military Medical Center in Washington, D.C.[157] Major Ray Miller or Captain Thomas J. Burns accompanied the president on those rare occasions when Graham was on special duty at Walter Reed. The staff of the White House Physician's Office remained meager: "the nurse [R.N.] was always there [at the White House] or on call. Mrs. Harrell was the nurse who was always there."[158]

Several presidents brought their personal physicians with them to the White House. In a reversal of the usual direction, Harry Truman brought his presidential physician back to Missouri, where Graham continued as the Trumans' family doctor. Graham operated on both Harry and Bess Truman in their retirement and treated the ex-president during his terminal illness.[159]

The most significant event of Graham's occupancy in terms of this historical narrative occurred during the summer of 1952, when Harry Truman became the first president to be hospitalized. After two days with a viral upper respiratory infection and fever, the president was admitted by Graham to Walter Reed on July 16, 1952. Truman's three-day hospital stay was uneventful and disclosed no significant complications.[160]

The Graham incumbency was notable for two additional reasons: his advocacy of a contentious political position and his appearance as a witness before a congressional committee that was investigating his trading in commodities. In a break from the presidential physician's customary silence on political issues, General Graham publicly supported the president's controversial national health insurance program. He made several speeches before groups that supported the Truman policy, a policy that was strongly opposed by the American Medical Association. His advocacy probably led to his future difficulties with the AMA.[161]

As a result, the American Medical Association thought that Graham was a socialist. In his oral history, the doctor gruffly responded, "I'm a social fellow; I'm very sociable whatever the hell I am.... I don't think I'm a communist, but I do not know what the hell I am other than a hundred percent good American."[162]

In early January 1948 Graham was subpoenaed to appear before a Senate appropriations subcommittee to explain his involvement in commodities trading. A political storm engulfed the physician after records disclosed that he had been a minor trader in grain futures at the same time that his president was accusing speculators of causing an increase in consumer food prices. Graham's responses were embarrassing and confusing, especially after an admission that his profit was $6,165, a more than doubling of his investment. In his congressional testimony, the White House physician pleaded ignorance and financial naivete as an explanation for this misadventure, and the investigation faded into the political miasma.[163]

After graduating from Creighton School of Medicine, Graham, repeating a practice from early in the century, took his postgraduate training in Europe. He trained in surgery in Vienna, Hungary, and the University of Edinburgh, but did not serve an approved American surgery residency. The May 1947 educational requirements for admission to the board examination of the American Board of Surgery was four years of surgery training in a hospital, presumably American but unstated, that was endorsed by the American Medical Association and the American College of Surgeons.[164] As a consequence, when Graham applied for specialty certification by the American Board of Surgery in 1950, the certification process was never completed.[165] President Truman blamed the AMA for delaying his physician's board certification and considered Graham's difficulties as political retribution for the president's advocacy of national health insurance. In January 1949 the president wrote the Surgeon General: "I understand that my physician, General Wallace Graham is being penalized by the American College of Surgeons because he is my physician. I don't like it."[166] The American Board of Surgery had been established in 1937,[167] and by 1950 "at least 50 percent of all full-time specialists were board certified, either by examination or through the board's generous grandfather clauses."[168]

The AMA continued to give Graham grief when he practiced in Missouri. This organization strongly discouraged his setting up a medical clinic in Kansas City, and Graham abandoned his efforts to do so.[169]

Like other presidential physicians both before and after, Dr. Graham published his memoirs. But, in contrast, his memoir concluded with his war experiences until he met President Truman in May 1945.[170, 171]

Chapter 8

Physician Anecdotes
The Returnee, the Academic, the Consultant and the Defendant, 1953–1981

The stories of four less conspicuous physicians merit attention in this narrative. Their experiences are significantly instructive and illuminant to merit this modest detour from strict chronology. Two (doctors Tkach and Lukash) served lengthy apprenticeships as assistant White House physicians before their eventual elevation to physicians to the president; two others (doctors Hurst and Riland) served as medical consultants to the White House. One monitored Lyndon Johnson's cardiac status and the second treated Richard Nixon's musculoskeletal problems. The members of this quartet participated in presidential care between 1953 and 1981, often in a secondary and almost always in an unpublicized role; their experiences may not be as dramatic as those of the military keepers of the stethoscope profiled in Chapter 7 or of the super specialists in Chapters 9 and 10, but their contributions to this tale of the presidential physicians should not be neglected. White House physician was but one identity for career military doctors Tkach and Lukash, who filled other roles during their professional careers. The Washington stories of doctors Hurst and Riland may broaden an appreciation of the nuanced and diverse roles that the physician-consultants play in ongoing presidential medical care.

First to be profiled is the Returnee: Air Force flight surgeon Walter Tkach, who served two discontinuous tours of duty in the White House physician's office, an unusual experience in this organization's history. Dr. Tkach served inconspicuously as assistant to the personal physician of President Dwight Eisenhower (1953–1961),[1] and in 1969, after an absence of nearly eight years, was appointed as the presidential physician to Richard Nixon. During Tkach's first tour Howard Snyder dominated Eisenhower's professional care together with prominent medical consultants Paul Dudley White, Leonard Heaton and Thomas Mattingly.[2] The written record of Tkach's active involvement during Eisenhower's several medical crises is almost a blank page, with only the following single reference: On the morning of June 8, 1956, the president experienced an intestinal obstruction. An increasingly concerned Snyder, unable to contact doctors Heaton or Mattingly, temporized as Eisenhower became more distended. "Snyder … and his assistant physician, Dr. Walter Tkach, tended to the president with a cup of tea, heating pads of the abdomen and feet, and a small enema."[3]

After a brief period in the White House of the newly elected John Kennedy, Tkach transferred to active air force duty and was stationed at air force commands both in the continental United States and overseas, including a tour as command surgeon at the headquarters of the Seventh Air Force, Tan Son Nhut Airfield, Vietnam.[4] Subsequently, Colonel Tkach distinguished himself in military operations in Vietnam, for which he was awarded the Bronze Star medal.[5] The newly elected Richard Nixon, a friend of Tkach's, which friendship probably dated back to the days of Nixon's vice presidency under Eisenhower, returned the command flight surgeon to Washington as his presidential physician.[6] The circumstances of Tkach's departure from the Kennedy administration are not clear. One report implied that he departed because of dissatisfaction with the policies of the new Democratic administration[7]; a second indicated that he had been overworked as he staffed the employee health clinic, apparently his principal medical responsibility. He told the incoming Dr.

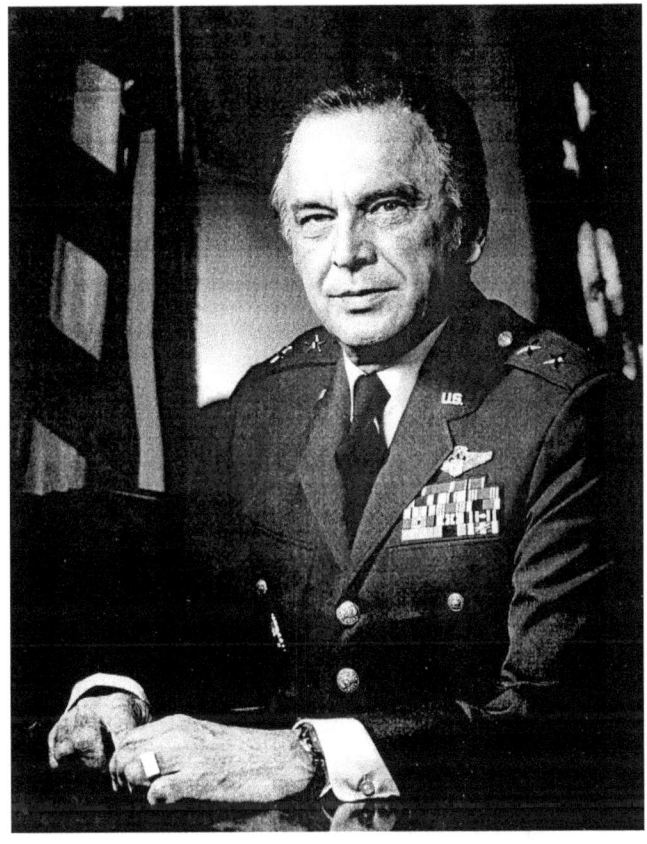

Walter Tkach. Major General Dr. Walter Tkach, who served two discontinuous tours in the White House Medical Unit, first as an assistant White House physician during the Eisenhower presidency, later as the personal physician to President Richard Nixon. (Courtesy National Archives and Records Administration)

Travell that he had not had as much as a week's leave in eight years![8] Another tale suggests that the newly inaugurated president may have been the facilitator for the doctor's departure. Early on, Kennedy had instructed his doctor Dr. Janet Travell, "Do not be in a hurry to choose an assistant."[9]

In the past, politics has often embroiled White House physicians in its cauldron, especially at times of presidential ill health.[10] It is hardly a source of astonishment that Richard Nixon, a skilled practitioner of the craft of politics, entangled his personal physician, Dr Tkach, in its web at least twice. The results of the president's annual physical exam were scheduled for release at the end of 1970, a year of antiwar turmoil and a weakening economy. As a counter, Nixon desired to program the announcement for his political benefit. Accordingly, he directed Ron Ziegler, his press secretary, to "Let Dr. Tkach give them the results.... He should say that his major concern about the president's health is that he does not get enough recreation, does not have the relaxations of others in the office.... He should say that the president's daily work schedule is the most backbreaking that he has ever observed in a public figure. He should point out, nevertheless, that the president remains in excellent health due to very Spartan habits.... I think Tkach could do it with complete credibility."[11] However, Tkach's credibility was spared since the doctor, apparently oblivious to the president's political coaching, instead "gave a pretty straight medical report. This led to great concern on the P's [Nixon] part."[12]

A second instance occurred shortly after President Nixon's resignation on August 8, 1974. In the tradition of other presidential physicians, Grayson and Graham, who had continued to follow their respective patients in retirement, Dr. Tkach accompanied Richard Nixon to his retirement home in San Clemente, California. In his case, the length of post-presidential care was brief but controversial. Nixon resigned amid political turmoil of the highest order—an impending impeachment—and accompanying physical distress. The crux of the health issue was a worsening case of lower leg phlebitis and venous thrombosis, a likely precursor to significant pulmonary damage. Some surmised that Nixon's ill health was the cause of his pardon, that President Ford wished to spare his predecessor any further medical harm.[13]

Dr. Tkach accompanied Nixon to the ex-president's California home, and proceeded to issue a series of dramatic medical announcements to the press in which his patient's prognosis was portrayed as dire. One example was that while the ex-president was not terminal, "it will take a miracle for him to recover."[14] The *New York Times*, inherently skeptical of all things Republican, hinted in an editorial that Tkach's announcements were politically inspired, if not professionally unethical. Its editors opined, "...it is odd to find his ... doctor conveying details to the public press before they have even been reported to the patient's wife. This is precisely what.... Walter Tkach admits to when he freely provided *Newsweek* with medical information that he says was withheld from Mrs. Nixon, 'for fear of frightening her.' Any family would be entitled to question such unprofessional behavior from its doctor...."[15]

There was a documented reciprocal friendship and loyalty between this president and his physician, a not uncommon occurrence. Richard Nixon was in attendance at both Tkach's bachelor party in Washington and his wedding in San Clemente. The widowed doctor married C.A. Gaillard, who was the former conference director at the Nixon Western White House.[16] Moreover, Tkach, an air force colonel when he returned to the White House, was promoted by the president to brigadier general in 1970 and then to major general in 1972.[17] Additionally the president awarded General Tkach the Distinguished Service Medal for his service as the physician to the president.[18]

Last, Walter Tkach was the last personal physician to the president to practice without certification by a specialty board.[19] All his successors in that post, commencing with the most immediate, Dr. William Lukash, have been certified as diplomats of one medical specialty board or another.

The next to be profiled is the Academic: Navy doctor William Lukash was superbly trained: Medical school at the University of Michigan, an internship year at Wayne County Hospital, Detroit, three years of an internal medicine residency at the Great Lakes Naval Hospital, climaxed by a two-year fellowship in gastroenterology at the Philadelphia Naval Hospital.[20] The quality of his education was reflected by board certification by the American Board of Internal Medicine, by further internal medicine sub-certification in the specialty of gastroenterology,[21] and by his academic and administrative status as the chairman of the department of gastroenterology at Bethesda Naval Hospital, a respected teaching hospital.[22] Perhaps the proximity of Bethesda to the White House made Lukash an attractive candidate to serve as an assistant White House physician. He simultaneously held both appointments for six years until Gerald Ford appointed him as the physician to the president in 1974. Lukash's academic production as an educator and a specialist in gastroenterology in teaching hospitals had been robust: participation in twelve research projects, 12 oral presentations at national medical meetings, fifty-seven published scientific articles, and authoring three books and monographs.[23]

William Lukash was one of the longest-serving doctors in the White House physician's office, serving continuously under presidents Nixon, Ford and Carter. He served from 1966 until the inauguration of Ronald Reagan in January 1981.[24] His transition from part time academician to a family physician was successful, since Jimmy Carter reappointed him as his personal physician upon succeeding Gerald Ford. Modern history records only a rare situation when the physician to the president did not relinquish this position conterminously with his patient's retirement. An example was Presley Rixey, who successively served presidents McKinley and Theodore Roosevelt.[25] Lukash was kept on despite the change in the new president's party affiliation from Republican to Democratic. A third instance occurred in 2017 when Navy Captain Ronny Jackson remained the presidential physician when the presidency shifted from Democrat to Republican. However, it has not been uncommon for an assistant physician to be promoted to presidential doctor by a succeeding administration.

Lukash's obituary reflected the change in course in his professional focus: "Becoming a White House Physician meant changing from a specialist into a family doctor. He likened his new role to that of a country doctor."[26] Lukash resumed his academic career upon his 1981 resignation from the navy; he became medical director of the preventive medicine section at the Scripps Clinic and Research Foundation in California.[27] Between 1964 and 1974, Lukash authored or coauthored more than thirty-one articles

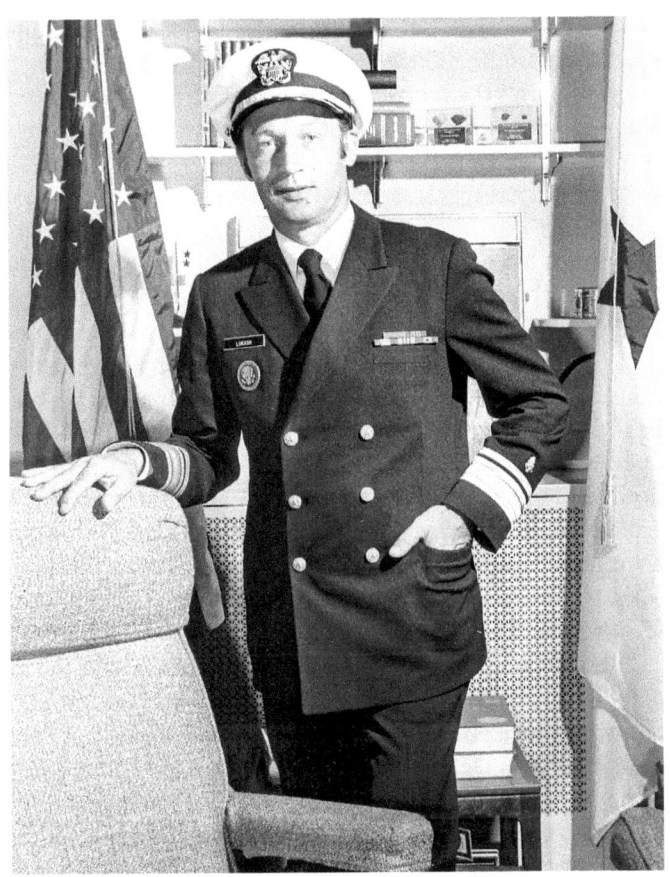

William Lukash. Admiral William Lukash was presidential physician to Gerald Ford and Jimmy Carter. He relinquished a distinguished academic career as a gastroenterologist for a general medicine practice as physician to the president. (Courtesy of the Bureau of Medicine Library and Archives)

on esophageal, gastric and pancreatic diseases These appeared in prestigious medical journals including *The New England Journal of Medicine*, *American Journal of Gastroenterology* and the *Journal of American Medical Association (JAMA)*. As a general practitioner fulfilling his responsibilities as presidential physician, Lukash published but single articles in 1976 and 1979.[28]

In other respects, the nature of Lukash's tenure was typical. He retired from the navy at age 49 as a rear admiral. He was dispatched from Washington by Richard Nixon to monitor the health of family members and prominent personages. He flew to Indiana University Medical Center to attend the operation of the president's daughter, Mrs. Julie Eisenhower; during which a benign ovarian cyst was successfully removed.[29] On May 15, 1972, presidential contender and Alabama governor George Wallace was severely injured by an assassination attempt at a campaign rally in Laurel, Maryland. Interested in the well-being of his political rival, Nixon sent his assistant physician to Wallace's operating room. Dr. Joseph Schanno, the operating surgeon, recalled: "'...Don't look now, but Nixon's physician is looking over your shoulder!' It was Dr. William Lukash.... I looked up and there was this tall, rather good-looking guy in a surgical gown. 'Are you a surgeon?' I asked. 'No. I do gastroenterology as an internist.' I said 'Well, for God's sake, if you see me doing anything wrong, tell me! By the way,' I added, 'you can treat me for my ulcer when this thing is over with!' We later became good friends."[30]

Lukash also called Dr. John C. Lungren late in the evening of September 11, 1974, on behalf of the newly inaugurated Gerald Ford to inquire about Richard Nixon's worsening lower leg phlebitis.[31] Lungren had just arrived at the ex-president's temporary residence in Palm Desert, California, after Nixon had requested his medical attention. Dr. Lungren was a Long Beach, California, board certified cardiologist who previously had a physician-patient relationship with Nixon and had conducted Nixon's official preinaugural physical examination in January 1969.[32] Lungren took over the ex-president's care, which proved to be consequential, complex, and above all, controversial. Thrombosis and pulmonary damage complicated the phlebitis and required two hospitalizations, an operation and a lengthy program of anticoagulation to resolve. The controversy resulted from Lungren's medical opinion that the ex-president, his patient, was far too ill to testify in Washington, D.C., as a witness in the various Watergate criminal trials. As a result, the cardiologist's integrity, judgment, and competence were questioned by the press, politicians, and even colleagues in the medical profession.[33] Lungren's record of his recollections of his treatment of ex-president Nixon is a recent addition to the bookshelf containing memoirs of other physicians who have treated presidents.

One lesson to be learned from this episode is that an ex-president, at least in the case of Richard Nixon, is personally responsible for his medical and hospital bills. Nixon paid out of his own pocket for his two 1974 hospitalizations at Long Beach Memorial and for Dr. Lungren's professional services.[34]

While presidential physician Dr. Lukash became a swimming and tennis partner of both Ford and Carter,[35] his companionship with President Carter was so tight that Carter conceded that any White House physician would be unable to recommend that Section 4 of the Twenty-fifth Amendment to the United States Constitution be properly invoked. Section 4 details the procedures for replacing a medically disabled president against his will. In his address to the opening session of the elite panel to restudy the applicability of the amendment, Carter said, "I am familiar with White House physicians. I know that this is a very difficult question for White House physicians.... In the four years I was in the White House, I did not have a closer, more intimate personal friend than Bill Lukash. He and I played tennis against each other. We were just about equal. He and I fly-fished together. We went cross-country skiing together. We watched movies together. We jogged together. There could not be a closer relationship between any person and his physician than between me and Lukash. When I was defeated, he chose to retire."[36]

Next, the focus will be upon the consultant: The academically talented Dr. J. Willis Hurst served as a consultant to the White House physicians during Lyndon Johnson's presidency (1963–1969). He was Johnson's cardiologist before, during, and after his presidency. Dr. Hurst was a naval medical officer and chief of cardiology at Bethesda Naval Hospital when then Senator Johnson was admitted with a severe heart attack in 1955.[37] Thereupon, Hurst assumed the care of Johnson's cardiac problems for the duration of his lengthy hospitalization; he continued in this role during LBJ's senatorial career and his vice presidency (1961–1963). Subsequently Dr. Hurst became a frequent consultant in cardiology during the Johnson presidency, frequently traveling to the District of Columbia and to the Johnson ranch in Texas from his teaching position at Emory School of Medicine in Atlanta.[38]

Dr. Hurst continued to add to his illustrious professional career at Emory until his death at age ninety. At age 35, he was chairman of the school's department of internal medicine. He authored 66 books and 460 scholarly articles, and traveled the world as a consultant cardiologist, occasionally at the behest of a U.S. president.[39]

Hurst flew unannounced to Washington from New York City to examine Johnson on November 22, 1963, the night of the Kennedy assassination. Dr. Janet Travell, the deceased Kennedy's presidential physician, urgently requested that Johnson's cardiologist examine the newly sworn-in president as reassurance that Johnson's health was equal to the responsibilities of his new office.[40] In a subsequent interview Hurst acknowledged that the new president "…has done beautifully" since his heart attack eight and a half years previously.[41] Subsequently the cardiologist's consultation was part of the reports of the president's annual physical examinations and the evaluation of his cardiac tolerance for the gall bladder operation occurring during his presidency.[42] In July 1968 the national press remarked upon the Johnson-Hurst close relationship by noting that Dr. and Mrs. Hurst had accompanied the Johnsons to church while houseguests at the White House.[43]

Dr. Hurst was compensated for his travel expenses when he attended LBJ, but he never rendered a bill for his professional service, explaining, "…my relationship was as both a physician and a close friend of the entire family…. I never thought of being paid for my services because of the close friendship with all the Johnson's."[44]

An occasional perquisite of a White House consultancy is government-sponsored overseas travel. While vice president, Johnson asked his cardiologist to accompany him on numerous official visits to foreign countries. Senegal, Iran, Turkey, Pakistan and many European countries were among the destinations.[45] Referring to his frequent trips, Johnson suggested to Hurst: "I believe it would be wise for you to sign up with the naval reserve. Then when I call you to come on a trip, you will be on duty when you leave home and go off duty when you return home."[46]

Johnson employed his legendary persuasive powers to cajole his cardiologist into succeeding Janet Travell as his presidential physician. The doctor had been invited to spend a weekend as a White House guest, where the president inquired, after discussing

Hurst's children and future grandchildren, "Don't you want them to remember you as the White House Physician?" Hurst, unwilling to relinquish a challenging academic career at a top-level medical school, resisted his patient's lengthy arguments, inducements and offers. In perhaps a final attempt, on Sunday morning Johnson and Hurst attended church where one of the president's favorite ministers preached on the responsibility of American citizens to serve their country when the opportunity arose.[47]

Many years later Hurst recalled: "I was offered the position of White House physician when.... Dr. Travell left the position. I recommended Dr. George Burkley to President Johnson. I explained to him that he did not need a cardiologist every day and that I needed to see many patients to retain my skill. Dr. Burkley served as the White House physician very well and welcomed me at all times. We worked well together. He often called me when Johnson had a cold or any other minor problem. I hoped the president would forgive me for not accepting his offer. Later he indicated that he did forgive me but he didn't forget it."[48]

And last, the subject is the Defendant. The White House activity of a second consultant, Dr. Kenneth Riland, follows a different plot line. This doctor administered muscle-relaxant treatment to President Richard Nixon approximately twice monthly. The physical reason for this therapy was unclear, since presidential physician Walter Tkach claimed that the president had no backache or other skeletal trouble.[49] The tale of this medical consultant is of interest in two respects. Dr. Riland not only was the first of only four osteopathic-trained physicians to attend to the health of a sitting president, but also was the only doctor who treated a president to be criminally indicted! In April 1973 Riland was indicted on charges of income tax evasion. He was alleged to have avoided $39,000 in taxes in patient fees that he failed to report as income. Reimbursements for Nixon's treatments were a component of Riland's unreported income.[50]

Osteopathy, like homeopathy, emerged in nineteenth-century America as an alternative to the dominant orthodox practice of medicine. It was similar to homeopathy in its skepticism with the exuberant, often toxic drug dosage regimes of regular physicians, but differed from homeopathic practice by its total exclusion, at least initially, of all ingested medicinals from its treatments.

Unlike homeopathy, osteopathic medicine is totally American in its origins. It developed over a number of years, beginning in the 1870s by Andrew Taylor Still, the son of an itinerant doctor, preacher and farmer. Still learned medicine through an apprenticeship with his father, but after practicing in the traditional mode for a time, he became disillusioned with regular medicine over the toxicity and the inefficacy of its treatments. Instead, he synthesized major components of magnetic healing and bone setting into his own unique doctrine. Magnetism held that the effects of disease were due to the obstruction or imbalance of the bodily fluids. This hydraulic deficiency was caused by misplaced bones, especially of the spinal column, which interfered with the nerve supply that regulated the foremost body fluid, the blood.[51] Still's therapeutic methodology was based predominantly on practice rather than on textbook theory. It was the practice of a trained osteopathic doctor to locate by palpation a skeletal abnormality, defined as the *lesion*. Once identified, the practitioner would be able to diagnose which organ or organs were affected, and deduce which vessels or nerves might be inhibited. The disease would then be treated by manipulation.[52]

Still established his base in Kirksville, Missouri, where he established an infirmary in 1889. Three years later he organized the American School of Osteopathy

(AOA) there. The proprietor charged his students $500 apiece for several months of personal instruction. At the conclusion of this period of instruction, the American School of Osteopathy conferred the degree of doctor of osteopathy (D.O.).[53] It was at about this time that Still named his therapeutic creation: "I began to think over names such as allopathy, hydropathy (and) homeopathy." This led to "start out with the word *os* [bone] and the word pathology, and press them into one word—*osteopathy*."[54]

It wasn't long before tension developed between the *lesion* osteopaths who restricted their medical practice to structural diagnosis and manipulative therapy and the *broad* osteopaths who refused any constriction of their practice, since both political and practical reasons compelled that the spectrum of osteopathic medicine be broadened. First the curricula of the osteopath colleges were expanded to include the teaching of obstetrics and surgery; then, in 1912, despite opposition by its founder, adjuncts such as hydrotherapy, corrective exercise, diet and food, chemistry, and medical therapeutics were integrated into osteopathic education.[55]

However, the battle to introduce pharmacology and the teaching of the *Materia medica*—the branch of medicine that deals with drugs, their sources, preparations, and uses—into the curriculum was both protracted and bitter. Initially, many of osteopathy's adherents agreed with its founder, Still, that orthodox drugs were toxic, vile and disgusting; but students in osteopathic colleges required exposure to information about pharmacologic agents in their courses in surgery, obstetrics and practice. Moreover, in certain states applicants required instruction in *Materia medica* in order to obtain an unrestricted medical license. The 1918–1919 influenza pandemic significantly hastened the trend toward *Materia medica*'s inclusion, since orthodox physicians, employing harsher remedies to combat the infection, consequently produced a much higher mortality rate among their patients than osteopathic doctors, who avoided such remedies. It was not until 1929 that the American Osteopathic Association (AOA) officially supported an unlimited scope of practice, including acceptance of drug and medicinal therapy.[56]

After 1930 the most distinctive feature of osteopathic practice and the characteristic that more than anything defined its identity, manipulative treatment, began to diminish in usage. Both institutional changes and scientific advances were causes. A 1954 AOA mail survey discovered that only 44 percent of osteopath respondents answered that 50 percent or more of their patients received manipulation.[57]

Orthodox medicine and especially its institutional spokesman, the American Medical Association (AMA), attempted to diminish, if not erase, the influence of osteopathic medicine in the United States. In his landmark report, *Medical Education in the United States and Canada*, Abraham Flexner acquiesced in evaluating the then extant eight osteopathic medical colleges, and applied to them the same standards as he did to orthodox and homeopathic institutions. In his review Flexner discovered damning inadequacies in faculty, laboratory facilities and clinical opportunities in all eight institutions, concluding that "no one of the eight schools is in a position to give such training as osteopathy itself demands." In further excoriating commentary, Flexner wrote: "Their catalogues are a mass of hysterical exaggerations, alike of the earning and of the curative power of osteopathy."[58] However, Flexner's analytical skill far exceeded his ability to prognosticate, since he predicted, referring to osteopathy among others, that "there is no question that in the end the medical sects will disappear."[59] Almost 100, as osteopathic medicine flourishes, Flexner's reputation as a seer has correspondingly wilted.

For decades the medical establishment sought to impede full licensure for D.O.s by lobbying for combined rather than separate osteopath state licensing boards, and later for the adoption of a single test in the basic sciences to be taken prior to an actual licensing examination.[60] After increasingly adept political maneuvering by the osteopathic establishment had thwarted these attempts, the AMA pursued a policy of amalgamation wherein D.O.s would shed their uniqueness and independence and become subsumed entirely under the M.D. rubric. Initial success occurred in California when, in 1962, all osteopaths were allowed to exchange a D.O. for an M.D. suffix, and the osteopathic medical college in Los Angeles converted to an M.D. degree conferring school.[61]

However individual, institutional and organizational osteopathic medicine outside California withstood amalgamation and forced the AMA to adopt yet another strategy—poaching. In the late 1960s rules were changed to permit D.O. students to transfer to M.D. colleges, to accept D.O.s as members in county and state M.D. medical societies and in the national AMA, and to authorize specialty boards to examine D.O.s who had completed an AMA-approved residency program.[62]

When Dr. Riland became the first osteopathic doctor to enter this history, the osteopathic therapeutic approach was well-established. In 1965, D.O. hospitals became qualified for reimbursement under the Medicare program for seniors, and in 1966 Secretary of Defense Robert McNamara, for the first time, ordered the armed services to accept qualified osteopaths as military physicians and surgeons.[63] Although osteopaths constituted 3–4 percent of the total physician population between 1900 and 1960,[64] its share of graduates climbed to 5.9 percent in 1972.[65] There were still only seven osteopathic medical schools in 1972, but D.O. hospitals, numbering 260 in 1945,[66] continued to increase. Additionally, eleven osteopathic specialty boards had been established, prior to 1960, whose applicants received training in 389 separate programs.[67]

The relative importance of osteopathy to United States medical care increased during the succeeding half-century. In 2022, the number of osteopathic medical schools burgeoned to forty-four.[68] Its number of graduates reached 7,303, or 25.8 percent of the combined M.D/D.O. graduating class of 28,354.[69]

Kenneth Riland was the personal physician and friend to New York governor Nelson Rockefeller, who paid him a retainer of $1,000 monthly plus additional money for extra services. Riland was a graduate of the Philadelphia College of Osteopathic Medicine, joined the United States Steel Corporation, where he became its chief physician in 1958. The governor appointed him doctor to the New York State Public Health Council and Mental Hygiene Council, and later initiated the founding of the New York College of Osteopathic Medicine in 1977. Riland was a cofounder of this school and was chairman of its board when he died in 1989.[70]

Perhaps at the suggestion of Rockefeller and national security adviser Henry Kissinger, who was another patient of Riland's, the osteopath traveled to Washington twice a month to treat Nixon. He also accompanied Nixon on his trips to China and the Soviet Union.[71] In March 1974, the federal government charged Riland with secretly funneling fees, received from treating Nixon and Rockefeller between 1966 and 1970, into private savings accounts in order to avoid listing them as income on his federal tax returns. Court papers revealed that the doctor failed to report $4,516 received from the government for his presidential treatments. The federal vouchers made out to Riland had been signed by General Walter Tkach.[72] Apparently this medical consultant deviated from the tradition that nongovernmental physicians requested to treat a president did not charge for their professional services. On May 11, 1974, at the conclusion of a 43-day trial, Dr. Kenneth Riland was acquitted on all five counts of the federal indictment, and consequently was able to resume his active practice.[73]

Chaos and confusion were about to explode the tranquility of the White House physician organization as a series of ill-prepared presidential physicians were unable to deal effectively with an assassination and an assassination attempt, political subterfuge, chronic illness, and a series of acute medical emergencies. A set of strange appointments of presidential physicians contributed to the chaos, and civilian-military medical disputes arose, although less public than those occurring 100 years earlier.

CHAPTER 9

Civilian Interlude, Part I
Medical Chaos in Camelot

In December 1961 a meeting of President Kennedy's cast of doctors was called at the Kennedy estate in Palm Beach, Florida. Doctor Hans Kraus was the one professional performer to have been purposely eliminated from the dramatis personae by its leading actress, presidential physician Janet Travell. Kraus's biographer recounted the subsequent drama: "Kraus's blood continued to boil when he reached the Kennedy compound. In front of everyone there, Kraus lambasted Travell again, and then he turned his criticism on the President. He reminded Kennedy of their agreement, and concluded, 'I won't treat you again if she touches you.'"[1]

The military's monopoly of the White House physician's office was frequently sundered during the thirty-two-year span between the inaugurations of John F. Kennedy in 1961 and that of Bill Clinton in 1993. For fourteen of these years, a civilian doctor filled the role of the presidential physician.

All were medical specialists without recent experience in handling either the day-to-day commonalities of a general practice or the instantaneous decision making required in a medical emergency, of either traumatic or organic causation. Janet Travell was a pharmacologist/physiatrist; Dan Ruge a neurosurgeon; Burton Smith a urologist; and Burton Lee III a hematologist-oncologist specializing in the treatment of malignant lymphomas, that is, cancers arising in lymph nodes.[2] All except Travell possessed medical specialty certification. The stories of their selection will underscore the eclectic and idiosyncratic methods of choosing the presidential doctor, which until recently had been the rule rather than the exception.

Their White House tours of duty were replete with medical emergencies—the assassination of Kennedy; the near fatal shooting of Ronald Reagan; Reagan's urgent operation for colon cancer; and the cardiac collapse of George H. Bush while jogging at Camp David. There was also plenty of controversy—contention over the appropriate therapy for Kennedy's chronic back pain; the nonuse of the Twenty-fifth Amendment after Reagan's near-fatal wounding; its misuse at the time of his extensive colon surgery; and Burton Lee's unfortunate use of politically correct criteria for medical practitioners' use of the clinical laboratory.

Travell, Smith and Lee III knew their presidential patients prior to their selection as White House physician, suggesting that familiarity and patient comfort were of paramount importance in their selection as presidential physicians. Travell and Smith had actually treated John Kennedy and Ronald Reagan respectively before either man was president; Lee III was a Yale classmate of Nicholas Brady, President Bush's treasury secretary and had long known Bush socially. Doctor Loyal Davis, Nancy Reagan's stepfather, personally persuaded his former partner, Dan Ruge, to become his son-in-law's physician.

The outspoken and independent Dr. Lee rebelled against the evolving tradition that the duties of the leading White House physician constituted a full-time responsibility. He commented, "I have the liberty in this office of doing many other things that interest me besides the day-to-day activities of the medical unit."[3] He infrequently accompanied President Bush on trips, proclaiming that the military doctors on Lee's staff were better equipped than he to handle this responsibility. Yet his presence was usually noted on the president's important journeys abroad. Janet Travell likewise avoided much of Kennedy's domestic travels and was absent on that fateful November day in Dallas.

The office of the White House physician gradually expanded during these three decades as more military physicians, nurses and ancillary personnel were required to fulfill its increasing responsibilities. After the attempt on his life, Ronald Reagan determined that full medical coverage should be extended to his potential successor, the vice president, for the first time. Thereupon Daniel Ruge commenced ongoing care for Vice President Bush and his family. Ruge later estimated that 40 percent of his unit's time was spent on the care of the vice president's family.[4] Fortunately military physicians were around to resolve the problems left by these civilian doctors: George Burkley after Travell, John Hutton after Smith, and Lawrence Mohr after Lee.

The selection of Janet Travell was remarkable. Not only was she the first nonmilitary doctor since Charles Sawyer forty years earlier and only the second civilian since the time of the Pillars of the Profession a century previously to be named physician to the president, but she also became the first woman to hold this position. Moreover, her tenure became a crucible that boiled over from both political pressures and professional conflict. These threads tie this doctor into the fabric of this chapter.

Janet Travell was one of several controversial White House physicians who enjoyed the perquisite of publishing their White House experiences. After she left the White House, her autobiography, *Office Hours Day and Night*, appeared in print and described her personal and professional history, including the difficulty of a woman's entry into medical school. Her 1926 Cornell graduating class contained only nine women among its sixty-three graduates.[5]

From the perspective of the twenty-first century, at a time when approximately 50 percent of all graduating American medical students are women, it was certainly unexpected that so few female physicians had served in the White House. Aside from the ministrations of Susan Edson,[6] only two other women had treated presidents in the White House prior to 2000: physicians to the president Janet Travell (1961) and Eleanor C. Mariano (1993).[7] Indeed, female physicians had cared for sitting presidents for a shorter duration of time than have homeopaths. In this regard, until the millennium, this narrative was distinctly discordant from the story of the twentieth-century progress of women in American medicine.

Stereotypical concerns about female physiology, endurance, and emotional sensitivity had long discriminated against the acceptance of women as either medical students or as practicing physicians.[8] Interestingly, until 1900 female doctors were relatively more acceptable to the American than to the European medical community. In 1900 there were more than 7,000 women physicians in the United States compared to 258 in England and only 95 in France.[9] Between 1880 and 1900, women increased their share of the medical profession in the United States from 2.8 percent to 5.6 percent; they constituted an even greater percentage in urban areas, as, for example, 18.2 percent in Boston and 19.3 percent in Minneapolis.[10]

It has been suggested that a significant reason for the nineteenth century differential advantage for American as opposed to European women is due to the entrepreneurial character of American society in contrast to the governmental domination of social and economic developments then present in most European countries. The nineteenth century's increase in female physicians in the United States was mostly a result of their enrollment in the sectarian (homeopathic, eclectic) and woman's medical schools that together applied an element of competition to American medical education.[11] In 1852 the National Eclectic Medical Association voted openly for a policy of coeducation[12] and the openness of American homeopathy to women has already been examined.[13] Samuel Gregory in 1848 opened the Boston Female Medical College, the first medical college for women in the world and the predecessor of the eventual seventeen female medical colleges in America.[14]

Coeducational training in regular medical colleges arrived slowly; prior to 1880 only ten regular schools admitted women. The University of Michigan decided to admit female medical students in 1870,[15] but medical coeducation became widely respectable only in 1893 after the newly formed Johns Hopkins School of Medicine in Baltimore commenced admitting women on the same terms as men. Prominent women of that city, who eventually raised $500,000, a sum necessary for the school to open its doors, insisted on this policy as a prerequisite for their fund-raising.[16] This policy was not without opposition within the Hopkins medical community; the prominent pathologist William T. Councilman immediately resigned in protest and accepted a position on the Harvard Medical School faculty.[17] This institution did not admit women until 1945.[18]

The closure and consolidation of American medical schools at the turn of the twentieth century, which coincided with the preparation and release of the Flexner report, significantly reduced the number of medical graduates, both male and female. There was a 37 percent decline in the number of new graduates between 1904 and 1915.[19] As the numbers of medical graduates shrank, the numbers of female graduates shrank disproportionately. Institutional discrimination, the availability of new professional fields for educated women, and the higher expense in both time and money required for an increasingly vigorous and lengthy medical education have all been recognized as factors in this decline.[20] The total number of women medical students in 1909 dropped to 921 from 1,419 fifteen years earlier.[21] In addition, onerous discrimination in postgraduate training severely limited the professional opportunities for woman doctors. In 1921, of 482 general hospitals approved for internships, only forty admitted female interns.[22]

However, beginning in the 1960s, for a variety of reasons, the ratio of female to male medical students began to rise. In 1959–1960, women represented 8.4 percent of medical students while the class of 1996–7 was 40 percent female.[23] The 2003–2004 incoming class for the 126 accredited M.D. American medical schools contained 8528 women (49.8 percent of entrants).[24] In 2020, for the first time, more women than men graduated from medical school (10,578 women and 10,343 men). In 2022, the trend continued with 10,782 women vs. 10,202 U.S. M.D. graduates. In 2022, women accounted for 55.6 percent of all matriculants in AMA-accredited medical schools.[25]

This trend will be confirmed in a later chapter with an analysis of the sex of present and recent WHMU physicians.

Travell's gender apparently was no handicap, since she led a varied and successful career as a physician prior to her first meeting with then Senator John F. Kennedy. It encompassed research in the Cornell department of pharmacology,[26] the teaching of medical students, and a private practice that first emphasized cardiology, and then increasingly physical medicine.[27] Eventually she became a consultant to industry in ergonomic design and achieved some fame as an expert in the design of rocking chairs.[28] Travell retained a hallowed place among massage therapists and chiropractors as the author of the two-volume tome *Myofascial Pain and Dysfunction*.[29] This text, coauthored with David Simons, was first published in 1983 and has recently been reissued.[30]

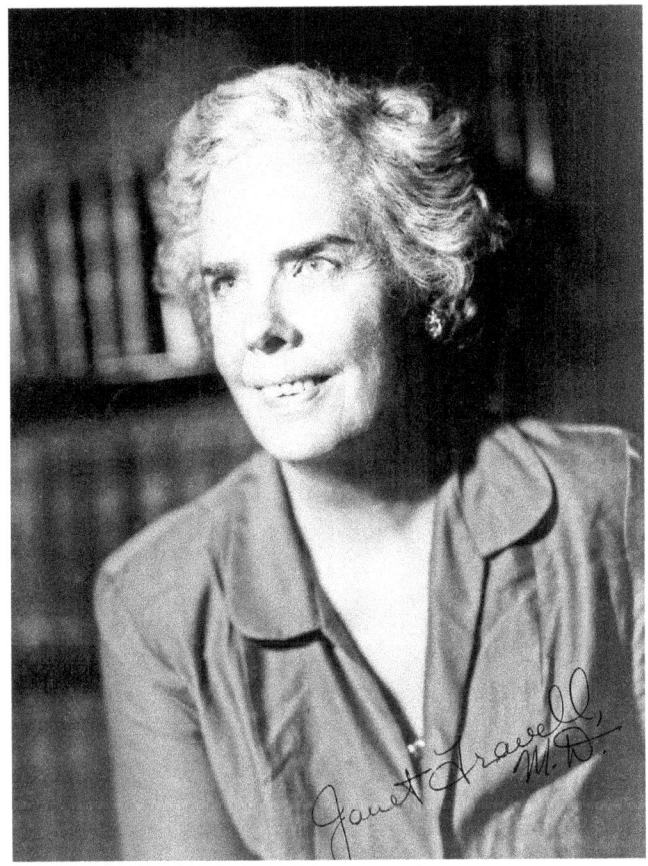

Janet Travell. Dr. Janet Travell, physician to President John Kennedy was embroiled in a serious controversy over her treatment of the president's back problem. She was also the first woman to be named the president's physician. (National Library of Medicine)

It was Travell's expertise in the treatment of back pain that led to her meeting Senator John F. Kennedy (JFK) in consultation in May 1955.[31] The senator previously had undergone three major surgeries on his back, which failed to alleviate his intractable chronic back pain. The Kennedy political apparatus, preparing for an eventual presidential campaign, had shrouded the future candidate's medical condition, especially his diagnosis of Addison's disease, with subterfuge, secrecy, and deceit.[32]

Travell apparently passed the Kennedy scrutiny, both with respect to her competence as a physiatrist and as an ally who could both be trusted and be used politically. Consequently, there ensued a long period of wooing Dr. Travell, not only by JFK but also by the entire Kennedy family. She was invited on trips to the Kennedy retreats at Hyannis port and Palm Beach.[33] Moreover, Dr. Travell was awarded a professional perquisite—travel as a lecturer for the Joseph P. Kennedy Foundation for Retarded Children.[34] Additionally, she may have been flattered by the solicitation not only of her medical but also of her political advice. Travell recorded the content of one 1956 discussion with

Kennedy as what "was the potential of his health in relation to the stringent responsibilities of the Presidency."[35]

Travell responded positively to these blandishments in a series of disingenuous remarks, both private and public, that masked the candidate's diagnosis of Addison's disease. In a July 21, 1959, medical statement requested by the Kennedy campaign, she wrote, "In 1943, when the PT boat which he commanded was blown up, he was subjected to extraordinary severe stress in a terrific ordeal of swimming to save his men. This, together with subsequent malaria, resulted in a depletion of adrenal function from which he is now rehabilitated."

She continued: "Concerning the question of Addison's disease … this disease was described by Thomas Addison in 1855 and is characterized by a bluish discoloration of the mucous membranes of the mouth and permanent deep pigmentation or tanning of the skin.… Senator Kennedy has never had any abnormal pigmentation of the skin or mucous membranes; it would be readily visible."[36]

In a conversation with the doctor, Kennedy's brother-in-law, Sargent Shriver, complained, "They claimed that he is living on drugs—cortisone," to which Travell responded helpfully, "Well that's right. Jack hasn't taken cortisone for years. He does take some relatives of cortisone; they are not drugs … [but] hormones that are natural constituents of the body."[37] Travell also cowrote a misleading medical report that was released at the Democrat nominating convention in 1960. The content of this report was paraphrased by a Kennedy spokesman: "With respect to the old problem of adrenal insufficiency, as late as December 1958, when you had a general checkup with a specific test of adrenal function, the result showed that your adrenal glands do function."[38] The pathologists who performed the Kennedy autopsy in 1963 could not visibly identify either of his adrenal glands during their postmortem examination. This finding documented that there had indeed been a history of extreme adrenal deficiency.[39]

In 1960 Senator Kennedy was involved in a very tough Democratic fight with Senate majority leader Lyndon Johnson for the Democratic Party nomination; subsequently he was involved in an extremely close presidential election against Vice President Richard Nixon. It is unclear what the outcome of either of these contests might have been if the question of the candidate's Addison's disease had been handled forthrightly. In an acknowledgment of her skill in successful misdirection, historians place Janet Travell in the same league as Cary Grayson and Ross McIntire as pennant-winning medical dissemblers.[40]

The day after his January 1961 inauguration JFK rewarded Travell by selecting her as his personal physician.[41] Thereby she became the first woman to serve as personal physician to the president of the United States. It would be another thirty years before a second female physician, Dr. E. Connie Mariano, became the personal physician to President Bill Clinton. Travell, then fifty-nine, gladly relinquished her New York consultative practice and moved to Washington, D.C. Thus, she traded her active Manhattan practice for the prestige of governmental employment with the meager annual salary of approximately $20,000.[42]

By the time of the Travell era, the White House Medical Unit had evolved to include two physicians, with a third to be added shortly. The personal physician to the president served as the senior White House physician, and it became the practice but not the rule since the Harding presidency for a second physician from the military to be assigned as the assistant White House physician. It was assumed that the professional opinions and judgments of the personal physician to the president would take precedence in any decision involving his care. On February 1, 1961—by arrangement with the surgeon general of the United States Navy—Captain George G. Burkley was named Assistant White House physician to Dr. Janet Travell and director of the White House Dispensary.[43] Burkley had previously served since 1956 as a backup physician at Camp David whenever President Eisenhower stayed there.[44] Then, as now, the selection of a personal physician had been a private political decision by the president and was not subject to congressional approval.

In addition to herself, Travell's staff consisted of Burkley, two navy chief corpsmen, a technician, a civilian nurse in the Dispensary, a navy nurse in Travell's office, and Travell's secretary, for a total of eight personnel.[45] Her medical domain consisted of a three-room office/examining room suite opposite the president's elevator on the ground floor of the White House and a dispensary in the Old Executive Office Building. At the time of her appointment, there was no X-ray equipment on-site. Travell improvised to remedy this situation, converting space that adjoined the Dispensary waiting room. (This area had been used to clip newspaper articles.) In it Travell installed screened massage tables and X-ray equipment. She expropriated a large closet that had stored the presidential flags for a dark room to develop X-rays.[46]

Travell's routine was to indicate her availability by remaining in her White House office until Kennedy passed by in the evening on his return to his private quarters. She was constantly informed of the president's whereabouts but did not accompany him on his daily movements and was not always present for his domestic travel, although Burkley was. JFK requested that Travell see members of the White House staff as well as visitors who had pain of clinical significance.[47] She also attended to the medical needs of Jackie Kennedy and the two Kennedy children.

Early in his administration Kennedy circumscribed Travell's role: He

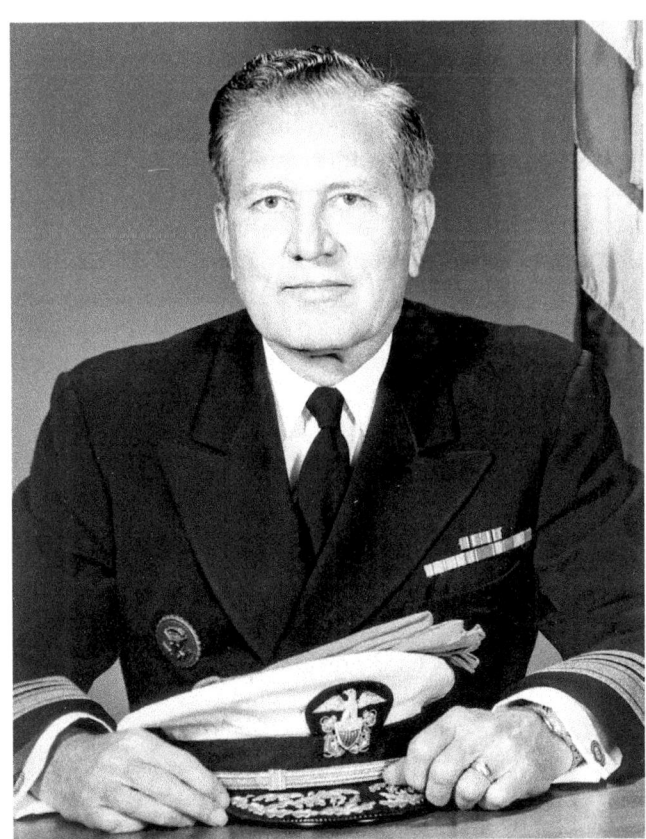

George Burkley. Navy Physician Dr. George Burkley, while assistant White House physician, was instrumental in bringing Dr. Hans Kraus to the White House to treat JFK's back. (Courtesy of the Bureau of Medicine and Surgery Library and Archives)

directed her never to make a statement about Medicare because national health insurance was an especially contentious political issue at the time.[48] Whether by presidential directive or by self-imposed discretion, White House physicians, with uncommon exceptions, have refrained from commenting upon public policy matters. They have relinquished any commentary into the hands of the surgeon general of the Public Health Service.[49] Furthermore, Kennedy limited Travell's medical authority when he ordered her to avoid any commitment to a hospital to plan for his hospitalization should that become necessary.[50]

Kennedy's hypersensitivity regarding his public image, i.e., that of a young, vigorous, and very healthy president was a prime determinant in the way he both organized and concealed his medical care. It may even have compromised his personal security since he shunned having any physician near him at all times, especially in public.[51] It also influenced the White House physician's location in presidential motorcades. In 1961 Travell insisted that Dr. Burkley ride in the Secret Service car directly behind the president's. Kennedy vetoed that suggestion.[52] As a consequence, assistant White House physician Burkley was placed in a distant VIP car in the Dallas motorcade and only caught up with the mortally wounded president in the Parkland Hospital emergency room.[53]

The organization for the delivery of health care to President Kennedy was dysfunctional, as five different physicians (doctors Travell, George Burkley, Eugene Cohen, Hans Kraus and Max Jacobson) either simultaneously or at different times orbited around the ailing president. Biographer Richard Reeves colorfully summarized this situation: "Doctors came and went around Kennedy. In a lifetime of medical torment, Kennedy was more promiscuous with physicians and drugs than he was with women."[54] Reeves thus succinctly identified a root cause of the confusion and conflict that characterized the tenure of Janet Travell, the titular presidential physician who came to lose control of Kennedy's health management. Her professional forte, the treatment of back pain, was first challenged and then discarded by her colleagues. Second, she was not consulted during the ongoing ministrations by the unorthodox Dr. Max Jacobson from New York.

The White House physician command and control system, so effective when a president's medical care is directed by a military physician, did not function for the civilian Dr. Travell. Deficiencies in continuity and communication resulted. One is left to imagine the nature of an alternative Kennedy narrative if an authoritarian McIntire or Snyder had been in charge.

Travell's primary medical responsibility was the management of JFK's back pain, which she had treated for years with numerous procaine injections.[55] Her rationale was that the commonly used procaine anesthetic would relieve the pain produced by myofascial strain.[56] Her therapeutic plan was the injection of procaine into defined "trigger points" of her patient's back skeletal musculature, in the belief that these same back muscles, in chronic spasm, would somehow be restored to their normal resting lengths.[57] Janet Travell and Dr. Hans Kraus were among a small group of practitioners who pioneered the "trigger point" theory. These were identified as small hard lumps of dead tissue located deep within muscle whose presence produced myofascial pain. Treatment to eliminate these lesions consisted of repeated painful jabs of an oversized needle to disintegrate the tissue. Dr. Travell's use of procaine as an anesthetic was her own modification of this painful therapy.[58] Unfortunately Kennedy's near-disabling pain persisted despite as many as three injections a day.[59]

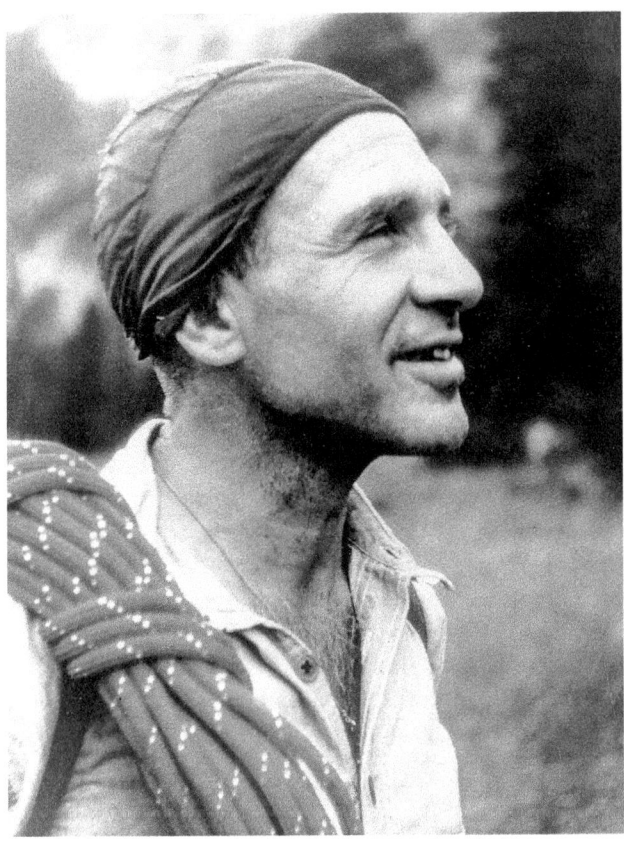

Hans Kraus. Physiatrist Dr. Hans Kraus at the Grand Tetons in 1959, two years before he became a consultant to treat President Kennedy's back pain. (Courtesy of Hans and Medi Kraus Collection)

Dr. Burkley, increasingly apprehensive over the potential ill effects of Travell's treatments, engaged in ever more frequent disputes with his titular superior over their use. He was fearful of both procaine's addictive effect and its potential to atrophy the president's back muscles.[60] His concerns were shared by Dr. Eugene Cohen, JFK's civilian endocrinologist, who knew a specific physician who might resolve their medical dilemma. Cohen knew Dr. Hans Kraus both professionally and socially and highly respected him. As a result, the endocrinologist called his fellow New Yorker in June 1961 to invite a second opinion. Kraus declined this invitation for several reasons, but the principal one was his ethical reluctance to usurp a patient from another physician.[61]

The professional impasse over the president's musculoskeletal treatment persisted while his back problems worsened. Eventually Burkley, with Cohen's complete support, insisted that Travell obtain a second opinion, specifically with the eminent New York physical medicine specialist, Dr. Hans Kraus. Travell resisted, but Dr. Burkley determinedly set aside any customary physician deference and threatened either to call Dr. Kraus himself[62] or to inform the President.[63] Kraus, unlike Travell, was certified by the American Board of Physical Medicine and Rehabilitation.[64] Perhaps, Travell, already forty-six years of age when this specialty board was established in 1947, had decided against sitting for its qualifying examination.[65]

Travell finally acquiesced, and upon the presidential physician's formal request for a second opinion Kraus examined the president in the White House in October 1961. The examination revealed to Kraus that the president was a musculoskeletal wreck! The doctor completely rejected Travell's treatments and instead recommended three weekly one-hour physical therapy and exercise sessions.[66] Further, he bluntly warned JFK that the president would become a cripple unless he subscribed to this exercise program. Kraus, Teutonic and decisive, insisted that a patient-physician contract be agreed to by the president. This agreement, previously alluded to, bound Kraus, the physician, to fly from his New York City office to the White House to personally treat his patient three times weekly, to train three White House therapists to supervise Kennedy's two other weekly sessions, and to be available to personally treat any emergency anywhere at any time. The patient's responsibilities, in addition to a complete adherence to his exercise regimen, included the granting of total control over his musculoskeletal therapy to Kraus, the elimination of any therapeutic interference from any other doctor, and the promise that only Kraus could seek a second opinion.[67] As a further precaution against any future meddling, both Kraus and Eugene Cohen warned the president that Travell was a threat to his well-being.[68] Finally, Kraus informed JFK that if there should be any deviation from their agreement, Kraus would dismiss the president as his patient.[69]

Kraus was born in Trieste, then part of the Austro-Hungarian Empire. The Kraus family's wealth and connections permitted refuge in Zurich, where they sat out World War I in perennially neutral Switzerland. The preceding is of little interest except that while in Zurich Kraus's father employed a struggling Irish writer to tutor his son in the English language. James Joyce, the writer, taught Hans and other wealthy families during the day and wrote his masterpiece, *Ulysses,* at night.[70]

Kraus's medical degree was bestowed by the University of Vienna where he graduated in 1930. He continued postgraduate training there where he selected "fracture surgery," now known as orthopedics, as his specialty. After his training Kraus practiced orthopedic surgery at the University of Vienna Hospital and opened an office practice that increasingly treated an athlete clientele. But Hans Kraus realized that he and his family "flunked the Hitler test." Although his parents had been baptized as Christians, both had a Jewish parent. Connections, wealth, and planning placed the young medical doctor Hans on a Trieste-bound train on the same day in 1938 that Hitler's army marched into Vienna. His immediate family also escaped to the United States, where they settled in an affluent New York City suburb.[71]

Kraus was welcomed as a member of the orthopedic service of New York's prestigious Columbia Presbyterian Hospital. However, he soon changed his professional interest to rehabilitation and sports medicine and became acknowledged as an expert in the field. Together with a colleague he developed the Kraus-Weber test to determine the level of physical fitness. Together with Weber he developed a series of strengthening and loosening muscle exercises. In 1952 he produced the first of many medical papers that claimed that Americans, both children and adults, led lives devoid of sufficient activity, which made them vulnerable to a myriad of chronic illness. His prescription was fitness through exercise as the essential element for physical and emotional well-being.[72]

Of all the members of President Kennedy's constellation of physicians, Kraus alone possessed a specialty board certification; his was physiatry. Kraus had been appointed to Eisenhower's President's Council on Physical Fitness, later receiving the Distinguished Service Award from this organization, and served as the medical adviser on physical fitness to the YMCA. In later years many dubbed this practitioner, a longtime associate professor of clinical physical medicine and rehabilitation, the father of sports medicine in the United States.[73]

Kraus commenced his care of JFK in October 1961; as agreed upon, he personally supervised muscle-strengthening exercises in the White House gymnasium three times a week. He continued his active oversight, albeit on a somewhat reduced schedule, until the end of the Kennedy presidency.[74] Kraus continued the tradition of physicians treating the presidents, which required him, if not to lie, to at least shade the truth in describing his medical care. Kennedy and his physiatrist "agreed to describe the therapy as

Chapter 9. Civilian Interlude, Part I

exercises improving the president's condition from very good to excellent."[75] JFK, determined to perpetuate the false Camelot image of a supremely healthy athlete, demanded that Kraus seek no publicity for his presidential treatments and that all press inquiries be directed to press secretary Pierre Salinger for an appropriate political response.[76] Additionally, the president, fearing that the phones may have been tapped, installed secure red lines in Kraus's New York City apartment, office, and upstate country home to assure that the president and patient would have secure direct access. Moreover, whenever doctors Burkley, Kraus and Cohen wished to confer concerning the president's health, pay phones were always used.[77]

Dr. Eugene Cohen, Kennedy's endocrinologist, was a New York colleague of both Travell and Kraus, and like other physicians in Kennedy's entourage commuted from New York to the White House, Hyannis Port, and Palm Beach whenever the president beckoned. He was a longtime professor of endocrinology at the Cornell School of Medicine. Interestingly, Professor Cohen was certified neither in internal medicine nor in its subspecialty, endocrinology.[78] Travell claimed that she was responsible for introducing Cohen to Senator Kennedy, but the endocrinologist eventually allied with Burkley in deposing her.[79]

Travell's memoir is silent regarding the turmoil that led to Kraus's selection. Claiming that she was responsible for the change in the president's therapy, her only reference to the White House situation was, "I had known Dr. Kraus for years, through a mutual interest in the relief of painful muscle spasms by vapocoolant sprays, and I had first asked him to see President Kennedy late in the summer of 1961 at Hyannis Port."[80] Travell was intent upon maintaining her control. She attempted to establish that she was Kraus's superior by meeting him at the airport whenever he landed to treat Kennedy. Finally, in December 1961, after JFK had experienced a relapse, Travell called a press conference to announce that she was convening a meeting there of the president's entire staff of physicians. As described above, Travell's attempt to exclude Kraus from this meeting misfired with disastrous results for her standing with the president.[81]

From then on Kennedy's treatment was under the effective oversight of the civilian Kraus and the military assistant White House physician Burkley. Travell was permitted to administer procaine shots only with the authorization of either Kraus or Burkley.[82] Her loss of responsibility was to remain confidential, but speculation about her standing was inevitable. Articles in prominent newspapers reported that she had been fired or had offered her resignation.[83] However, the president politically needed to placate Travell in order to prevent her from leaking information about his health. He kept her on as White House physician and continued to identify her publicly as the principal physician in charge of his health care.[84] One Kennedy biographer characterized the situation in the following manner: "It was easier to let her stay on and retain her dignity, than to turn loose a discontented physician eager for revenge through her pen."[85]

Travell was thus without a say in managing the president's health during the latter part of the Kennedy presidency. In June 1963, she could not even order medical services from Walter Reed National Military Medical Center for anyone at the White House without Burkley's approval.[86] According to then Captain George Burkley, in late 1961, "the President specifically stated in the presence of another individual that I was his physician and that I alone was to take responsibility for anything that was indicated." He continued, "The President never had any doctor treat him, except with my cognizance."[87] Fortunately for JFK, the untoward physical consequences of his politically motivated selection of

Travell as his presidential physician were reversed, and even she agreed that his orthopedic problems were greatly alleviated by the new therapeutic regime.[88]

Kraus's therapeutic plan was successful to the extent that "by September of 1963, it was clear even to Burkley that Kennedy was cured."[89] The doctor continued to be available for his patient; government planes often flew Kraus to Kennedy's side whenever his consultation was required. In 1963 Kraus was on a mountain-climbing vacation in Italy when his patient suffered a mild leg injury while playing golf. A White House plane was dispatched to return Kraus to Washington the following day.[90] Kraus's dedication to his presidential patient was in part a way to express gratitude to the United States for welcoming his family as émigrés from Nazi-controlled Europe. He never mentioned to Kennedy payment for his medical service. Indeed, after a year Kraus wrote to Evelyn Lincoln, the president's secretary, to request reimbursement only for his travel expenses. Kraus never charged the president or the government for his time and treatments.[91]

A second example of Dr. Travell's lack of command over the White House medical office was the bizarre episode involving New York doctor Max Jacobson. While still a senator, John Kennedy, freelancing for alternative cures for his back pain and for stimulants for his hormonally deprived system, happened upon Upper East Side Manhattan physician Max Jacobson. Jacobson had a wide following among portions of the New York artistic and celebrity set for his "energizing" injections. His grateful patients named him "Doctor Feelgood."[92]

The German-born Jacobson received his medical degree in 1924 from Friedrich Wilhelm University in Berlin. He, a fugitive from the Nazis like Kraus, immigrated to the United States in 1936 and established an office practice in New York City. Since 1946 Jacobson was without staff privileges at any hospital. Instead, he referred patients to other physicians when the need for hospitalization arose. It is unknown whether he had received any formal postgraduate medical education after medical school.[93] The doctor was extremely grateful to the United States. When Kennedy insisted that Jacobson accompany him to Europe in 1961—"Will you rearrange your schedule…. You can send a bill"—Jacobson replied that he would come, but never would he send a bill, "…not to the leader of a country that made it possible for him and his family to escape Nazi Germany before the war."[94]

Candidate Kennedy was first introduced to Jacobson during the 1960 presidential campaign by his friend Charles Spalding.[95] Thus commenced a bizarre doctor/patient relationship.[96] In September, just prior to his crucial television debate with his opponent, Richard Nixon, Kennedy slipped into Jacobson's Manhattan office that had been cleared of patients just before his arrival. After taking a brief medical history, "Dr. Feelgood" administered an injection whose effects were a disappearance of pain, enhanced alertness, and an increase in energy.[97]

Unknown to Travell, his presidential physician, Kennedy continued to be injected by Jacobson after becoming president. According to White House gate logs, the doctor made more than thirty visits to the White House during Kennedy's brief incumbency.[98] The doctor's pilot for these White House office visits was another Jacobson patient, well-known photographer Mark Shaw. Shaw "…owned a twin-engine Cessna. The two of them shuttled back and forth between New York and Washington on presidential call."[99] The doctor frequently was summoned at times of foreign or domestic stress, including James Meredith's forcible entry into the University of Mississippi in September 1962.[100]

The most infamous of Jacobson's engagements was his surreptitious trip to Paris, Vienna and London in June 1961 in order to treat the president for fatigue and diminished energy. The focus of the trip was a critical Vienna summit meeting with the Soviet leader, Nikita Khrushchev. Jacobson injected Kennedy frequently on this journey; one injection was administered just moments before the president was scheduled to have his initial meeting with the communist leader.[101] Jacobson and his wife were not listed as members of the official presidential party and instead were roomed with the president's military attachés. To maintain secrecy, the Jacobsons were flown separately to Paris, the only passengers on an Air France jetliner![102]

Eventually, the president's brother, Attorney General Robert F. Kennedy, seized one of Jacobsen's treatment vials and had it analyzed. Testing disclosed that "Dr. Feelgood's" treatments contained amphetamines and steroids in high concentrations.[103] Thereupon the attorney general unsuccessfully attempted to dissuade his brother from continuing Jacobsen's injections. The doctor continued to treat the president for the duration of Kennedy's truncated presidency; Jacobson flew to Palm Beach for his final treatment on November 15, 1963, just prior to the trip to Dallas.[104]

Dr. Travell initially was oblivious to Dr. Jacobson's interloping medical care of her primary patient,[105] and she does not mention Jacobson in her autobiography.[106] However, "Dr. Feelgood's" frequent appearances in the presidential living quarters had become so obvious that she dared to seek out and accost her competitor there.[107]

A December 1972 *New York Times* article brought attention to Dr. Jacobson's amphetamine-dispensing practices. It reported that each month his practice purchased enough of the stimulant to inject 100 fairly strong doses of 25 milligrams of amphetamine daily. His active practice included such luminaries as singer Eddie Fisher, author Truman Capote, composer Allan Jay Lerner, influential congressman Claude Pepper, and playwright Tennessee Williams. The *Times* investigative article further disclosed that the aforementioned Mark Shaw had died as a result of an amphetamine overdose.[108] A wave of unfavorable publicity was ignited, resulting in a two-and-a-half-year investigation by the New York State Board of Regents into Jacobson's dispensing practices. Finally, in April 1975, "Dr. Feelgood's" license to practice medicine was revoked. He died four years later.[109]

On February 13, 1964, twelve weeks after Lyndon Johnson's accession to the presidency, Pierre Salinger, his press secretary, confirmed a tandem arrangement by announcing that the White House medical team of Travell and Burkley would continue their joint responsibility to "handle medical problems in the Executive Mansion. Both Dr. Travell and Dr. Burkley bear the title of 'A Physician to the President.' Both had offices at the White House and are on call around the clock."[110]

The scope of Dr. Travell's duties during the Johnson administration is unclear, but she seemed to have developed an affinity for Lady Bird Johnson and the Johnson daughters. Travell was the physician on "The Lady Bird Special" 1964 campaign train and took care of the staff and others who accompanied Mrs. Johnson.[111] Travell remained at the White House through Johnson's successful election and designed suitable seat and backrests for LBJ. Travell left the White House on March 31, 1965, shortly after Johnson's successful election campaign, in order to write her autobiography and to resume her active career in teaching, writing, and scientific investigation.[112] Previously Kennedy had secured for her the title of associate clinical professor of medicine at the George Washington University School of Medicine.[113] Travell died in 1997 at the age of 96.[114]

Burkley continued as Johnson's White House physician for the remainder of his presidency and was promoted to vice admiral in 1965. In August 1961, six months after his appointment to the White House, Kennedy promoted Burkley from captain to rear admiral.[115] The generosity of presidents toward the rank of their trusted military physicians has been a constant theme of this narrative.

Chapter 10

Civilian Interlude, Part II

The Specialist Physicians of Presidents Reagan and George H. Bush

On Saturday, July 13, 1985, President Ronald Reagan underwent an extensive two hour and fifty-three-minute operation at Bethesda Naval Hospital to remove a cancer of his right colon. As Reagan underwent general anesthesia, presidential authority was transferred by letter to Vice President George H. Bush under an aberrant interpretation of the Twenty-fifth Amendment to the U.S. Constitution.[1] That same evening three presidential aides—attorney Fred Fielding, chief of staff Don Regan, and acting press secretary Larry Speakes, anxious for the president to regain his constitutional powers—arbitrarily devised a test to determine whether Reagan had fully recovered his mental acuity: his ability to read aloud a two-sentence statement reclaiming his office.[2]

Shortly after 7:00 p.m. the three aides approached the president, who was awake but still numb from the waist down. Attorney Fielding recalled, "When Reagan looked at the letter, he blinked his eyes and faltered.... Don Reagan and I looked at each other and decided that maybe we were a little premature." However, the president then asked for his reading glasses and read the passage aloud. In this way, he passed the test devised by his aides, who discussed the letter with him and offered to bring it back in a couple of hours for his signature. But Reagan replied, "Heck no, I don't want you to wake me up later, I'll sign it now." In this unorthodox manner, Ronald Reagan recovered his presidential authority from George Bush after an interval of seven hours and fifty minutes.[3]

Curiously, the opinion of the president's personal physician in the White House, Dr. Burton Smith, a board certified urologist, had not been solicited by this trio in arriving at this medical decision. Political concerns trumped the solicitation of any appropriate medical insights from Smith, the second of President Reagan's three personal physicians during his two-term tenure.

After Ronald Reagan was elected president in November 1980, the Reagans asked Nancy Reagan's stepfather, the prominent and crusty Chicago neurosurgeon Dr. Loyal Davis, to select the White House physician. Davis importuned his former partner, neurosurgeon Daniel Ruge, to take the position. After some reluctance on Ruge's part, Davis finally persuaded him with this argument: "Because you won't let anybody do foolish things to Ronnie."[4]

Doctor Ruge was an eminent Chicago neurosurgeon and the author of two widely recognized textbooks on spinal cord injury and spinal cord disability.[5] Until 1976 he was a professor of neurosurgery in Chicago, where his professional and personal character was much admired. A former student described his mentor as gracious, funny, very capable, and as someone who went out of his way to assist medical students in their careers.[6] Ruge, deciding to devote his time to public service, had relocated to Washington, D.C., where he was deputy director of spinal services at the veterans' administration hospital when he accepted his new role as presidential physician.[7]

When Ruge arrived at the White House, the doctor discovered no mission statement, no table of organization, and no standard order of procedure for the White House physician's office. The only available records were the personal records of those staffers who had stayed on. There was no budget dedicated to the operations of the White House Medical Unit; funding flowed as needed from the head of the White House Military Office. Ruge was grateful to Admiral Lukash, the White House physician for presidents Carter, Ford, and Nixon, for an orientation prior to President Reagan's inauguration, thereby somewhat smoothing his transition.[8]

Dan Ruge was an unassuming person who had not been and did not become a personal friend of the Reagans. The lack of a close relationship may have been detrimental to the appropriate use of the Twenty-fifth Amendment on presidential disability when the president was shot in March 1981. Ruge did not believe in the general practitioner approach to presidential care. Rather he considered it his mission to provide first-rate medical care for Reagan, not to render it himself in the White House.[9] He made free use of eminent physician consultants both military and nonmilitary, believing correctly that no doctor would refuse to become a consultant for an ailing president.[10] When the president went to Bethesda Naval Hospital for his checkups, Ruge told the attending physicians there that the president was their patient until the moment that the helicopter wheels left the ground for the return trip to the White House, at which time he again became Ruge's patient.[11]

Ruge saw the president frequently, giving Reagan his allergy shots every few weeks.[12] In a routine similar to Janet Travell's, Ruge kept the door of his office ajar to view the president's daily comings and goings from the White House family quarters to the Executive Office Building. If he felt that the president needed to see him, he stood outside his office so that Reagan would stop by on his return that evening from the Oval Office.[13]

In an interview, Ruge commented that caring for the president is "vastly overrated, boring, and not medically challenging."[14] He famously described the job as "strictly blue-collar."[15] As evidence of the low prestige of the position, Ruge was not invited to state dinners, but sat in his White House office in his tuxedo.[16] Ruge complained to Burton Smith, his successor, that he would someday write a book called *Kitchens I Have Eaten In* while waiting around for the President.[17]

Despite his disparaging assessment of his status Dr. Ruge was able to expand significantly the role of the White House Medical Unit. He arranged for continuous health care for Vice President Bush, Bush's family, and his staff. Medical care for the vice president and family remains an integral component of this unit's mission to the present time. Second, Dr. Ruge expanded the military medical staff by making the White House their permanent assignment. William Lukash, his predecessor, rotated military physicians onto his staff on a temporary basis, and then rotated them back to their permanent stations. Ruge's organizational pattern remains in place to the present.[18]

Unfortunately, Ruge is most famous for the failure to invoke either Sections Three or Four of the Twenty-fifth Amendment in March 1981 after Reagan was severely wounded in an assassination attempt. A ricocheted bullet from the gun of John Hinckley became embedded in the president's left lung. Ruge accompanied the president to the George Washington Hospital emergency room and, as was his practice, deferred to the medical decisions of the George Washington physicians.[19] Two months into the Reagan presidency, procedures had not yet been worked out between Ruge and the president's closest advisers regarding the appropriate implementation of the amendment's disability clauses. Consequently, as confusion reigned in the White House, staffer Richard Darman hid the authorization forms for implementing the amendment in his office safe.[20] No members of the White House staff consulted the White House physician regarding either the president's cognitive ability or the possible relevance of the amendment.[21]

All the attending hospital doctors and Ruge agreed that George Washington staff physician Dr. Dennis O'Leary should be the sole spokesman in detailing the medical news concerning the president's operation and postoperative course.[22] O'Leary wrote all the press releases after consultation; he then shared the statement with Ruge, who occasionally made a rare correction. He subsequently presented the statement to the assistant press secretary, Larry Speakes who would release it to the media.[23]

Ruge's successor, Dr. Burton Smith, previously had actively solicited appointment as Ronald Reagan's presidential physician. Smith was yet another medical specialist who somehow was selected to function as a family practitioner in the White House. Smith, a California urologist, had treated the bladder and prostate problems of Ronald Reagan for fifteen years and had operated upon the then governor of California for an enlarged prostate in June 1967.[24]

Upon Reagan's election in 1980, Smith, aware that the incoming president's private doctor in California, John Sharpe, was in poor health, put himself forward for the position of presidential physician. Using his personal friendship with William French Smith, who was unrelated, the Reagans' personal attorney and future United States attorney general, Dr. Smith sent a letter to Reagan, suggesting "that it would be a privilege for me, and helpful to him, if I became his White House Physician."[25] Ronald Reagan graciously telephoned Smith to inform him that Loyal Davis had already made arrangements for the White House physician.[26]

Smith was determined to remain under consideration. He asked the president elect for tickets to the 1981 inauguration and flew to Washington for the ceremony on the same chartered plane that carried the Reagan children.[27] Smith, trying to show his availability, again flew to Washington in March 1981 to meet Daniel Ruge, and accompanied Ruge and his presidential patient to Bethesda Naval Hospital for a urologic evaluation. Smith journeyed once more to Washington in March 1982 to oversee yet another urologic examination of the president.[28] Finally Ruge, acknowledging the hints, asked Smith if he would have interest in serving as his replacement if Reagan decided to run again. In July 1984, after yet another transcontinental flight, Burton Smith met with Ronald Reagan in the Oval Office and was asked by Reagan to become the White House physician shortly thereafter.[29]

A press release dated January 4, 1985, announced the appointment of Dr. Smith to be physician to the president. It stated that the appointee had practiced urology in California since 1951, was a graduate of the University of Southern California School of Medicine, and had done graduate training at Jefferson Medical College. He was board certified in urology and past chief of urology at St. John's Hospital, Santa Monica.[30]

Smith agreed with his predecessor that the White House physician's office lacked the respect that its important functions deserved. As an example, the president's doctor was frequently stationed in a garage when President Reagan attended diplomatic functions.[31] By 1985 Smith's White House Medical Unit had reached a complement of fourteen in addition to himself. It included Colonel John Hutton, a general surgeon recruited by Dan Ruge, and three internists, navy lieutenant commanders Kenneth Lee and Ronald Savage, and air force major Robert Gasser. Doctor Savage also was a cardiologist. The latter three tended to the medical needs of the Bush family, while Smith and Hutton were responsible for the Reagans. The burgeoning complement of medical personnel required a table of organization. In response, Smith appointed Hutton as his chief of staff of the White House Medical Unit in an initial step in its bureaucratization.[32]

Smith stated that his personal responsibility was "to serve the President and the First Lady, and the relatively few people who worked [for them] in the White House, such as ushers, cooks, flower arrangers, curator, valet, maid, etc." His professional service also was sought, albeit uncommonly, by the president's top advisers for minor medical complaints, e.g., Attorney General Ed Meese with a sore throat, and presidential chief of staff Donald Regan with an earache. Prior to a presidential trip overseas, Smith administered the required vaccinations to the president and his accompanying staff.[33]

Smith's day in the White House commenced with his standing outside his office door at 9:00 a.m. to view the president on his way to the Executive Office Building. In this way he indicated his availability should Reagan wish to chat, and to announce that certain immunizations were due.[34] Smith's memoir proudly proclaimed that he was one of only two persons to accompany Reagan wherever he went, the other being the military officer with the nuclear "football." Smith also boasted that he was the only person who could be alone with the president in the oval office.[35] After Reagan's colon surgery in 1985, Dr. Smith slept in one of the guest suites on the third floor of the White House during the president's recovery period.[36]

The urologist advanced several innovations in presidential care. One was a formalization of the pre-advance and advance medical preparations for a presidential trip abroad. Under these arrangements a member of the White House physician's office personally assessed the adequacy of the foreign medical facilities, and corrective measures were taken to assure the presence of first-rate care in case of a presidential medical emergency.[37] This requirement led to Smith's commandeering aircraft carriers to be stationed offshore during Reagan's trips to Bali and Grenada.[38] Second, Smith instituted emergency drills with the Secret Service[39] and required all his staff to be advanced trauma life support (ATLS) and advanced clinical life support (ACLS) certified.[40]

Dr. Smith believed in collegial decision making. His conviction was that medical decisions be "done by a committee within the White House. We discussed it, added our input, and then made the decision. We'd go out to Bethesda with him and work together in concert, so there is not one head, never has been, and I'm sure never will be."[41]

However, Smith's tenure was less than a success. His planning for the possible invocation of Articles Three and Four of the Twenty-fifth Amendment was either ineffective or absent. Confusion over its appropriate invocation reigned in the White House at the time of the president's diagnosis and surgical treatment of colon cancer in July 1985.[42] When asked about the effects of sedation prior to a colonoscopy, Smith compared it to drinking one or more martinis.[43] In his published account of the Reagan presidency, the acting presidential press secretary, Larry Speakes, criticized Smith's counsel, claiming that any decision whether to transfer authority to the vice president was hampered by the inadequacy of Smith's advice, a urologist who "couldn't articulate much about medicine outside his specialty." Consequently, the president's advisers circumvented Smith and consulted with Dr. John Hutton for a realistic assessment of the effects of anesthesia during a colonoscopy.[44]

Speakes and his staff often disdainfully referred to Smith as "a celebrity doctor," and, as noted above, the doctor's counsel was bypassed in the discussions regarding the Twenty-fifth Amendment prior to Reagan's subsequent colon resection.[45] Smith stated defensively that he was too busy with other things and left this important matter to Reagan's chief of staff, Don Regan.[46]

The doctor's worth, in the opinion of Larry Speakes, declined even further after the latter's credibility with the Washington press corps suffered as a result of the sloppy reporting of the president's skin cancer. An innocuous basal cell carcinoma was removed from Reagan's nose shortly after his colon surgery. Dr. Smith, apparently cowed by the strong-willed Nancy Reagan, became complicit in preventing the press, including Larry Speakes, from discovering the true story. According to Speakes, "Both Mrs. Reagan and Smith denied to reporters that a biopsy was being performed, and the tissue sample ... was sent to the lab under a false name. The name on the pathology report was Tracy Malone, who was identified as a white female, age sixty-two. Tracy Malone actually was a military nurse assigned to the White House Medical Unit, and to put her name in the same age bracket as the President, they added nearly forty years to her true age."[47]

Notwithstanding their complicity on the president's nose surgery, Mrs. Reagan felt much more comfortable with John Hutton, Smith's deputy, than with the presidential physician in confronting the health crises that afflicted both Reagans during this period. In her memoirs, Nancy Reagan made frequent references to "John" (Dr. Hutton) as being available, supportive, and reassuring; in the same volume, Burton Smith's name does not appear even once.[48] The embattled Burton Smith relinquished his position to John Hutton in December 1986. His stated reason for his resignation was the necessity to return to California to attend to ill members of his family.[49] However, one wonders whether the previously listed problems and a general dissatisfaction with his advice provided more compelling reasons.

Smith's successor and the third personal physician during the Reagan presidency was Army Colonel John Hutton, a board certified surgeon. Prior to his selection as a White House physician, Hutton was chief of surgery at Walter Reed National Military Medical Center, and held the appointments of clinical professor of surgery at both George Washington School of Medicine and the Uniformed Services University of Health Sciences.[50] A factor in Dr. Smith's departure may have been Nancy Reagan's discomfort over the appearance of intimate physical details in the mainstream press after her husband's colon operation. At her orders, treating physicians were forbidden to speak to the press and medical statements were to be released through the White House press operation.[51] Consequently, during his tenure Colonel Hutton almost always communicated his medical findings to the public through the White House press office.[52]

Nancy Reagan was uncomfortable, sometimes severely distressed, by Drs. Ruge and Smiths' medical attention to her husband. But she developed both a respect for, and friendship with John Hutton. He frequently visited the Reagans during their California retirement, and served as an unofficial medical adviser to the couple. "A couple of afternoons a week, the doctor took Ronnie to a driving range where he hit golf balls."[53]

An unusual practice developed during the Reagans' final years in the White House, and that was the delegation of significant elements of their medical diagnosis and treatment to teams of physicians from the Mayo Clinic in Rochester, Minnesota. Dr. Hutton apparently acted as liaison with the Mayo physicians, but the Washington military/civilian medical establishment otherwise was bypassed. This departure from tradition may have been a result of Mrs. Reagan's desire to control the flow of medical information, the Reagans' long relationship with the clinic, a longtime friendship with Dr. Oliver Beahrs, a distinguished Mayo surgeon, or a combination of these factors.[54]

Mayo Clinic doctors flew to Washington on at least four occasions to perform a colonoscopy, a cystoscopy, and a major prostate surgery on the president, and a radical mastectomy upon the first lady. All the operations were performed at the Bethesda Naval Hospital. At the time of the major prostate surgery in January 1987, two urologists, two anesthesiologists and a pathologist, together with all their surgical equipment, flew from Minnesota to Bethesda.[55]

The unusual nature of these arrangements precipitated many questions over payment. The White House press secretary responded to reporters' inquiries by saying that the president had opted out of the federal government's Medicare plan for seniors, and instead intended to apply his Blue Cross-Blue Shield insurance policy from the California legislature's retirement system to pay his medical bills. The press secretary declined to discuss the fees charged by the Mayo Clinic physicians, who, as civilian consultants, were free to charge the president for their professional services. Speakes stated that "It was a personal matter," and continued that the doctors "are certainly not being flown at government expense."[56] However, Speakes may have been misinformed since, at the present time, the travel expenses for medical consultants to the president are reimbursed by the government.[57]

At about this time, one of the infrequent appearances in this history occurred: that of a woman physician attending a president. Dr. Diane Colgan, a board certified plastic surgeon, then serving as a navy captain at Bethesda Naval Hospital, cosmetically repaired a surgical excision on President Reagan's nose.[58] An indolent skin tumor, a basal cell carcinoma, had been removed that required the skill of a plastic surgeon. Dr. Colgan previously had removed a similar tumor from the lip of first lady Nancy Reagan.[59]

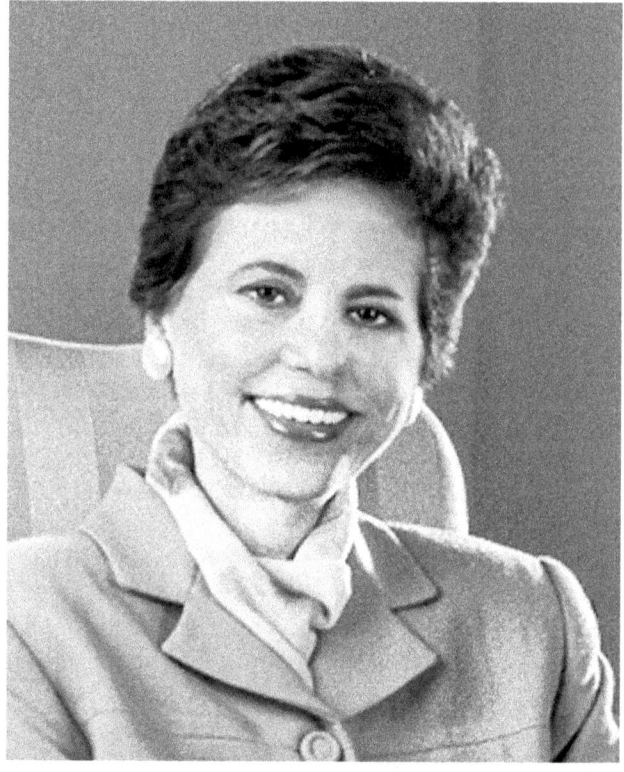

Diane Colgan. Diane Colgan, a navy plastic surgeon, who operated on the face of both President and Mrs. Reagan. (Courtesy of Diane Colgan, M.D.)

Two years after Burton Smith's departure, another Burton, Burton Lee III, was appointed as the president's physician. Lee was a friend of President George H. Bush.[60] Nicholas Brady, Bush's new treasury secretary and Lee's Yale classmate, introduced the two men during a 1980s fishing trip.[61] Lee, a graduate of Yale and Columbia Medical School,[62] specialized in oncology. He had practiced for thirty years at New York's Memorial Hospital where as an expert in the treatment of lymphomas he had written more than 120 research articles.[63]

Doctor Lee previously served on Ronald Reagan's AIDS commission.[64] He initially wanted to be appointed Bush's surgeon general but his proabortion stance disqualified him from that job.[65] Lee then wished to expand his duties as physician to the president to include the formulation of policy as special assistant to the president for health care. George Bush originally agreed to this proposal but the arrangement was withdrawn prior to Lee's arrival at the White House.[66]

Burton Lee was not from the tradition of retiring, unobtrusive White House physicians who, except at the time of a medical emergency, were rarely seen and even more rarely heard. The outspoken Dr. Lee criticized other physicians (they complain too much and drive around in Mercedes)[67]; medical academic centers (they emphasize research over patient care)[68]; the AMA ("should act less than like a union protecting their members' pocketbooks")[69]; and the test-ordering practices of physicians (medical resources should be rationed, especially unnecessary and expensive laboratory tests and surgical procedures).[70] In a February 1992, interview with *The New York Times,* Lee even suggested that his patient, the president, was dyslexic.[71]

The purview of presidential physicians and other doctors serving in the White House Medical Unit has not included commentary on health policy or contemporary medical issues. Their role has been distinctly separated from that of the surgeon general of the Public Health Service, whose function has been to serve as the president's physician spokesman for these matters. Dr. Ruge opined that a key aspect "of the job include(s) learning to stay out of the range of news cameras and otherwise 'being unobtrusive.'"[72] Both Wallace Graham and Burton Lee departed from this tradition with untoward consequences.[73]

Lee imposed his philosophical views upon the care of the president with unfortunate results. In one instance the doctor severely limited the screening panel of laboratory tests performed as part of George Bush's routine checkups. Thyroid function tests, considered routine by most physicians but a wasteful exercise by Lee, were not performed. Consequently, the president's hyperthyroidism was not diagnosed until he collapsed while jogging at Camp David with a significant cardiac arrhythmia that was a result of thyroid malfunction.[74] Characteristically, Lee was not in attendance when this event occurred and an assistant White House physician treated Bush.

It was Lee's intention to upgrade the job from the low esteem he perceived it to have, "so that when I leave here—eight years from now—it is one of the premier health policy positions in the nation."[75] Lee continued to envision himself as a key player in the formulation of national health policy, stating that he hoped that the future job description of the position, in his words, would include just that: "the President's physician empowered him not only to provide medical advice, but also to formally provide influential advice on key health-policy issues of our time."[76] The routine responsibilities of daily oversight of the president's well-being were left to members of his staff (then numbering sixteen, including three other physicians, all military, physician assistants, nurses, and medical corpsmen),[77] while Lee spent more than half his time attending medical meetings and conferences around Washington, D.C.[78] Thus this presidential physician infrequently accompanied the president on domestic plane trips or on Camp David weekends.[79]

Lee was dismissive of his predecessors in his office, controversially stating that "looking back over the people who have held my position, I'm not overcome by any sense that they were top-of-the-line intellectuals or had any particular qualities that would allow them to make completely momentous decisions. I think people in my office would need to remember humility a little bit."[80] Lee announced that his background had highly qualified him to serve effectively as physician to the president for the following reasons: Lee was a friend to the president, and was trusted by the first family. In contrast, Reagan's physicians had not been close friends, and Mrs. Reagan was the determining voice regarding medical consultations. Second, Lee was a civilian and was able to act independently and call upon the best physicians, military or nonmilitary, for consultation. Third, Lee had the requisite academic and clinical skills that permitted him to stand up to VIPs—presumably the president and the president's advisers—when making the appropriate medical decision.[81]

Burton Lee offered to stay on during the Bush-Clinton transition, but he became involved in a controversy over an unlabeled vial of allergy medicine. During the White House mayhem at the onset of the Clinton administration, Lee was requested to administer an allergy injection to the new president. The doctor refused, claiming that he was only practicing good medicine, since the medicine vial did not bear President Clinton's name as the patient. Lee subsequently charged that Clinton fired him over this incident.[82]

A second version detailing Lee's departure from the White House claims that the doctor lingered in his White House office in the hope that the new president would nominate him as surgeon general. Senior White House physician Colonel Lawrence Mohr, in tandem with the White House Military Office, finally persuaded Lee to leave. Lee's position as physician to the president was a political appointive position whose incumbency expired with the inauguration of a new president.[83] President Clinton did not offer Lee a position in his administration.

In retrospect, the White House experiences of the four twentieth-century civilian physicians, profiled in these two chapters, can be viewed historically as mere eddies within a mainstream current. The course of its history is more accurately reflected by the present-day White House Medical Unit. For example, the current model for selecting the physician to the president is the promotion of one of the existing military members of the White House Medical Unit. This model had been used previously, most recently during the "Civilian Interlude." Rear Admiral William Lukash had joined the White House medical staff during Lyndon Johnson's administration. He then became assistant physician to President Richard Nixon, and upon Nixon's resignation in 1974 he was selected as Gerald Ford's presidential physician. He was retained in this role by Jimmy Carter.[84] The selection of Bill Clinton's and George W. Bush's presidential physicians has followed in this tradition.

Moreover, at present, generalists have replaced specialists, any whiff of political intervention has been lessened significantly, the table of organization has been closely followed, and attention to the terms of the Twenty-fifth Amendment has been increased.

Chapter 11

Twenty-First Century Presidential Physicians

The Doctors Who Treated George W. Bush, Barack Obama, Donald Trump and Joe Biden

George W. Bush

George W. Bush was elected to a second presidential term in 2004. He was succeeded by Barack Obama, who served for served for eight years (2009–2017). Donald Trump became president in 2017 and was succeeded by Joe Biden in 2021.

Air Force doctor Richard (Dick) Tubb cared for the medical needs of the Bush family for their entire eight years in the White House. Colonel Tubb, a WHMU physician, was promoted to Physician to the President in January 2001. His WHMU service had commenced in June 1995 and lasted until his retirement from the Air Force in August 2009.

Tubb's thirteen-year, seven-month tenure as a White House physician is one of the longest on record. Previously, Air Force General Walter Tkach also had performed as a White House doctor (Eisenhower/Nixon), although non-continuously, for thirteen years, seven months. Historically, the record for WHMU longevity was established by Navy Admiral William Lukash at over fourteen years (1966–1981) of service during the Johnson/Nixon/Ford/Carter administrations. However, Dr. Kevin O'Connor, presently the presidential physician for Joe Biden, is posed to establish the record for tenure in the WHMU. O'Connor previously had treated Biden during his eight years as Barak Obama's vice president (2009–2017). Earlier, in 2006, Tubb had invited O'Connor to join the WHMU to address President G.W. Bush's back issues. Should Joe Biden serve out his first term, this doctor would set the record (fifteen years) for longevity as a White House Physician.

Richard Tubb, a Wisconsin native, was board certified in family medicine. He was an Air Force flight surgeon whose expertise was so respected that he taught flight medicine and evacuation at many air force bases in the United States and abroad. The National Aeronautics and Space Administration (NASA) twice recommended Tubb for consideration as an astronaut. Although not selected for a space mission, this was a further acknowledgment of his qualifications and expertise.[1]

"Tubb's immediate priority as physician to George W Bush was to build the trust relationship that is the foundation of medicine, with his new patient and his family."[2] Richard Tubb was a meticulous and very careful physician. His term as presidential physician for the two term Bush presidency is specifically notable for his detailed preparation for and conduct during the annual presidential medical examinations and second, his formulation of and strict adherence to exact and defined protocols with respect to the Twenty-fifth Disability Amendment during this president's two colonoscopies. Thereby, Dr. Tubb became the first presidential physician to appropriately acknowledge and implement section three of the Twenty-fifth Amendment to the United States Constitution. His protocol for the transfer and subsequent recovery of presidential powers set the standard and was subsequently followed by Dr. O'Connor several years later.[3]

The doctor worked closely with Dr. Ken Cooper during the two-term presidency. Cooper, the pre-presidential Bush physician for twelve years, was the director of the Cooper Clinic in Dallas, Texas. Cooper was an early advocate of preventive medicine, e.g., treadmill tests on healthy males, and a promoter of aerobic exercise.[4] Tubb planned Bush's first presidential and all subsequent presidential physicals with Cooper. Together they oversaw the complete physical examination and all diagnostic procedures by the many relevant specialists. All examining doctors, together with Drs. Tubb and Cooper, signed the final report, the results of which were released to the press and public through the White House press secretary.[5] Tubb did not appear at the post exam press conference; he considered such an appearance a very bad idea although previously some occupants of his position had welcomed them. He believed that such news conferences before a demanding and confrontational White House press corps might be treacherous, as would be proven by Drs. Ronny Jackson and Sean Conley years later.

Tubb's second enhancement of presidential care was the development of careful protocols for the constitutional transfer of power during presidential disability. Polyps of the colon, identified as tubular adenomas by pathologists, are benign tumors that over time may become malignant. Colon polyps had been removed during George Bush's pre-presidential annual physicals in 1998 and 1999. Dr. Tubb knew beforehand that the standard of care required that George W. Bush needed periodic colonoscopies during his presidency. Consequently, the doctor prepared for the anesthesia protocols to be in place during President Bush's two colonoscopies during his eight-year presidency. His preparations will be scrutinized in detail in the subsequent chapter on the Twenty-fifth Amendment.[6] Except for a torn meniscus, the forty-third U.S. president presented no other urgent medical issues to his physician. Tubb accompanied the departing Bushes to their Texas ranch when the president retired in January 2009. The doctor was rewarded with a promotion to brigadier general at the conclusion of his White House tour.

Dr. Tubb as part of the president's "response bubble" was with Bush and a WHMU nurse during the 9/11 attack, just days after his first physical, in the motorcade, the Florida schoolhouse, *Air Force One*, the "bomb shelters," and at his side in the "days and weeks following."[7] "Tubb made the decision, aboard *Air Force One* to begin prophylaxis with the antibiotic ciproflaxin for the president and later at the White House for the key presidential principals and staff.' This proved prescient when just a week later, anthrax ... joined 9/11 in the headlines of the 24 hour news cycle."[8]

Tubb accompanied the departing Bushes to their Texas ranch when the president retired in January 2009. The doctor was rewarded with a promotion to brigadier general at the conclusion of his White House tour. Despite being "stratified to a very low coronary risk profile" during his annual presidential physical in 2001, Bush underwent coronary artery stenting on August 6, 2013, at age sixty-seven.[9] At the time of this writing in 2023, George W. Bush remains in good health.

Barack Obama

Barack Obama's health remained excellent; any medical issues were both routine and insignificant during his two-term presidency (2009–2017). Obama was under the careful care of Navy Captain Jeff Kuhlman, a long-time veteran of both naval medicine and the White House Medical Unit, who was promoted to the post of presidential physician in 2009. Kuhlman retired from military service at the end of Obama's first term; he was succeeded by another Navy physician from within the WHMU. Captain Ronny Jackson remained the physician to the president during Obama's entire second term and for the early years of the succeeding Trump administration.

Four complete physical examinations were completed during the Obama presidency, in 2010, 2011, 2014, and 2016. All reports confirmed that the president was in excellent physical condition. Jackson's 2014 report stated that "the president's overall health is excellent. All clinical data indicate that the president is currently healthy and will remain so for the duration of his presidency."[10] All medical examination reviews were released through the White House Press Secretary. Following the example set by their predecessor Dick Tubb, neither Dr. Kuhlman nor Dr. Jackson discussed their physical findings at a press conference until January 2018.

Jeffrey Kuhlman, his father a college physics professor, was an intelligent and a quick achiever, completing college in 24 months at age nineteen. He graduated from Loma Linda University School of Medicine and was certified in family medicine. In 2000, while serving as senior flight surgeon of the presidential helicopter squadron at Andrews Air Force Base, the doctor was assigned to the White House Medical Unit.

Dick Tubb, his senior officer at the WHMU, supported Kuhlman's application for the highly competitive full-time out service training with the Navy. Between 2003–2005, Kuhlman both obtained a Masters of Public Health from Johns Hopkins, and achieved board certifications in the specialties of Occupational Medicine and Aerospace Medicine.[11] The first four years of the Obama presidency were tranquil with no medical emergencies. The Obamas were safe and Barack Obama achieved a personal goal of smoking cessation.[12]

Kuhlman departed the White House after Obama's first term, in contrast to predecessors Drs. Mariano and Tubb, who served for the entirety of Presidents Clinton and Bush's respective two terms each. Perhaps he left after his service in the WHMU of twelve years, seven months, was deemed to be enough. His subsequent career has been spent in practice and senior administrative roles in Florida's Advent health system.[13] Although Jeff Kuhlman and his successor Ronny Jackson mutually respected the other's medical opinion, social friction entered their once cordial relationship.[14]

Navy Captain Ronny Jackson became Physician to the President and director of the White House Medical unit in 2013 upon his predecessor's retirement. Previously, Jackson was the assistant to Kuhlman since the beginning of the Obama presidency.

Jackson, an affable Texan, was a Navy doctor. His Lone Star roots grew sturdier with a B.S. from Texas A&M University[15] and a Doctorate of Medicine from the University of Texas (Galveston).[16] He was board certified in emergency medicine and was on duty with the Second Marines in Iraq when he was called to the White House for a job interview.[17] During the Obama presidency, he treated not only President Obama, but also Michelle Obama, the couple's two daughters, Mrs. Obama's mother, senior White House staff, and members of the Cabinet. Jackson professed that he got along very well with the Obama family.[18]

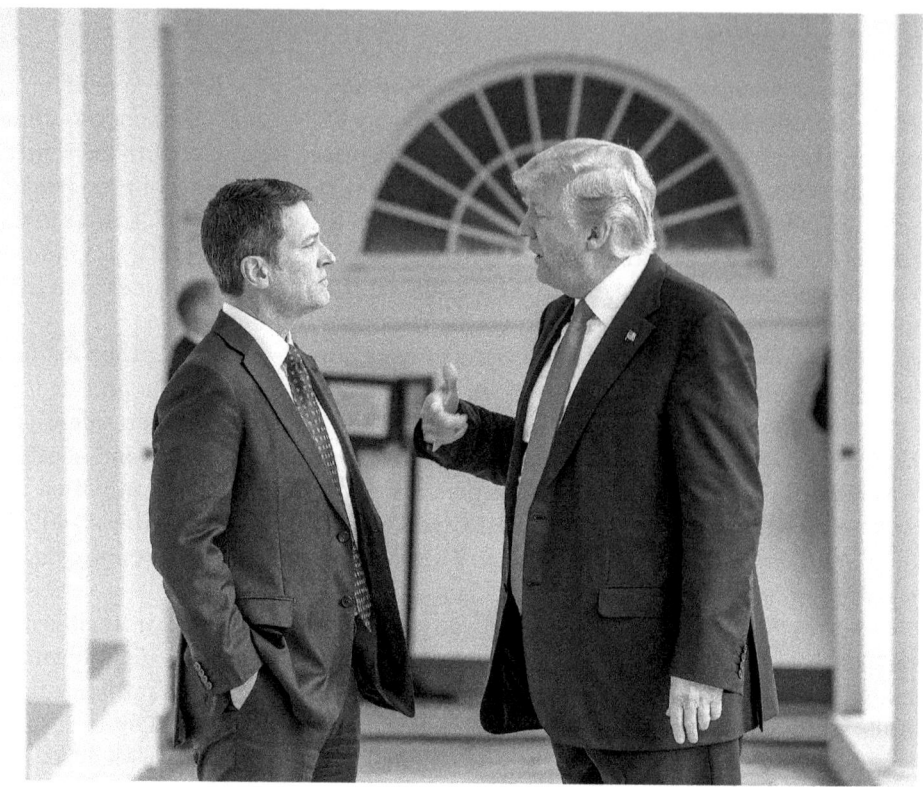

Ronny Jackson. Dr. Ronny Jackson with President Donald Trump. Dr. Jackson served as physician to Presidents Barack Obama and Donald Trump. His nomination to become a cabinet secretary was rejected before he was elected twice as a Representative to the U.S. Congress. (Courtesy of Dr. Ronny Jackson)

Donald Trump

Donald John Trump was inaugurated as the forty-fifth U.S. President in January 2017. Trump, seventy years and seven months of age on his Inauguration Day, became the oldest first-term president since Ronald Reagan at that time. However, when Reagan was sworn in at his second-term inauguration, his age was almost seventy-four.

Two Navy doctors, Captain Ronny Jackson and his successor Commander Sean Conley, served as Trump's presidential physicians. The Trump transition team, familiar with Dr. Jackson's previous WHMU's experience during the Bush and Obama administrations, convinced this doctor to remain as the new president's personal physician, but only for a six-month period.[19] However, Donald Trump and his new doctor, Captain Ronny Jackson, soon discovered that they got along extremely well. Both possessed vocal, direct, frank, controversial and somewhat flamboyant personalities. Consequently, Jackson's tenure was extended by mutual agreement.[20]

Under Jackson's leadership, the staff of the WHMU expanded from sixty-five to seventy-two personnel. Meanwhile, its complement of nurse practitioners was reduced, to be replaced mainly by physician Aassistants (PA); emergency medicine became the dominant specialty among White House doctors.[21]

Jackson designated himself as the Physician to the President and not the Director of the White House Medical Unit, and thereby limited his mission to solely furnish health care to the president, First Lady Melania Trump, their teenage son Barron, and Mrs. Trump's parents. He interpreted his professional responsibility to be separate from the multiple responsibilities of the other members of the WHMU. As a solo actor, he became detached from the organization, leadership. and personnel assignments of his White House medical colleagues. His reimagined job description subsequently caused trouble with his former WHMU physician associates. WHMU physician Jennifer Pena, assigned to the care of Vice President Pence and family, "accused Jackson of overstepping his authority and inappropriately intervening in a medical situation involving the second lady." Furthermore, she charged Jackson "…as potentially violating federal privacy rights by briefing White House staff and disclosing details to other medical providers—but not appropriately consulting with the vice president's physician (Jennifer Pena)."[22]

During Trump's tumultuous tenure, his physician was confronted by persistent and insistent partisan charges that Donald Trump, his patient, was mentally and emotionally unfit to fulfill the duties of president, and consequently that the incumbent president should be removed from office according to Section 4 of the 25th Amendment of the United States Constitution.[23] A number of partisan newspapers, cable, radio and television media, opposition politicians and even several psychiatrists decried the president's supposed psychological and emotional inability to perform his constitutional responsibilities. Psychiatry professors Bandy Lee of Yale and John Talmadge of the University of Texas conspicuously critiqued the president's mental capacity.[24] Because neither had examined the patient in question, they substantially violated the American Psychiatric Association's code of ethics.[25]

Ronny Jackson sought to dispel these accusations during a combative January 16, 2018, press conference held immediately after the 45th president's initial physical examination. Jackson reported that Trump received a perfect thirty out of thirty score on a common dementia screening exam called the *Montreal Cognitive Assessment*.[26] The presidential physician concluded that his patient was mentally sound, and deemed him fit to fulfill his executive responsibilities as commander in chief.[27]

As a consequence, Dr. Jackson apparently made enemies both among segments of the news media and among the political establishment: "What I didn't realize at first that was that was the day I got the Trump stamp on me. That was the day I became public enemy number one for the Far Left and the liberal press."[28]

Shortly afterward, in April 2018, President Trump nominated his physician to become Secretary of Veterans Affairs. This was a cabinet position that required senatorial approval. Opposition to Jackson's nomination was both intense and widespread. Democrat Senator John Tester, chairman of the Senate Veterans Affairs Committee, was to schedule hearings on Jackson's appointment. However, the hearings never occurred because the nominee waited while both resistance and reservations to the appointment mounted. The principal objections were internal complaints delivered to Tester from within the White House Medical Unit. Dr. Jennifer Pena, the designated physician for Vice president Pence and his family was identified as a principal accuser of Jackson.[29] Any consideration of the nominee was torpedoed and the appointment was withdrawn. Tester neither interviewed nor met with Dr. Jackson.

The nominee was confronted by a barrage of accusations: that he handed out sleeping pills (Ambien) on overseas trips as though they were candy, leading to his nickname "Candy man." It was further alleged both that Jackson presided over a hostile work environment, and that he was prone to drinking while on duty. Last, he was accused of crashing a government car while inebriated.[30] Subsequently, the Inspector General of the Defense Department launched an investigation. Throughout this process, President Trump actively supported his physician.[31] Additionally, Jackson angrily responded, "The allegations against me are completely false and fabricated. If they had any merit, I would not have been selected, promoted, and entrusted to serve in such a sensitive and important role as physician to three presidents over the past 12 years." Consequently, Jennifer Pena resigned as the Pence family physician, departed from the WHMU, and resigned her military commission.[32] As a further development, Ronny Jackson withdrew his nomination from consideration by Tester's committee; he returned to the White House not as the physician, but instead as assistant to the president. Soon after, Jackson retired from the White House and from the Navy, but not before he was promoted. Instead of selecting the practice of medicine or accepting an academic appointment, in a unique decision by a prior presidential physician, Jackson immediately decided to pursue a political career from his home state of Texas. He was elected in 2020 and reelected in 2022 to serve as the representative from the Texas Thirteenth Congressional District.[33]

Navy Commander Doctor Sean Conley ascended to the post of presidential physician when his predecessor abruptly resigned to pursue his cabinet nomination. Thereby, Dr. Conley became the first Doctor of Osteopathy (DO) to become Physician to the President.

Sean Conley was a victim of either bad luck or bad timing. Both tradition and regulations stipulated that the Physician to the President should hold the rank of colonel or its Navy (USN) equivalent, captain (pay grade O-6).[34] However, Conley remained a navy commander (O-5) for the duration of his tenure. Unfortunately, at the time of his promotion, the flag rank (navy captain or army/air force colonel) became no longer automatic. In 2017, the number of flag rank billets across the military was reduced by 25

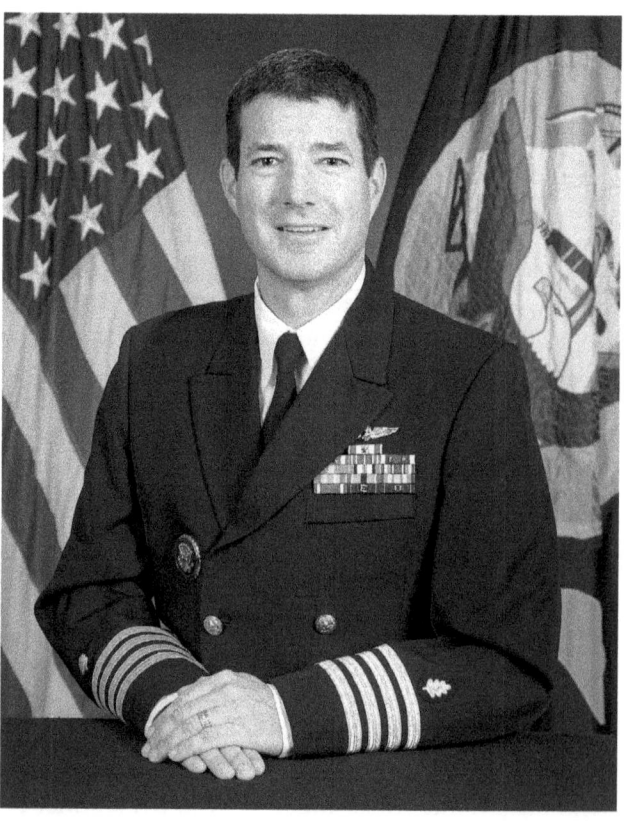

Sean Conley. Dr. Sean Conley was the first Doctor of Osteopathy to become physician to the president. He was President Donald Trump's doctor during the president's Covid illness. (Courtesy of Navy Captain Sean Conley)

percent (NDAA2017). Dr. Conley became Donald Trump's doctor a year later, in 2018.[35] It was only several years later and after his departure from the White House that Conley was finally promoted to Navy Captain.[36]

Sean Conley, a Pennsylvania native, graduated from the Philadelphia College of Osteopathic Medicine and completed a residency in emergency medicine at the Naval Medical Center Portsmouth. Conley saw service overseas in Afghanistan and aboard the aircraft carrier USS *Carl Vinson*. In 2016 while serving as the Senior Medical Officer Research Director of Emergency Medicine at Portsmouth Navy Hospital, he was competively selected for assignment to the White House Medical Unit. He was stationed in the WHMU for only a year before he became Physician to the President.[37]

Moreover, it may have been bad timing that Conley's White House career coincided with the last two- and one-half years of Trump's tumultuous presidency. The press and political opposition were not restrained from continuing their anti–Trump bias. Moreover, their antagonism remained toward Dr. Jackson, Conley's predecessor. It had emerged after Jackson's previous confirmation of the president's mental acuity, and only escalated during this physician's unsuccessful and embarrassing nomination battle. Perhaps, Sean Conley became the unfortunate recipient of the Deep State's misplaced enmity. Therefore, Dr. Conley was medically in charge when Donald Trump was hospitalized with Covid during the close of the 2020 presidential election campaign.

Therefore, Conley was very new to the WHMU when he became Donald Trump's physician. The first two years of his medical stewardship were tranquil, other than the controversy dredged up by his prescription of hydroxychloroquine as prophylaxis at the onset of the 2020 Covid pandemic.[38]

Dr. Conley was a neophyte to Washington politics and, admittedly lacking either experience or training in public relations, he always relayed any medical information regarding President Trump to Press Secretary Kayleigh McEnaney and Chief of Staff Mark Meadows for public release. Consequently, he was both unaware and unprepared for the confrontation with the press that occurred when he had to brief the reporters at Walter Reed National Military Medical Center when Donald Trump was hospitalized with a symptomatic Covid infection.

In a heated and hostile exchange, the Washington press corps forced the doctor into several factual errors in his presentation.[39] The conflicted and confusing situation was compounded by Meadows' contemporaneous "off the record" discussion with favored reporters. Meadows' remarks seriously undercut Conley's credibility. Later, the Chief of Staff regretted that he did not step in to correct any misinformation out of concern that the press would doubt the White House Medical Unit. He later characterized his reluctance as an "enormous mistake."[40]

The coronavirus (Covid-19) pandemic had raged both internationally and in the United States since March 2020. On September 27, 2020, on the day of his scheduled television debate with Democrat nominee Joe Biden, Trump was confronted with a positive Covid test. A few hours later a confirmatory test was negative; consequently, the initial test result was considered to be a false positive. But, for the next four days, the president displayed appreciably less energy until both Melania and Donald Trump tested positive on October 1.[41]

"Trump in rough shape, pale, exhausted, and nearly asleep on his feet." In the president's words, "I have lost so much strength … the muscles are just not responding." At the White House Dr. Conley initially treated with rednisivir,[42] dexamethasone, regeneron,[43] and oxygen. But that evening Trump was hospitalized at Walter Reed National Military Medical Center in Bethesda, Maryland. In a statement Conley attempted to reassure the nation: "In consultation with this group (of medical consultants), I recommended that we bring the president up to Walter Reed as a precautionary measure to provide state of the art monitoring ... days 7–10 are the most critical...."[44] In contrast, Meadows judged that the doctors were medical and not political, that Dr. Conley was trying a little too hard to paint a rosy picture, and was coming very close to "jading the truth."[45] However, the president recovered rapidly and was released from the hospital a few days later.

Unfortunately for Dr. Conley who had addressed the press and public with full transparency, his reward by reporters was castigation and skepticism. He was accused of misleading the public about Trump's Covid-19 diagnosis.[46] CNN reporters amplified the press criticism with the headline, "Trump's White House doctor facing fresh scrutiny over Covid test timeline."[47] President Biden replaced Conley as physician to the president the day after he was inaugurated.

He accompanied the Trumps to their retirement home and left the WHMU but continued in the Navy. In a conversation with the author, Conley noted his frustration with the WHMU organization, opining that the "greatest challenge was who was in charge ... a splitting of responsibility..." Although the military side ruled doctors, non-physicians ruled the WHMU.[48] With the departure of Ronny Jackson, there was an immediate and often nebulous shifting of responsibilities.

Both Drs. Conley and Jackson were appalled by their treatment at the hands of the Washington political establishment and the Capital press corps. Sean Conley reacted with frustration as he shortly thereafter left the White House to prefer the anonymity of an academic appointment at the United States Uniformed Services Medical University. The mild-mannered physician characterized his treatment as "unfortunate."[49] Conversely, Ronny Jackson sought vindication in anger. He resigned from the Navy, ran for Congress, and in 2020 was elected, and in 2022 was reelected to the House of Representatives from Texas with an overwhelming majority. His memoir, *Holding the Line*, was published in 2022. Therein, he presented his side of the story and condemned his critics, several of whom had been his medical colleagues. Congressman Jackson has been a consistent vocal critic of President Joe Biden's fitness for office.

Joe Biden

Former vice president and senator Joseph Biden was elected the 46th U.S. President in November 2020. On his January 2021 Inauguration Day, Biden, at seventy-eight years, two months old became the oldest person to hold the office, surpassing President Ronald Reagan, who was seventy-seven years old when he left the White House.

Biden was elected U.S. Senator from Delaware at age twenty-nine and only reached the constitutional age limit of thirty just a few weeks before his inauguration. Although trained as an attorney, Biden's vocation was politics; he served continuously as senator from Delaware for decades until Barack Obama selected him during his seventh senatorial term as his vice president. Biden was vice president for two terms (2009–2017).[50]

Personal tragedy afflicted Biden's family life. His first wife and infant daughter were killed in a car crash early in his political career. His first marriage also begat two sons, Beau and Hunter. Beau Biden, the older son, had a laudable career in the military and elected Attorney General of Delaware twice. Beau died in his forties from a malignant brain tumor, a glioblastoma multiforme.[51] Biden remarried; his wife Jill achieved a doctorate in education. Their marriage has been long and apparently happy, and produced Ashley, a daughter. Hunter's and Ashley's adult lives have been both psychologically difficult and politically explosive.

Joe Biden, now an octogenarian, did not escape medical illnesses. In 1987, he was twice operated on for the excision of cerebral artery aneurysms, one of which had ruptured and bled into his brain. Moreover, he has been diagnosed with atrial fibrillation, hyperlipidemia, seasonal allergies, and benign prostatic hypertrophy.[52]

The president selected Kevin O'Connor, long his personal doctor, to be his presidential physician. Dr. O'Connor received his medical degree from the New York College of Osteopathic Medicine and his specialty training in Family Medicine at The Mountainside Hospital in New Jersey. Thereupon he joined the U.S. Army Medical Corps.[53]

His military service was active, overseas, and combat experienced. He saw duty as a flight surgeon and as a hyperbaric medical officer for some of the nation's most elite units, including the 82nd Airborne Division, the 75th Ranger Regiment, and a special mission's unit within the U.S. Army Special Operations Command ... "He was instrumental in rethinking Department of Defense trauma procedures to develop innovative point of wounding strategies that addressed the unique needs ... of wounded combatants in hostile settings."[54]

O'Connor was serving at a Colorado army hospital where he was available to manipulate George W. Bush's orthopedic issues. Dick Tubb appreciated O'Connor's osteopathic skills and brought him onto the WHMU in 2007. During the Obama eight-year presidency, Jeff Kuhlman and Ronny Jackson successively served as presidential physicians, while O'Connor oversaw the medical care of Vice President Biden's family. He served in that capacity for eight years and meanwhile became very attached to the Bidens. There is no record of any medical care provided to the vice president during this period.[55]

O'Connor left the WHMU and retired from the military when Donald Trump was inaugurated. He remained in the nation's capital city to serve as an associate professor at its George Washington School of Medicine and its director of executive medicine. Meanwhile, as a civilian, he continued to serve as the Biden family doctor.[56]

O'Connor resigned his commission as an army colonel in 2017. When he reentered the White House as Biden's personal physician, he was a civilian. Moreover, he became only the second individual to serve non-continuously as a White House physician. Previously, Air Force General Walter Tkach was a physician in both the Eisenhower and Nixon White Houses. An eight-year hiatus occurred between his tenures in the White House. In contrast to O'Connor, the general did not resign from the military during the interim.

O'Connor's relationship with the WHMU appears untroubled because he does not concern himself with its operations or scheduling of personnel. The confused lines of authority that Sean Conley experienced may have altered since as a civilian, O'Connor is not subject to the military command structure, through neither the WHMU nor the WHMO (White House Military Office). The matter was touched upon briefly during a post-inaugural interview with a colleague: O'Connor said he "had a great team to work with...." Further in a personal interview, he suggested that his policy of openness and respect with colleagues has made cooperation with the WHMU smooth and fluid. Dr. O'Connor follows his predecessors' practice of greeting the president each morning from his office door as the chief executive exits the elevator from the second-floor personal quarters. He also checks in with Joe Biden toward the end of the day but does not shadow his patient. Secret Service is in continual electronic communication with the physician during the day in the event of an emergency. O'Connor accompanies the president on almost all foreign trips and occasionally on domestic journeys.[57]

O'Connor's medical care of Joe Biden prior to his inauguration and during the first two-and-a-half-years of his presidency included treatment of an ankle fracture and the administration of Covid tests and vaccine boosters.[58] He oversaw the 46th president's physical examination in November 2021. At the time the White House physician declared Joe Biden, "fit for duty, after investigating (the patient's) persistent cough and stiffened gait."[59] An individual benign polyp (tubular adenoma) of his colon was discovered during this physical examination. A subsequent colonoscopy under anesthesia noted no additional polyps. According to section 3 of the 25th Amendment, the vice president temporarily held the executive powers of the presidency.[60] The results of a cognitive test were not reported.

On July 21, 2022, President Biden tested positive for Covid-19. His physician wrote in a letter, released by the White House, that Biden was experiencing only mild symptoms including a runny nose and fatigue "with an occasional dry cough." The physician continued, "The President is fully vaccinated and twice-boosted, so I anticipate that he will respond favorably, as most maximally protected patients do." Unfortunately, positive tests persisted for many days before resolution.[61] In June 2023, sharp-eyed reporters of the Washington press queried the assistant press secretary about the distinct strap lines that appeared on the president's face. Only then did the press office admit that Biden wore a CPAP (continuous positive airway pressure) machine to ward off sleep apnea.[62]

White House Physician Kevin O'Connor has remained the rare administration official for whom press anonymity has been habitual, permanent, and perhaps mandatory. He apologized in a text to this author, "Sorry to be so conservative.... I am very conscientious not to be the story." The Physician to the President was not available to the press at the conclusion of both President Biden's annual comprehensive examinations. Instead, this physician chose to release a statement through the Presidential Press Secretary. O'Connor's press unavailability became starkly apparent during Biden's protracted bout with the Covid virus during the summer of 2022. His medical bulletins were delivered to the press and public through daily written statements to the press secretary. When the Washington press corps demanded to speak with a physician, another administration doctor appeared, not O'Connor. The reasons proffered for Dr. O'Connor's absence were unsatisfactory.[63] O'Connor dismissed such criticism as press carping, stating that his reporting on Joe Biden's medical matters were the "most transparent in history."[64]

After Biden underwent dental surgery in June 2023, which forced him to avoid several scheduled meetings, O'Connor again avoided the press. A reporter from the New York Post commented, "In a break from historical practice, the White House press office has not allowed O'Connor to field press questions on Biden's health."[65] As Joe Biden serves out his presidency, his doctor will set the record (15 years) for longevity as a White House physician.

Chapter 11. Twenty-First Century Presidential Physicians

Presidential health care during the first two plus decades of the twenty-first century is notable for the first appropriate applications of section three of the 25th Amendment, a worsening partisanship of the White House press congeries, its open skepticism and hostility toward selected presidential physicians, and a public conflict between White House physicians reminiscent of the Bliss-Baxter contretemps in the aftermath of the James Garfield assassination.

CHAPTER 12

The White House Medical Unit Continues to Evolve

On August 3, 1998, President Bill Clinton rolled up his shirt sleeve in the White House map room. Thereupon, in the presence of an FBI agent and a prosecutor from the office of the Whitewater independent counsel, Dr. Connie Mariano, the physician to the president and the senior White House physician, drew a vial of the president's blood.[1] The DNA obtained from this blood sample provided the key evidence that embroiled Clinton in a long political struggle that culminated in his impeachment by the United States House of Representatives. Involvement in this medical procedure was as close as contemporary presidential physicians have come to the political process. As future physician to the president, Brigadier General Richard Tubb would explain, "I'm the background guy. That's really my role here. Not policy, not politics."[2] Dr. Ronny Jackson, in his memoir, *Holding the Line* several years later expressed the unspoken rule of confidentiality regarding private political talk—to never disclose anything overheard while in the presence of the president. "You really are like a fly on the wall. They know you're in the room, but they do not hold anything back."[3]

After a period of idiosyncratic civilian leadership, the medical presence within the White House has evolved into its present form as an apolitical, professionally focused, tightly structured, military staffed, health maintenance organization. One indication of its present bureaucratic structure is the acceptance and usage of its official designation as the White House Medical Unit (WHMU).[4] Navy Captain E. Connie Mariano, President Clinton's personal physician, has been credited with transforming the unit, in the opinion of one observer, into "the world's benchmark for the health care of the world's leader." She, too, considered the "transforming the organization into a topnotch, well-respected unit seen as the standard for other countries" her proudest accomplishment in her nearly eight-year tenure.[5]

During Dr. Mariano's tenure, the designation White House Medical Unit (WHMU), previously used occasionally, came into general and common usage although formally designated neither by Congressional legislation nor bureaucratic rule.[6] The WHMU is only one of eleven units under the command of the White House Military Office (WHMO). The WHMO oversees 2,200 military personal attached to the White House, who staff, in addition to the WHMU, the White House Communications Agency, the White House Staff Mess, Camp David, *Air Force One*, and *Marine Helicopter Squadron One*.[7]

In the course of the last three decades, its staffing has varied both in total numbers and in medical specialties. The WHMU consists of physicians, nurses, physician

Chapter 12. The White House Medical Unit Continues to Evolve

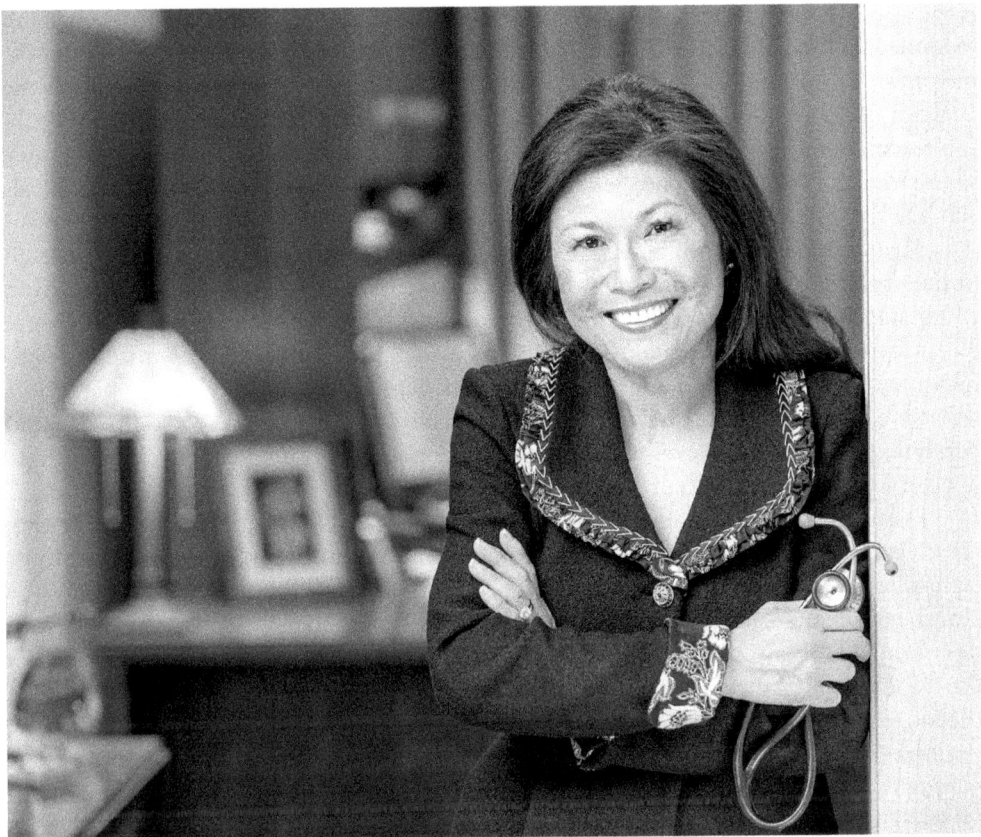

Connie Mariano. Navy Rear Admiral Dr. E. Connie Mariano was the second woman physician to the president. She served as physician to President Bill Clinton for most of his two-term presidency. (Courtesy of E. Connie Mariano, M.D.)

assistants, medical technicians, secretarial and other support staff. During 2013–2019, its staff expanded from 25 to 62 total personnel. The number of physicians totaled nine, usually three from each military service, with emergency medicine becoming the most common medical specialty. Registered nurse practitioners (9 or 10 at one point) were gradually replaced by Physician Assistants (PAs), who at one point totaled 16 in number.[8]

The unit's increased organizational complexity and complement of medical personnel require the following definitions. All physicians who serve in the White House are designated *White House Physicians*, The White House physician with the longest tenure is named the *Senior White House Physician*. The *Physician to the President* is a political appointee of the president. This appointee may be a civilian but since 1993 has been most often a military doctor. However, President Biden selected Dr. Kevin O'Connor, a civilian, to provide his medical care. Because this physician provides ongoing personal care to the president, it is only appropriate that the president, as is the prerogative of any patient, personally selects this doctor. This appointment is not subject to congressional approval. Obviously, the *Physician to the President* is also a *White House Physician*. During the less complicated times of presidential administrations from the distant and not so distant past, the title of *White House Physician* was often synonymous with *Physician to the President,* a congruence now rendered defunct due to the WHMU's expanded responsibilities and its enlarged complement of physicians. The administrative head of the WHMU holds the title of *Director of the White House Medical Unit*. Additionally, the physician to the president may also serve, either concurrently or sequentially, as the *Director of the White House Medical Unit*. Connie Mariano, Dick Tubb and Ronny Jackson often combined these roles. However, the combined burden became too onerous, so the Medical Director is now held by a second person, who may be a nurse or a physician's assistant.[9]

Medical Consultants include any physician who is selected either by the physician to the president or by the president himself for medical care. This title has no basis in either statute or administrative code. Medical consultants far outnumber White House physicians during the course of a presidency; they may be civilian or military doctors, may have a major and ongoing role in presidential care, or may simply perform a one-time, minor function. Several presidents have arranged for their pre-presidential personal physicians to travel to Washington for occasional medical check-ups. These doctors also fall under the rubric of medical consultant.[10]

Presidents Bill Clinton, George W. Bush, Barack Obama, and Donald Trump selected their presidential physicians from among the military White House physicians already assigned to the White House. The process that selects the military White House physicians is both complex and rigorous. When a vacancy occurs, the three military branches, army, navy and air force, nominate candidates who are then screened by the Department of Defense and by the White House Military Office of Security. After a thorough review of each nominee's qualifications has narrowed the field of candidates, the finalists are invited to the White House for a demanding series of interviews by members of the WHMU and others. A top-secret security clearance must be established for each candidate early in the process. Selection is made by a member of the WHMU, usually the physician to the president. Burton Lee personally interviewed Dr. Mariano before he approved her application as a White House physician.[11] Navy captain Gerald Cox, White House physician from 1999 to 2001, was offered the position after an interview with then presidential physician Dr. Mariano.[12]

Military physicians of the WHMU usually serve for two years. However, the length of their tours frequently is extended.[13] Navy captain Eleanor ("Connie") Mariano served as a White House physician for eight years (1992–2001); Rear Admiral William Lukash was a doctor in the executive mansion for fourteen years (1966–1981).[14] The present physician to the president, Dr. Kevin O'Connor, is a civilian who retired from the U.S. Army Medical Corps. O' Connor is not unknown to Joe Biden, since as an WHMU colonel he previously had treated Vice President and Mrs. Biden and was their private practitioner during their temporary retirement from the political stage.[15]

During her tenure, Mariano revised the criteria for selection to the WHMU. Currently White House physicians are selected from the ranks of board certified internists, family practitioners, and emergency room physicians. All are generalists who have been trained in acute or emergency medicine rather than the more narrowly focused specialists who staffed the unit during several previous administrations.[16] At the onset of the twenty-first century, medical knowledge has burgeoned so dramatically that board certification in a medical specialty that attests to additional training in depth in more focused areas of medical information has become a near necessity to practice medicine in the United States. A board certified physician has completed postgraduate education in that specialty, lasting up to seven years, and has successfully passed an examination designed to assess the knowledge, skills and experience required to provide quality patient care in that specialty. Specialization—another bureaucratic imperative—acknowledges that it is impossible for anyone to master the technical skills, body of information, and clinical experience that comprise today's broad practice of medicine. The American Board of Medical Specialties (ABMS), formed in 1933, is the umbrella organization that oversees America's medical specialty boards, which presently number twenty-four.[17] The American Board of Medical Genetics, established in 1991, is the most recent specialty to be recognized.[18] Emergency medicine, officially recognized by the ABMS as a medical specialty in September 1989, became the twenty-third certifying board.[19] The state of American medical practice has evolved to a point that the ABMS estimates that approximately 90 percent of all presently practicing physicians are board certified.[20] All White House physicians attend continuing medical education meetings and lectures to assure that they maintain both their board credentials and licensure.[21]

In a recent interview Mariano discussed the expanded responsibilities of the WHMU.[22] The unit's overriding duty is the provision of continuous, twenty-four-hour health care for the president, the first lady, and their sub-adult children. To accomplish this, a White House physician, usually the president's doctor, may shadow the chief executive during his working schedule, and a nurse or physician's assistant remains on-call overnight in the White House, except during periods when the threat level is elevated. During these times a physician remains in the White House around the clock.[23] White House physicians also are available to provide continuous twenty-four-hour care for the vice president, his spouse, and his subadult children.[24]

Mariano's tenure at the White House included the organization of six annual physical examinations of President Clinton, the oversight of his rehabilitation after he tore a knee tendon in Florida, and the aforementioned forensic phlebotomy during the Monica Lewinsky affair. During Mariano's tour as presidential physician, she took fifty-one trips abroad and visited close to 100 foreign countries. In a traditional acknowledgment of loyal medical service to the president, she was promoted to rear admiral when she completed her tour of duty in 2021.[25]

The WHMU is heavily committed to advance and pre-advance planning for all presidential trips, both foreign and domestic. Recent presidents have been hyperkinetic in their travel activity, and as a result advance missions now account for a major part of the WHMU's effort. Planning for foreign travel includes health risk assessments for the locations to be visited (e.g., altitude, temperature, air quality, endemic disease risk, etc.), liaison with the state department and medical representatives of the host nation, and on-the-ground inspection of all the sites and locations to be visited. An initial planning mission, or pre-advance trip, is usually scheduled several months prior to the presidential visit to determine whether the host country can meet the basic requirements of the WHMU.[26] A White House physician may be a member of the team dispatched to these foreign venues in order to make an initial determination as to whether their available medical resources are capable of handling a presidential medical emergency.

Since the advance medical team determined that there were no medical facilities capable of attending to a medical emergency, a deployable hospital was set up on hospital runways in several countries during President Clinton's 1998 trip to sub–Saharan Africa.[27] Approximately two to four weeks before the president departs upon a previously announced overseas trip, an advance WHMU team, consisting of a physician and a nurse, arrives at each foreign location to intensively coordinate the medical support required for the arriving presidential party. Upon arrival, the presidential physician and nurse who traveled with the president customarily hand off the on-call medical responsibility to the advance contingent to allow for their rest.[28] To support the peripatetic Bill and Hillary Clinton, the WHMU was required to provide pre-advance and advance planning for an average twenty-five foreign venues annually.[29]

Several members of the WHMU routinely accompany the vice president on all their domestic and overseas trips. In addition, a White House physician attends the first lady on all her foreign travels. Independent foreign travel became a distinctive feature of Hillary Clinton's eight years as first lady. Clinton, then identified by a newspaper reporter as "the most traveled first lady in American history,"[30] dedicated considerable space to her globe-trotting in her recent autobiography, *Living History*.[31] Kazakhstan, Uzbekistan, Nepal, Mongolia, Bosnia, and the countries of sub–Saharan Africa comprised some of the exotic destinations she visited. White House physician and emergency medicine specialist Dr. Robert Darling was assigned to accompany Clinton on some of these trips in order to provide the expert acute care that many of these underdeveloped countries lacked.[32] First Lady Laura Bush most likely has established the record for travel, forty-six foreign trips and 212 days abroad during her husband's two-term tenure.[33]

Medical care for the vice president and his wife has been provided during recent administrations, and a specific WHMU doctor may be assigned, e.g., Dick Tubb for the Gores, O'Connor for the Bidens, and Jennifer Pena for the Pences.

White House physicians also staff the urgent care clinic in the Eisenhower Executive Office Building (EEOB), formerly called the Old Executive Office Building (OEOB) across the street from the West Wing of the White House. Urgent and even routine care is provided for the 2200 members of the White House Military Office who are on duty at the White House complex.[34] Since the ever-expanding civilian White House staff had overburdened these facilities, a recent attempt was made to restrict medical care at the clinic to military patients only. However, no staff member who walks through the door is refused service.[35] President Richard Nixon moved the clinic from its historical location on the ground floor of the West Wing of the White House to the EEOB, where it remains. Nixon, more comfortable working in the EEOB than in the Oval Office, insisted that a medical unit be nearby during his workday.[36]

As the doctors who are most available, White House physicians provide on-site emergency medical care for White House staff, visitors, and tourists. Chest pain, fainting spells, and minor traumatic injuries among tourists routinely require medical attendance. On the rare occasion, the need for immediate physician intervention may be more dramatic. On November 14, 2004, a fifty-two-year-old man attempted to immolate himself just beyond the gate of the White House as he repeatedly shouted, "Allah! Allah!" According to a television news report, "White House doctors joined uniformed Secret Service personnel in administering first aid until the emergency service technicians arrived." The injured man then was transported to the Washington Hospital Center burn unit.[37] Occasionally assistance by the WHMU has been offered to others during presidential and vice-presidential travel. During a 2004 campaign appearance in Lansing, Michigan, Vice President Dick Cheney dispatched his physician to assist a supporter who had fainted.[38]

In his memoir, *Holding the Line*, Ronny Jackson elaborated on the "proxy care" he proffered to the key members of the president's staff since, by extension, he would be taking care of the president. He provided urgent treatment in their offices, or in house

Chapter 12. The White House Medical Unit Continues to Evolve

calls. It included the delivery of medicines, and on occasion, the delivery of IV fluids or medications. He called it concierge executive medicine.[39]

A recent addition to the WHMU's list of responsibilities has been emergency medical care for members of the president's cabinet. After Attorney General John Ashcroft became acutely ill with gallstone pancreatitis in March 2004, White House physician Daniel Parks was called to Ashcroft's home to perform an examination.[40] The attorney general developed abdominal pains severe enough to cancel an appearance at a news conference where he was to announce terrorism convictions. Upon returning home to recuperate, surmising that his abrupt illness was merely "stomach flu," he had become progressively ill to the point that emergency attention became necessary.[41]

Previous chapters of this narrative demonstrated that a president occasionally has dispatched a White House physician to care for a foreign dignitary. A recent instance was when Bill Clinton directed his personal physician, Connie Mariano, to consult at the Mayo Clinic in Minnesota at the bedside of Jordan's King Hussein.[42]

The WHMU is charged with complying with the Twenty-fifth Amendment on Presidential Disability and Succession. It is the responsibility of the physician to the president to advise the selected officials regarding any medical disability and furthermore to provide recommendations regarding its implementation to the vice president, the cabinet, and the president's legal counsel. This crucial responsibility will be addressed and analyzed in the following chapter.

An unusual and uncommon activity of the WHMU is the provision of dental and even veterinary care to the White House. The White House dentist is chosen from the dental staff at Bethesda Naval Hospital. A military veterinarian from Fort Myer, Virginia, is available to tend to the first family's pets.[43] The recent euthanasia of Spot, the Bush family's aged English springer spaniel, on the recommendation of a veterinarian, received extensive press coverage.[44]

Recent presidents, perhaps appreciative of the time-consuming nature of their personal medical well-being, have not burdened their physicians with political or health policy matters. this task is generally delegated to the Surgeon General, a political appointee. During the Covid pandemic (2020–2022), the Administration's political/medical spokesman was Dr. Anthony Fauci from the National Institutes of Health. As Ronny Jackson, presidential physician to both G.W. Bush and Obama, wrote, "It wasn't my job to have a political opinion; it was my job to make sure the president of the United States was alive and healthy."[45] This separation has not always the case. For example, Harry Truman's physician, Wallace Graham, was an attendee in at least one high level White House political gathering.[46] Moreover, Graham was encouraged to enter the health insurance debate, with unhappy consequences. And President William Howard Taft (1909–1913) did not hesitate to commandeer his personal physician, Army major Matthew Delaney, into a conference with the surgeon generals of the army and navy to determine whether a politically well-connected banker merited a compassionate medical release from federal prison.[47]

The WHMU staffs a number of facilities, the most important of which is the presidential physician's suite on the ground floor in the main section of the White House. It is located just below the state floor which contains the president's living quarters. It consists of the presidential physician's office and an adjacent examination room, both located across the hall from the president's private elevator. The president receives any on-site medical care at this location. Other WHMU sites include the Naval Observatory, which is the vice-presidential residence in Washington; the previously mentioned dispensary in the Old Executive Office Building; a dental office in the basement of the White House; a medical clinic at the Camp David presidential retreat that is a fully equipped and supplied outpatient clinic. The last venue is staffed by navy corpsmen to provide medical assistance to the military and civilian personnel assigned there, which the WHMU augments the staffing whenever the president is in residence.[48] Other supervised locations include inpatient suites at Bethesda Naval and Walter Reed hospitals; a medical annex aboard *Air Force One*; and additional airborne on-board trauma centers and operating room facilities whenever foreign countries are unable to provide such contingency services during presidential trips abroad.[49] In a colorful narrative, Reagan's physician, Burton Smith, related such an example: "When the president scheduled a one-day trip to the tiny island of Grenada more than a year after the U.S. invasion ... we checked the local medical facilities and found them to be extremely primitive. So, we created our own definitive care capability right there, because the closest first-class hospital was in Miami, and it would have taken nearly three hours to get him there in *Air Force One*. So, I had a helicopter landing ship, a kind of baby aircraft carrier, stationed less than ten minutes offshore. It had an excellent medical setup which we augmented with extra doctors, laboratory, and X-ray equipment."[50]

National security concerns have significantly affected presidential routine, particularly influencing the proximity of the physician to the president. The presidential physician often closely accompanies the chief executive during the daily work schedule, often shadowing the president in close proximity to his Secret Service detail. As an example, the presidential physician is the only individual other than the First Couple to exit the front door of *Air Force One*. All other members of the presidential staff, including the chief of staff, leave from the rear door of the airplane. In contrast to past practice a White House physician at present rides with the secret service in the car immediately following the president's in any presidential motorcade. But, in order to remain inconspicuous, the president's military physicians routinely wear civilian clothes instead of military uniforms.[51] The contemporary security environment explains the major commitment that the WHMU has invested in the planning for an appropriate and expeditious use of the disability provisions of the Twenty-fifth Amendment.

Bethesda Naval Hospital funds the WHMU and its facilities through the White House Military Office. The American taxpayer pays the salary of the presidential physician even when the physician is civilian rather than military. However, covered individuals are free to seek outside physicians and hospitals. As examples, Tipper Gore, the wife of Vice President Albert Gore (1993–2001), underwent thyroid surgery at the Johns Hopkins Hospital to remove a benign thyroid nodule,[52] and President George W. Bush's longtime family physician from Texas, Dr. Kenneth Cooper, played a prominent role in this president's annual physical examinations, serving as a medical consultant.[53] Governmental reimbursement for civilian consultants covers only their professional services, although many, including doctors Max Jacobson, Hans Kraus, J. Willis Hurst and probably Paul Dudley White, have performed their services gratis.[54] The selection of medical consultants is likely under the joint purview of the presidential physician and the presidential patient. It has been reported that Dr. Mariano had "...her own list of appropriate consultants from which she can draw, who have been approved by the president."[55] In the aftermath of Clinton's knee surgery and rehabilitation, his press secretary, Mike McCurry, illuminated the method by which contemporary presidents pay for

Chapter 12. The White House Medical Unit Continues to Evolve

their medical care. Clinton's consultant physician's bills totaled approximately $7,000, of which the president's government insurance plan paid 80 percent. The 20 percent co-payment, or approximately $1,400, was the responsibility of the president. Medical insurance deductibles and co-payments were a familiar reality for most of his constituents when confronted with medical bills. However, this president's extensive physical therapy treatments were provided gratis by the WHMU as a perquisite of the nation's chief executive, a benefit unavailable to the average citizen.[56]

The Presidential Physician works very long hours, under stressful conditions and often in very tense situations. Family life may be disrupted and marriages can sunder.[57] However, in addition to the prestige of the proximity to power, the doctor benefits from opportunities for travel and the likelihood of promotion. During Mariano's tour as presidential physician, she took fifty-one trips abroad and visited close to 100 foreign countries.[58] In the traditional acknowledgment of loyal medical service to the president, Mariano was awarded a promotion to rear admiral when she completed her tour as White House physician in 2000.[59] Subsequently, at the conclusion of their White House tours, physicians Dick Tubb and Ronny Jackson were both elevated to flag (Brigadier General and Rear Admiral rank).

During the past two decades three significant developments have occurred in the WHMU. These entail: the increased presence and prominence of Physician Assistants; the important role of female physicians; and, the fragmentation of the chain of command.

According to the American Medical Association, physician assistants (PA) always work under a physician's supervision, and are authorized to perform physical assessments, diagnose and treat illnesses, order and interpret tests, and assist in surgery. PAs also manage treatment plans, patient education, and coordination of care. Nurse practitioners (NP) depending upon state law, in addition to the scope of practice of a PA, may practice independent of a physician, and may prescribe pharmaceuticals.[60] In this regard, the trend in the WHMU mirrors the trend is physician practices nationwide. During Ronny Jackson's tenure, the number of PAs in the WHMU burgeoned from 6 to 16.[61]

Dr. Janet Travell (1961–8) was the first woman to practice in the White House; it was thirty years before Dr. Connie Mariano (1991–2001) became the second White House Physician. During the past three presidencies, women have appeared more frequently within the WHMU ranks, although none became the president's physician. However, Jennifer Pena, the eighth female doctor in the WHMU, served as the physician to Vice President Pence and his wife. Merlene Horan, Ingrid Pacowski Mulkerrin, Francesca Cimino, Jocelyn Robinson, Denise Whitfield, Jennifer Pena, Leslie Vojta, and Joanna Jackson became the 4th thru 10th WHMU women physicians. Four specialized in emergency medicine, the others either in family or internal medicine. Drs. Jackson and Whitfield assumed professorial appointments in California after their military discharges. Dr. Cimino, although remaining in the Navy, has achieved academic success in the Washington, D.C., area. Cimino, a mother of three, actively nursed one of her babies while serving in the WHMU.[62]

The numbers and complexity of responsibility at the WHMU has necessitated a divergence of presidential and first family care from the tasks of the WHMU so that no longer is it feasible for the Presidential Physician and the WHMU director to be a sole physician. The chain of command is separate. The president's physician is directed by the president; the other WHMU doctors are under the command of the WHMO director, often a nurse or physician assistant. This table of organization had the effect of Dr. Jackson's overseeing and countermanding Dr. Jennifer Pena's treatment of Mrs. Pence even though the physician did not fall under his purview. When I asked Dr. Sean Conley, he replied that his greatest challenge as President Trump's doctor was determining "who was in charge."[63]

It is apparent that the preservation of the president's health has become more comprehensive, increasingly complex, and more efficiently organized. In a word, it has become bureaucratized. It is also abundantly clear that the scope of the White House physician's responsibilities has been significantly broadened, especially with reference to the implementation of the Twenty-fifth Amendment of the United States Constitution. (See Chapter 13.)

CHAPTER 13

The Twenty-fifth Amendment and Its Impact on the White House Medical Unit

The Twenty-fifth Amendment to the United States Constitution deals with the issues of presidential succession and disability. It was first proposed in 1965, was quickly approved by the Congress, and was swiftly ratified by the requisite three-fourths of the states on February 23, 1967.[1] It has imposed a significant additional responsibility upon the White House physicians and has already been incorporated into the training and preparedness exercises of the WHMU. The presidential physician has been charged with the duty to recommend the implementation of section 4 of this amendment under clearly defined circumstances. Presidential physician Mariano explained: "Under the terms.... I play a significant role, as the president's physician, in determining medical disability and in advising the administration about the president's health."[2]

Two distinguished groups have convened panels of prestigious participants to consider, clarify, and conclude the intent and implementation of this amendment. The Miller Center for Public Affairs of the University of Virginia held forums from 1985 through 1993, whose proceedings have been published in four monographs.[3] A separate organization, the Working Group on Presidential Disability, held symposia at the Carter Center of Emory University, Wake Forest University, and the White House during 1995 and 1996.[4] Subsequently, political science professor Robert Gilbert edited a compilation of essays by the amendment's framers, previous and present presidential physicians, and other knowledgeable experts regarding its implementation.[5]

More recently, Fordham Law professor Robert Feerick published the third edition of his comprehensive history and applications of the Twenty-fifth Amendment.[6] A few years later, Brian Kalt's "Unable" focused on the law, politics and limits of its Section 4, its most controversial, and so far, its only invoked section.[7] In this chapter the evolution, provisions, and previous usage of the Twenty-fifth Amendment is discussed, to be followed both by an exposition of the dilemmas its utilization poses to the WHMU and by a discussion of possible solutions.

The series of significant illnesses that befell President Eisenhower and the subsequent assassination of his successor, John Kennedy, the latter event creating an unfilled vacancy in the vice presidency, were the immediate impulses leading to the Twenty-fifth Amendment. Kennedy, whose demise led to the elevation to the presidency of the incumbent vice president, was the eighth United States president to die in office. Additionally, another eight vice presidents either died or resigned prior to 1965. As a consequence, the vice presidency, established primarily to provide an assured and predictable replacement for a deceased president, had itself been vacant for 37½ of the Republic's first 168 years.[8] Although the departures of vice presidents Clinton, Gerry, King, Hendricks, Wilson, Hobart, Sherman and Calhoun were unfortunate—at least for them—the luck of the Republic prevented an even greater misfortune by providentially protecting the welfare of those presidents who served without an elected successor. Moreover, several presidents had been disabled while in office, and the fact of their disability had been masked not only from the electorate but also from members of the disabled president's own administration! Previous chapters profiled the complicity of several White House physicians in this politically expedient deception.

The Presidential Succession Act of 1947 sought to clarify the line of succession to the White House in the event of the death of the president when the vice presidency was unfilled. According to this act, the Speaker of the House of Representatives was designated to be next in line of succession, followed by the president pro tempore of the Senate (the most senior member of the majority party). Inevitable political conflict would have ensued if either of these incumbents represented a different political party than that of the deceased president.[9]

The Twenty-fifth Amendment contains four sections, which become progressively more complex in interpretation and enforcement. Sections one and two already have been verified by their appropriate use and do not involve the participation of a White House physician. Section one states: "In case of the removal of the president from office or his death or resignation, the vice president shall become president."[10] John Tyler in 1841 was the first of nine vice presidents to ascend to the presidency, when the office became vacant upon the death of President William Henry Harrison.

Section two has been implemented smoothly twice, in 1973 and 1974, to fill a vice presidential vacancy. "Whenever there is a vacancy in the office of the vice president, the president shall nominate a vice president who shall take the office upon confirmation by a majority vote of both houses of Congress."[11]

After the forced resignation of Vice President Spiro Agnew, Congressman Gerald Ford was nominated as vice president designate by Richard Nixon. The House and Senate quickly confirmed the nominee after brief hearings. After Gerald Ford succeeded to the presidency as the thirty-eighth U.S. president, upon Richard Nixon's resignation, Ford in turn nominated former New York governor Nelson A. Rockefeller as his successor.[12] The controversial Rockefeller underwent four months of congressional scrutiny before confirmation in December 1974.[13]

Sections three and four, however, require the intimate involvement of the presidential physician. A consultative role is required for the invocation of section three and a substantial, decisive, and possibly career-damaging involvement for the appropriate implementation of section four. Section three has been considered on at least eight occasions since 1982, but it has been invoked correctly only on three occasions. It declares that: "Whenever the president transmits to the president pro tempore of the Senate and Speaker of the House of Representatives his written declaration that he is unable to discharge the powers and duties of his office, and until he transmits to them a written declaration to the contrary, such powers and duties shall be discharged by the vice president as acting president."[14]

Chapter 10 of this book has already recorded the total disregard of section three by the members of the inexperienced Reagan administration at the time of the assassination attempt on March 30, 1981.

Prior to Reagan's colonoscopy in July 1985 that detected a cancer of the colon, Dr. Burton Smith attended a meeting with his assistant, Dr. John Hutton, chief of staff Don Regan, presidential counsel Fred Fielding, and acting press secretary Larry Speakes. The meeting was to determine the applicability of section three. Smith advised that its invocation was unnecessary since, although the president would be drowsy, "he could be roused at any time even though he might feel that as though he had just had two martinis."[15] As a result, section three of the amendment was not invoked. However, after a biopsy obtained at the colonoscopy detected cancer, extensive colon surgery was scheduled. President Reagan did submit letters to the speaker of the House and president pro tempore of the Senate that appointed Vice President George Bush as acting president. Yet Reagan sidestepped being the first to apply section three: "After consultation with my Counsel and the Attorney General, I am mindful of the provisions of Section 3 of the Twenty-fifth Amendment to the Constitution and of the uncertainties of its application to such brief and temporary periods of incapacity. I did not believe that the drafters of this amendment intended its application to situations such as the instant one."[16] Smith was not present when the appropriate letters were signed by the president after his surgery to regain the powers of his office.[17]

Presidents George H. Bush and Bill Clinton also underwent medical treatments that provoked consideration of section three. In 1991 Bush developed an extremely rapid heart rate, clinically known as atrial fibrillation, which was caused by a previously undetected hyperthyroidism. Control of the heart rate was initially intractable to medications and consideration was given to cardioversion under general anesthesia in order to normalize the heart rate. Since the president would have remained unconscious, a decision to institute a cardioversion would have initiated section three of the Twenty-fifth Amendment. As noted previously, certain segments of the press, and large parts of the public panicked over the possibility that Vice President Dan Quayle, much scorned by elements of both, would have the opportunity to be acting president. However, drug therapy was successful in controlling Bush's abnormal heart rhythm, and more dramatic treatment became unnecessary.[18]

In March 1997 President Clinton tore his quadriceps tendon while vacationing in Florida. Under spinal anesthesia, a two-hour operation to repair the tendon took place on March 14 at Bethesda Naval Hospital. Due to the selection of an anesthetic that would not affect the president's consciousness or his cognitive abilities, it became unnecessary to invoke section three, which would have turned presidential powers over to Vice President Albert Gore.[19]

President George W. Bush on June 29, 2002, correctly invoked section three for the first time when he temporarily transferred the powers of the presidency to his vice president, Dick Cheney. Bush was scheduled to be under sedation for several hours during a colonoscopy examination at Camp David. The transfer of power under the Twenty-fifth Amendment was authorized after consultation with the presidential physician, Colonel Richard Tubb, and the White House Counsel, Alberto Gonzales. The applicable letters relinquishing and then reclaiming the powers of the presidency were sent by fax from Camp David to Capitol Hill. The entire event passed without any political or medical incident.

Dick Tubb had foreseen that his patient would require a diagnostic colonoscopy under general anesthesia as part of presidential physical examination. A previous exam prior to his presidency had disclosed many benign polyps (tubular adenomas) in his colon. The president was a "polyp producer" whose large intestine required frequent cancer screenings. Concerned that the anesthetic Versed, commonly employed during these procedures, was a narcotic that might hinder the president's thought process for up to twenty-four hours, the doctor searched for an alternative, selecting Propofol. It had a very short half-life that permitted a rapid conscious recovery.[20]

Tubb carefully prepared for his patient's required screening large intestinal examination. He extensively reviewed the relevant scientific literature, consulted national experts and sought out neurologist opinion regarding an appropriate cognitive protocol. On a Friday evening, Dr. Tubb and his team assembled at the White House to perform a "dry run" using propofol and a protocol to test the patient's cognitive ability. The patient was Doctor Richard Tubb.[21]

Dr. Tubb had employed a neurologist to assess Bush's brain function as part of the president's first physical examination. This assessment would set the standard to determine when Bush regained the mental competence to perform the executive functions of the presidency. Armed with this comprehensive preparation, section three of the amendment was invoked. Bush regained presidential powers two hours and fifteen minutes after temporarily assigning them to Vice President Cheney.[22] A second colonoscopy was performed five years later in July 2007, again at Camp David, Maryland. The same protocols were adhered to as previously. Five benign polyps (tubular adenomas) were resected. The entire procedure was uneventful. This time the vice president was acting president for two hours, five minutes.[23]

Dr. Kevin O'Connor oversaw the third implementation of section 3 when President Joe Biden was anesthetized during a colonoscopy on November 20, 2021. Biden, too, possessed a history of colon polyps. A single benign polyp was removed. O'Connor reported through the president's press secretary, "Consistent with carefully planned and well-established practices, presidential powers were temporarily transferred to Vice President Harris in accordance with the 25th amendment, transfer of authority occurred at 1010 hours, and President Biden assumed presidential authority at 1135 hours." The criteria employed to demonstrate Biden's regain of cerebral function was not disclosed.[24] Richard Tubb apparently had established the proper presidential physician's protocols for application of section 3.

Section four has never been invoked, but the recent presidencies of Donald Trump and Joe Biden have provoked discussion in disparate quarters about whether it should be. The somewhat erratic and occasional controversial verbal and text messages of the former, and the age, unusual instances of physical debility, and frequent confusion of the latter have stimulated these conversations. These controversies will be addressed later in this chapter.

The section's ambiguities have occasioned much discussion.[25] The doctor-patient relationship and the corollary matter of the limits of patient confidentiality, if any, have been part of these conversations. A perusal of section four's text (below) demonstrates why this section may be controversial or confusing. The provisions for its implementation are definitely complicated.

> Whenever the vice president and a majority of either the principal officers of the executive departments or of such other body as Congress may by law provide, transmit to the president pro tempore of the Senate and the Speaker of the House of Representatives their written

declaration that the president is unable to discharge the powers and duties of his office, the vice president shall immediately assume the powers and duties of the office as acting president.

Thereafter, when the president transmits to the president pro tempore of the Senate and the Speaker of the House of Representatives his written declaration that no disability exists, he shall resume the powers and duties of his office unless the vice president and a majority of either the principal officers of the executive department or of any such body as Congress by law provide transmit within four days to the president pro tempore of the Senate and the Speaker of the House of Representatives their written declaration that the president is unable to discharge the powers and duties of his office. Thereupon Congress shall decide the issue, assembling within forty-eight hours for that purpose if not in session, If the Congress, within twenty-one days after the receipt of the latter written declaration, or if Congress is not in session, within twenty-one days after Congress is required to assemble, determines by two-thirds vote of both houses that the president is unable to discharge the powers and duties of his office, the vice president shall continue to discharge the same as acting president; otherwise the president shall resume the powers and duties of his office.

Writers of fiction have used section four's complicated imprecision to concoct many differing plot lines that involve a disabled president, reluctance to transfer power, or a vice president's disinclination to assume the executive functions of the presidency when the president is incommunicado or missing.[26]

The Working Group on Presidential Disability issued nine recommendations at the conclusion of its meetings. Its recommendation four both empowers and burdens the presidential physician:

> The assessment of impairment is a medical responsibility. The physician to the president is responsible, with the assistance of appropriate medical and nonmedical consultants, for determining and documenting the extent to which impairment might affect the cognition, judgment, behavior, and communication abilities of the president. The physician to the president should communicate and interpret these findings to the constitutionally designated decision makers responsible for determining presidential inability under the provisions of the Twenty-fifth Amendment.[27]

Although the physician to the president clearly has been assigned the responsibility of determining whether or not the president is medically impaired, it is likely that the presidential physician may find himself conflicted in fulfilling this task. The relationship between the president and his personal physician is likely to be one of extraordinary intimacy. In the past, a close social and personal relationship with the president has, as prior chapters document, dulled physician objectivity regarding the medical status of the presidential patient. No less a figure than ex-president Jimmy Carter has had serious doubts that a White House physician would divulge medical information under the appropriate circumstances, citing his close relationship with his presidential physician.

Significant conflict also resides in the military chain of command. In recent years, with only one exception (O'Connor) not only the presidential physician but all WHMU doctors have been military officers. The president is not only their patient but also their commander in chief, thereby able to exercise a two-track command upon his physician. One wonders whether a military doctor would have the courage to disobey a command of his superior officer. Additionally, it has become a tradition for presidents to reward their military physicians with a promotion to general or admiral rank at the conclusion of their loyal service. Could this persuade a doctor to rethink his responsibilities under this amendment?

The aforementioned conflicts were deemed insurmountable in a minority report of the Working Group. This report recommended the creation of a consulting commission on the health of the president. It ideally would be composed of a panel of dispassionate expert physicians who would, according to this report, "...provide consultative advice and support to the president's physician and ... report to the public on the state of the president's health in the event that the question of impairment arose." However, after considerable discussion, this opinion was rejected, and the final report of The Working Group hopefully concluded that a combination of the intent of the law, the knowledge of the provisions of the amendment, and the increased professionalization of the WHMU would assure that section four would be implemented correctly and appropriately. The Working Group correctly decided this matter in the view of the author.

A second difficulty with section four concerned the lifting of the veil of confidentiality that has always been an important feature of the physician-patient transaction. The tradition of confidentiality dates from the Oath of Hippocrates in the fourth century BC. The oath contains the following prohibition: "What I may see or hear in the course of the treatment in regard to the life of men, which on no account one must spread abroad, I will keep to myself, holding such things shameful to be spoken about."[28] Traditionally, an expectation of confidentiality has been critical in securing a patient's trust. Trust is necessary for a patient to confide significant but potentially embarrassing medical history.[29] But the increasing complexity of society has produced dilemmas regarding the balancing of the public good with an absolute privacy of information. The American College of Physicians Ethics Manual has stated: "The physician must not release information without the patient's consent, unless required by the law or if there is a duty to warn another. Confidentiality, like other ethical duties, is not absolute. It may have to be overridden to protect others or the public."[30]

Currently, the confidentiality privilege must be breached by law in the reporting of gunshot wounds, knife wounds, suspected child abuse, and the reporting of certain communicable diseases. Moreover, a 1976 court ruling in California held that a psychotherapist had the duty to protect individuals from patients who express intent to harm them.[31] Consequently, it should follow that the citizens must be protected from the actions of a president who might be unable to make appropriate life or death decisions. Confidentiality must be limited by the need for the protection of public safety and the public welfare, as Leonard Emmerglick elegantly summarized: "The protective privilege ends where the public peril begins."[32]

Recommendation three of the Working Group proposed that "a formal contingency plan for the implementation of the Amendment should be in place before the inauguration of every president."[33] Burton Lee, anticipating the appropriateness of this proposal, dealt with the issues of presidential disability and the transfer of power soon after George H. Bush was inaugurated in 1989. Lee met with the president, the vice president, the chief of staff, the head of the White House military office, the president's counsel, and the coordinator of White House operations. According to Dr. Lee, a common understanding of the issues of presidential disability was arrived at: "We decided the point man would be the chief of staff, and he would make all the arrangements. The counsel would draw up the requisite documents." Both the president and vice president agreed with this plan.[34]

Several years later, Dr. Mariano participated in the contingency meetings of the Clinton administration that were held to review the implementation plans in the case of presidential disability. Medical historians James Toole and Robert Joynt observed, "It was their feeling that they would definitely include the physician in those plans, in terms of determining the disability of the president should any illness, impairment, or disability fall upon him."[35] As a result, Mariano, shortly after selection as presidential physician, discussed the Clinton administration's Twenty-fifth Amendment plan with its chief of staff, legal counsel, and members of the Presidential Contingency Program, an organization run by the military whose main function is the preservation of the Office of the President.[36] Furthermore, Mariano ensured that the White House staff and the WHMU members were thoroughly informed regarding the Twenty-fifth Amendment. During her tenure, every WHMU exercise and emergency drill ended with the question: Should the Twenty-fifth Amendment be invoked?[37] All succeeding presidents together with their physicians and appropriate senior staff assuredly have continued this practice shortly after inauguration.

Presidents Donald Trump (2017–2021) and Joe Biden (2021–2025) continue to invite allegations of an inability to discharge their oath of office. Both were besieged by claims of disability by their political and media enemies. However, in the case of the 45th president, constitutional claims of disability were used inappropriately. Trump was not incapacitated but simply was accused of doing political bad things.[38] Moreover, his personal style was raucous, confrontational, direct, and occasionally offensive before and after he entered the White House. The refined tastes of the Capitol and media elites may have been repelled by the brash New Yorker's style.

Yale psychiatrist Dr. Bandy Lee was one of the first critics to propose that his personality traits might produce the "greatest possible harm." In 2017, she edited a book which contained twenty-seven essays by psychologists and psychiatrists that called this president "a clear and present danger."[39] In response, Dr. Maria Oquendo, president of the American Psychiatric Association, chastised Lee for breaching its "Goldwater Rule" that deemed it unethical and irresponsible to offer professional opinions on people who were not properly examined in person.[40]

In May 2017 after the President fired FBI Director James Comey, Deputy Attorney General Rod Rosenstein and FBI Assistant Director conspired to remove Trump from office. Rosenstein considered wearing a wire to record disabling or unconstitutional statements.[41]

Twenty-fifth Amendment concerns subsided somewhat after Presidential Physician Jackson publicized Trump's perfect score on the Montreal Cognitive Assessment for mental ability. However, cries of inability rose again during the last six months of his single presidential term. First during his hospitalization with Covid, and in the aftermath of the January 6, 2021, occupation of the U.S. Capitol Building.[42]

Joe Biden became an octogenarian in January 2023, becoming by far the oldest serving American president. His 2019 pre-presidential examination and his 2022 and 2023 presidential examinations when he was seventy-six, seventy-nine, and eighty years of age respectively did not contain any specific mention of his mental function. Cognitive test results were not revealed at the conclusion of any of these examinations.

Earlier, during the 2020 Democrat nomination contests or the 2020 presidential campaign, Biden's mental state was questioned, and suggestions of dementia were posed.[43]

During the initial more than three years of his presidency, Biden's verbal gaffes, non-recall of significant names, word salad in verbal communications and apparent lack of awareness continued. The press and political partisans looked the other way. But, in a break from the uniform media narrative, The *Washington Times* refused to characterize his incomprehensive mumblings and numerous gaffes as, "Oh, that's just Joe Biden's inherent political routine."[44]

Increasingly, the public became concerned about the president's mental health. An August 2022 survey by the *New York Post* found 56 percent of respondents were worried about Biden's mental health. A previous poll in September 2021 disclosed that 48 percent were not confident that he had the mental soundness to serve effectively as president.[45] Former Presidential Physician and current Texas Congressman Ronny Jackson together with other congressmen repeatedly has questioned Biden's cognitive ability to perform his responsibilities, while calling for cognitive testing.[46]

Two substantive areas of inquiry, arising from the above analysis of presidential disability and succession, require discussion. One concerns the psychological evaluation of a chief executive who may be crippled by a psychiatric illness. Chapter 14 probes this fascinating issue at length. Second, the health of the vice president has been an underreported and often neglected part of the American historical narrative. The telling of its story in chapter 15 may assist in completing the discussions of both the White House physician's duties and of the complexities of the Twenty-fifth Amendment.

Chapter 14

Psychiatry and the Presidency

In August 1974, during the last act of the Nixon impeachment drama, Nixon's son-in-law, Edward Cox, telephoned Republican Senator Robert Griffin to discuss Richard Nixon's mental state. "Cox sounded distraught. He was worried about the President's mental health. The President was not sleeping, and he had been drinking. The man couldn't take it much longer, Cox said. The President had been acting irrationally.... Cox continued: 'The President was up walking the halls last night, talking to pictures of former Presidents—giving speeches and talking to the pictures on the wall.'"[1]

More than a century earlier on Inauguration Day 1853, President Franklin Pierce, emotionally distraught for a very different reason—in his case, a family tragedy—felt compelled to include in his address a reference to the recent accidental death of his son: "It is a relief to feel that no heart but my own can know the personal regret and bitter sorrow over which I have been borne to a position so suitable for others rather than desirable for myself." He explained to the assemblage that his grief and the shock of the accident had left him both tired and "in an unfortunate state of mind."[2]

In any discussion of the appropriate application of sections three and four of the Twenty-fifth Amendment, presidential disability produced by cognitive, emotional, or psychological factors is considered, albeit gingerly and delicately. Mental disease traditionally has been and continues to remain a sensitive matter when the health of a public figure is at issue. Despite many instances of presidential mental distress, with one exception, psychiatry is a specialty that has not been represented among the expertise of the presidential physicians, although even more abstruse specialties such as neurosurgery, physiatry, and oncology have been.[3]

A recent conference convened to consider changes to the amendment heard the following critique of presidential physicians' competence in this area:

> ...that with all the expertise of the individuals who have served in this unenviable role, when it comes to mental disability, i.e., behavioral disturbance that might affect decisions, not one of those presidential physicians has had the necessary training in either psychiatry or neurology to assume the preeminent role that they have.[4]

"Should we have a psychiatrist in residence at the White House?" was a question posed to psychiatrist Dr. C. Knight Aldrich during a May 1992 seminar on presidential disability. Dr. Aldrich responded that "any president would benefit from having a professional counselor in whom he or she could confide and not fear that it would go any further." However, he concluded that political and personal reasons would conclusively negate any such possibility. In his view, the type of successful individual likely to achieve the presidency is unlikely to acknowledge the presence of those personal vulnerabilities that would benefit from such treatment.[5]

In this context, this chapter will explore the relevance of psychiatry to the implementation of the Twenty-fifth Amendment; examine the political effects of any whiff of mental disability upon the politician so tainted, correctly or not, by this scent; trace the development of American psychiatry as a medical specialty; and summarize those instances when a president may have suffered from mental or emotional impairment.

Mental illness may be the "elephant in the room" in any political discussion regarding the invocation of sections three or four. Neither of these sections precisely defines what is meant by disability, possibly because its framers foresaw that strict constitutional language might not be adaptable to either all future political circumstances or subsequent unforeseen advances in medical diagnosis and treatment. Gilbert concluded that presidential illness, psychological as well as physical, temporary as well as permanent, is at the core of both sections. As examples of the former he listed intense grief over the loss of a loved one, severe distraction caused by a protracted impeachment proceeding, severe dementia, and other unnamed major psychological disorders.[6] Abrams perceptively listed several conditions, relevant to this discussion, when these sections should be invoked: the use of psychoactive drugs in significant amounts, including narcotics, tranquilizers, amphetamines and barbiturates; death or serious illness in the patient's immediate family; and the diagnosis of Alzheimer's disease or of any progressive, mentally disabling conditions.[7]

Senator Birch Bayh, an author of this amendment, was skeptical about any expert's ability to determine whether a president was mentally unfit to perform his duties, since such a judgment would necessitate nearly continuous observations of the subject in interactions with others in different circumstances. In his opinion, the signs of mental illness are often transient, coming and going depending upon the environment, or gradual and insidious, and probably undetectable even to the presidential physician who sees the patient daily.[8]

An almost insurmountable impediment against the use of appropriate psychological diagnosis and treatment is the attitude of the president's closest advisers. They have a collective need for their leader to be perceived as wise, decisive, and in control. Illnesses that affect the leader's mental processes and emotional control would be perceived as especially threatening and might likely be concealed.[9] The testimony of at least one White House physician corroborates this: "We thought, collectively, that clearly a president who suffers from a situational depression, for example, and receives the proper treatment … may not be impaired to the degree that he can no longer perform his duties."[10]

A recommendation has been made to alleviate the potential conflict of a presidential physician who may have to make a medical determination about whether a sitting president is psychologically or emotionally disabled. The recommendation suggested that a group of impairment physician-specialists be selected or appointed *prior* to the formation of an incoming president's administration, to include two psychiatrists and two neurologists in addition to two internists with demonstrable expertise in hypertensive and cardiopulmonary pathophysiology, and the presidential physician.[11]

There is a good political reason for presidential staffs to consider a host of words, including "psychiatry," "psychological," "emotional," "paranoid," and "counseling," as pejorative when applied to their leaders. The national election campaigns of 1964, 1972 and 1988 provided proof of the damaging and diverting effects of these words.

Presidential candidates Barry Goldwater (1964) and Michael Dukakis (1988) lost their campaigns for the presidency for many reasons, but both had to contend with attacks upon their mental capacities. The overwhelming uproar over vice-presidential candidate Senator Thomas Eagleton's prior therapy for depression resulted in his resignation from the Democratic ticket in 1972; however, the hapless George McGovern undoubtedly would have lost the election even without this diversion. A further example which illustrates the stigma attached to this subject occurred during the consideration of Gerald Ford as the vice-presidential replacement of the disgraced Spiro Agnew. The former needed to refute an allegation that he had been treated by a psychiatrist.[12]

"Is Barry Goldwater psychologically fit to be President of the United States?" headlined an ad for *Fact* magazine that appeared in the *New York Times* in mid–September of the 1964 presidential campaign.[13] The magazine polled 12,356 psychiatrists for their answers to this question. Of the 2,417 responses it received, 1,189 psychiatrists answered this question with a "no," 657 with a "yes," and 571 claimed insufficient knowledge for an answer. *Fact* sought to buttress its negative view of the Goldwater candidacy with forty-one pages of selective hostile comments from its respondents. Both the American Medical Association and the American Psychiatric Association (APA) immediately assailed the poll. In a letter to *Fact*, the leaders of the APA wrote: "By attaching the stigma of extreme political partisanship to the psychiatric profession as a whole in the heated climate of the current political campaign, *Fact* has in effect administered a low blow to all who would advance the treatment and care of the mentally ill in America."[14] Afterward, the APA went further, issuing the so-called Goldwater Rule, which strongly advised its members that it was unethical for psychiatrists to offer a professional opinion unless the psychiatrist had personally conducted an examination of the patient and had been granted proper authorization for such a statement.[15]

Rumors floated about Michael Dukakis' losing presidential campaign that this Democratic candidate had been treated previously for depression. Dukakis refused to release his personal medical records following reports that he had sought treatment for depression after his brother Stellian died in 1973, and after his defeat in the campaign for the Massachusetts governorship in 1978.[16] Outgoing President Ronald Reagan, inadvertently or not, amplified the public discourse over the matter. In responding to reporters' questions regarding these rumors, Reagan responded, "Look, I'm not going to pick on an invalid." Both the Dukakis campaign and his personal physician were compelled to dismiss both the rumors and the departing president's remarks, thus diverting resources from the election campaign, at least temporarily.[17]

The singular event that extirpated all deferential reference to mental disease and psychiatry from White House political dialogue was the forced declination of the vice-presidential nomination by Senator Thomas Eagleton after he had been voted on by the 1972 Democratic national convention. Eagleton thereby became only the third man in American history to decline this nomination so offered.[18] Thomas Eagleton, a United States senator from Missouri and previously both the attorney general and lieutenant governor of that state, was compelled by mounting political pressure to exit the campaign a mere eighteen days after his selection.[19] On July 25, the then vice-presidential nominee revealed that he had been hospitalized three times between 1960 and 1966 for "nervous exhaustion and fatigue." He further disclosed the more politically damaging information that he had undergone psychiatric treatment in the form of electroshock therapy for depression on two or three occasions. He thereby claimed the dubious distinction of being the first national candidate to admit that he had undergone psychiatric treatment.[20]

After forcing Eagleton's departure, George McGovern, the doomed Democratic nominee, claimed disingenuously that Eagleton's health had not been a factor in the decision![21] Yet, a clamor had developed for Eagleton to leave, including a newspaper interview with Dr. M. Ostrow, past president of the Psychoanalytic Research and Development Fund. In that interview Ostrow concluded that Eagleton's history of mental illness limited his reliability and might impair his decision making.[22] Subsequent to this debacle, Eagleton was twice reelected as a U.S. senator from Missouri and authored two books on the Constitution.[23]

The controversy over whether a prior history of psychotherapy should eliminate one from national leadership reemerged a year later during Gerald Ford's confirmation hearings. In the first use of section two of the Twenty-fifth Amendment, Michigan, congressman Gerald Ford was nominated by President Nixon to replace Spiro Agnew as vice president, after Agnew's resignation. Congressmen questioned Ford, as well as psychiatrist Dr. Arnold Hutschnecker, over allegations that the doctor had treated Ford for emotional problems. Both testified that the allegation was false and that the two had but a single social contact at the doctor's New York office.[24]

A recent telephone survey of voter opinion disclosed that political attitudes toward candidates with mood disorders have not changed. The opinion poll reported: "In a telephone survey in July and August [2002], researchers interviewed 1,200 randomly selected adults. They found that 24 percent of respondents would not vote for a political candidate with a mood disorder, and an equal percentage 'might not vote' for such a candidate. Further, 25 percent said they believe that people with mood disorders are dangerous, can easily be identified in the workplace, and cannot form and maintain long-term, stable relationships. A fifth [19 percent] said that people with mood disorders should not have children."[25]

The combined accrediting organization, the American Board of Psychiatry and Neurology, was established in 1934. The relationship between what previously and presently have been commonly recognized as discrete but tenuously related specialties had been rocky, but a need to defend their respective professional turfs from encroachment by nonphysicians compelled their alliance. Elsewhere, as in the United Kingdom, members of these specialties maintain two separate and discrete accrediting organizations. In the United States, physicians who expect to practice psychiatry alone sit for the psychiatry examination; aspiring neurologists take a separate neurology qualifying test; and the few who desire a combined neuropsychiatry specialty practice are required to pass both the neurology and the psychiatry board examinations.[26]

Benjamin Rush, that near ubiquitous early American physician who has flitted about but has thus far escaped becoming stuck to this narrative, is considered the founding father of American psychiatry. Rush probably delivered the first lectures on mental disorders in America when he lectured Pennsylvania medical students on insanity. His talks were published in 1812 under the title *Medical Inquiries and Observations Upon the Disease of the Mind*, the first psychiatry textbook written on this continent.[27]

Until the late nineteenth century in America, psychiatrists were primarily superintendents of institutionally based asylums, while neurologists identified themselves with European scientific medicine and maintained office practices, principally in urban areas, and possessed their academic positions. Neurologists of this period considered themselves perfectly capable of handling mental illnesses. In the early decades of the twentieth century, psychiatrists began to look beyond the confines of mental hospitals and to begin to realign themselves with the broad practice of medicine. However, it was not until the 1930s that there was a marked improvement in the teaching of psychiatry in U.S. medical schools.[28]

A recent analysis of the frequency of mental illness in U.S. presidents appeared in the January 2006 issue of *The Journal of Nervous and Mental Disease*. Of thirty-seven presidents examined, a remarkable eighteen (49 percent) met criteria that suggested a diagnosis of a psychiatric illness at some time during their lives. Ten presidents (27 percent) manifested illness during their presidential terms; the authors suggested that in most of these cases, presidential job performance may have been impaired.[29]

Certainly, many past presidents suffered from emotional, psychological, and dependency problems which, in today's society, would have impelled most average citizens to seek counseling or psychiatric assistance. Manic depression (John Adams), chronic depression (John Quincy Adams and Abraham Lincoln), situational depression over the loss of a child (John Adams, John Quincy Adams, Franklin Pierce, Abraham Lincoln, and Calvin Coolidge), paranoid personality disorder (Richard Nixon), alcoholism (Franklin Pierce and Richard Nixon), amphetamine and steroid misuse (John Kennedy), and alleged sex addiction (Bill Clinton) have been identified as likely presidential disorders.

In a 1783 letter to Robert Livingstone, Benjamin Franklin famously described John Adams: "He means well for his country, is always an honest man, often a wise man, but sometimes and in some things, absolutely out of his senses."[30] In 1799 President Adams departed Philadelphia, the then capital city, for Peacefield, his Quincy, Massachusetts, home, where he remained for seven months before returning. While there he exhibited many of the classic symptoms of depression—loss of appetite, loss of weight, prominent irritability and testiness, apparent melancholy and anxiety over illness and death. While in this mood he launched prosecutions against two authors who had published attacks against his administration, and tongue-lashed Harvard students who traveled from Boston to wish him well.[31] Adams's second son, Charles, had become an alcoholic and was banished by his father.[32]

Adams's oldest son, John Quincy, the sixth president of the United States, had a decades-long engagement with depression. A major biographer wrote that in 1805 "... his mood soon sank into melancholia. Once again he heaped reproaches upon himself for what he called unmethodical and frivolous reading and study ... he claimed to see only mediocrity and failure ahead."[33] Later, about 1819, this biographer noted that "he wondered whether this susceptibility to distraction was one of the weaknesses which D. Rush, in his work upon the mind, describes as naturally leading to madness."[34] John Quincy Adams's presidency (1825–1829) has generally been considered both by historians and by Adams himself to have been an unsuccessful one. He experienced great disappointment, moodiness, an almost complete loss of appetite, loss of sleep, and a general apathy.[35] Finally, his biographer commented: "...the bitter disappointments and frustrations of both his presidency and his fatherhood had brought Adams near to mental and physical collapse ... he described an 'uncontrollable dejection of spirits.' He asserted that the depression was now so severe that he had begun to experience 'a sluggish carelessness of life, an imaginary wish that it were terminated.'"[36] Both presidents Adams, father and son, also agonized over having dissolute sons who died around the conclusions of their respective presidencies.[37]

The forgettable presidency of the nation's fourteenth president, Franklin Pierce (1853–1857), was marked by the accidental preinaugural death of the Pierces' sole surviving son, Ben, and by the president's chronic flirtation with alcoholism. Nichols's biography summarized the depth of Pierce's depression in semi-histrionic fashion: "It is difficult to express adequately the effect which this ... tragedy worked upon the President-elect. It became the fact of greatest importance in his life, troubling his conscience, unsettling him almost completely, and weakening his self-confidence for many months to come ... he was distracted and worn by heart-searching. Burdened with a dead weight of hopeless sorrow, he entered his office fearfully.... Much of the difficulties which he experienced in his administration during the next four years may be attributed to this terrible tragedy and its long-continued after effects."[38]

Pierce had long battled alcoholism and many authors assert that alcohol dependence followed him into the White House as he sought to deal with his depression. The most telling evidence for his dependence is found in an 1853 letter from John Forney to James Buchanan: "Pierce has had a fine reception but I deeply, deeply deplore his habits. He drinks deep. My heart bleeds for him for he is a gallant and generous spirit. The place overshadows him. He is crushed by its great duties and he seeks refuge.... His experience convinces me that a great mistake was made in putting him in at all."[39]

Calvin Coolidge was yet another president who suffered from depression over the death of a son. Coolidge, ascending to the presidency upon the death of Warren Harding in 1923, was elected in his own right as president in 1924. However, a personal disaster devastated Coolidge's psyche and damaged the efficacy of his presidency. The Coolidges' younger son, sixteen-year-old Calvin Jr. died from septicemia, an overwhelming blood infection, on July 7, 1924, just a few days after the family attended a baseball game together and enjoyed a cruise on the Potomac River.[40]

Robert Gilbert's analysis of the aftermath of his son's unexpected death concluded flatly that "Coolidge had entered into a state of clinical depression from which he never recovered."[41] In arriving at this conclusion, Gilbert matched Coolidge's symptoms with the American Psychiatric Association's criteria for the diagnosis of a major depressive episode. Coolidge, previously an ambitious and extremely conscientious public servant, became uninterested, disengaged, and withdrawn from his responsibilities. His eating habits were erratic, resulting in uncharacteristic weight gain. After July 1924 Coolidge slept up to eleven hours each night; additionally, a daytime nap, lasting up to four hours, became routine. He was always tired, worn out, and walked with a slow gait, in contrast to his previous dynamism. Indecisiveness, increased taciturnity, and frequent irrational temper tantrums also characterized his second term. Moreover, he became a hypochondriac, insisting that his physicians check his pulse twice daily.[42]

All four of these presidents grieved over the death of a child. According to Aldrich, "Grief reaction is one of the most responsive if not the most responsive to psychotherapy." This psychiatrist lamented the fact that President Coolidge did not have access to a psychiatrist, who might have assisted the president in controlling his depression and thereby resuscitating his presidency.

Abraham Lincoln's depression is well known[43] and was subjected recently to a book-length analysis by Jonathan Shenk.[44] The author traced the development of the president's depression (melancholy) through three periods. A severe clinical depression of Lincoln's young manhood characterized the first period. The second involved the treatments, mainly self-directed, mobilized to control and direct his depression. The third period was one in which his melancholy was fashioned in such a way as to contribute to Lincoln's accomplishments as a public figure.[45] Lincoln carried his depression with him into the White House. As president he told a friend that "he sometimes thought his only escape would be to hang himself from a tree."[46] After the Army of the Potomac's debacle at Fredericksburg, his face was depicted as "darkened with particular pain."[47] In the summer of 1863, Mary Lincoln's dressmaker remarked, "His step was slow and heavy, and his face sad."[48] An added psychological burden was the death of Willie, the Lincolns' favorite child in January 1862.[49]

Lincoln employed many devices to channel his depression in positive directions, which included poetry and humor. However, he also sought medical attention for his depressive symptoms. A journal article indicated that bed rest[50] and the ingestion of "blue pills," which probably contained mercury as its active ingredient, were the professionals' prescriptions for his melancholy.[51] A 1973 letter to the editor of the *American Journal of Psychiatry* opined that "he would probably have received antidepressants or electroconvulsive treatments if such therapy had been available then."[52] However, historians overwhelmingly have concluded that the sixteenth president of the United States managed his office very well without the intervention of any psychiatric assistance.

Richard Nixon, the thirty-seventh American president (1969–1974) and the only inhabitant of that office to have resigned from it, probably exhibited the strangest behavior of all during his lengthy political career.[53] Therefore, it is no surprise that this complex politician holds the somewhat dubious distinction of being one of the few presidents to have his psyche subjected to a psychobiography.[54] In this tome psychotherapists and historians Volkan, Itzkowitz, and Dod subjected Nixon's life to psychiatric analysis. Their chapter ten, "The Final Face: Enemies Everywhere," explored what they considered to be "Nixon's third face, that of his paranoid self."[55] They concluded that his decisions to install a taping system in the Oval Office, to establish the secret "plumbers" crew, and, finally, to authorize the Watergate cover-up all resulted from his paranoia.[56]

Paranoid personality disorder is characterized by the following: marked distrust of others, including the belief, without reason, that others are exploiting, harming, or trying to deceive him or her; lack of trust; belief of others' betrayal; belief in hidden meanings; unforgiving; and grudge holding.[57] This behavioral pattern has the potential, should it clasp a sitting president tightly in its grip, to lead to dangerous consequences. Jerrold Post voiced such fears: "During the last days of Watergate, the pressure on President Nixon was immense. According to memoir reports, he was drinking heavily and displaying paranoid and depressive symptoms, leading to fear that he might react in an aggressive paranoid manner, with grave international consequences."[58] Nixon's famous 1962 statement to the press after his California gubernatorial loss was characterized as paranoid by many: "One last thing. The last play. I leave you gentlemen now, and you will now write it. You will interpret it. That's your right. But as I leave you, I want you to know—just think about how much you're going to be missing. You won't have Nixon to kick around anymore, because, gentlemen, this is my last press conference."[59] Moreover, President Nixon maintained Enemies Lists that contained more than 200 citizens whom he considered to be threats to his political success.[60] Vanik's recent paper on the Nixon psyche concluded that the president had three faces: the public and grandiose, the suspicious and paranoid if the struggle to maintain the first is threatened, and the peacemaker attempting to integrate the first two.[61]

Reporters Bob Woodward and Carl Bernstein, *The Washington Post* chroniclers of

Watergate and admittedly no fans of the Nixon presidency, recorded many unflattering commentaries on this president's strange behavior: "Is the President off his rocker?" (Barry Goldwater)[62]; "Nixon said vile things about everybody—about bureaucrats, Congressmen, reporters, lawyers, Russians, Democrats, Easterners, ethnic groups, his own staff" (Fred Buzhardt)[63]; "If the President had his way, we'd have a nuclear attack every week" (Henry Kissinger)[64]; "Price never deluded himself about Nixon's darker instincts, his paranoia, the capacity for hatred, the need for revenge, the will to crush anyone he perceived as an enemy" (Ray Price).[65]

However, a recent comprehensive biographic review of mental illness in presidents did not cite Nixon as an example of a paranoid personality disorder. Instead, it identified alcohol abuse as the psychological disorder that afflicted Nixon during his presidency.[66] For the latter diagnosis there are many recorded examples. Summers' biography turned frequently to the theme of Nixon's drinking, while Nixon was president of a California young businessmen's club,[67] while vice president,[68] and during his forced exile from political office.[69] Future presidential aide John Erlichman described Nixon's drinking at the 1964 Republican national convention: "He was drinking hard and he lost it."[70]

Two years later, Erlichman, recruited by Nixon to join his campaign staff, informed Nixon of his difficulty with Nixon's drinking. Erlichman cautioned the future president that he did not want to involve himself in a campaign in which the candidate was not fully in control of himself.[71] Despite this admonition, Nixon continued his friendship with alcohol in the White House. After his television speech in April 1973 when Erlichman and other top aides resigned, Nixon made numerous late night and early morning phone calls in which his speech was slurred from alcohol.[72] Secretary of State Henry Kissinger was a rich source for quotes describing his leader's drinking habits: "Alcohol has alarming effects, even when he drank little," and later, "Two glasses of wine were enough to make him boisterous."[73]

Medical historian Kenneth Crispell remarked at a conference on presidential disability that "Nixon had a psychiatrist, which didn't help him much."[74] He was undoubtedly referring to New York psychotherapist Dr. Arnold Hutschnecker, who conducted a decades-long medical relationship with Richard Nixon. This physician/patient relationship had been well-known[75] but its psychiatric nature was only revealed in Anthony Summers' 2000 Nixon biography, *The Arrogance of Power*.[76]

The then senator Nixon first visited Hutschnecker's New York City Park Avenue office, most probably in late 1951, because of pain in his neck and back.[77] Nixon sought out the doctor after reading *The Will to Live*, the doctor's book on psychosomatic illness. Nixon publicly consulted Hutschnecker several times a year until 1955, when the doctor discontinued his combined internal medicine/psychiatry practice to focus entirely upon psychotherapy. Thereafter Nixon, then vice president, ensured the privacy of his visits, whether in New York or Washington, D.C.[78] The patient warned his physician against any disclosure of their relationship. He feared that any exposure would lead people to think that he "must be cuckoo or nuts."[79] After Nixon's 1968 presidential election victory, his aides severed this relationship, and the existence of any presidential psychiatric treatments is speculative.[80] However, Hutschnecker was identified in his 2001 *New York Times* obituary as "…the only mental health professional to have treated a president."[81] The doctor did make two public visits to the Nixon White House, ostensibly to discuss public policy issues.[82] Nixon renewed his psychotherapy after his resignation; his last meeting with Hutschnecker was at Pat Nixon's funeral in 1993.[83]

Dr. Hutschnecker was born in Austria and educated in Berlin, where his medical training occurred after World War I at the Friedrich Wilhelm University. He practiced medicine in Germany, but his public opposition to Adolf Hitler forced him in 1936 to flee Germany for New York City. He thereby joined noted émigrés and future presidential medical consultants Max Jacobson and Hans Kraus in escaping from Nazi tyranny.[84] His New York practice was successful and a number of celebrities sought his treatments.[85]

Hutschnecker received notoriety in the 1950s when he advocated that mental health certificates should be required for political leaders. He likened these to guarantees of mental competence in the same way as the Wasserman test for syphilis was performed as a guarantee for health before the issuance of a marriage certificate.[86] Hutschnecker also authored a *New York Times* opinion piece suggesting that personality evaluations for political leaders would proactively lead to successful conflict resolution.[87] In a later piece, he mourned the stigma of seeing a psychiatrist, writing, "To consider a branch of medical knowledge and practice with suspicion or condemnation is not merely an act of cruelty toward people in need, it is almost an act of negligence for a Government not to avail itself of the merits of this discipline."[88] He summarized this dilemma in a colorful and pithy quote: "It is safer for a politician to go to a whorehouse than to see a psychiatrist."[89] It is likely that the doctor's public proscriptions were influenced by his private treatments of patient Richard M. Nixon.

Twentieth century presidents John Kennedy and Bill Clinton may have had addiction problems. Kennedy's undisciplined use of amphetamines and steroids already has been recounted.[90] At least one psychotherapist was convinced that Clinton (1993–2001) was afflicted with a sexual addiction. Jerome D. Levin's *The Clinton Syndrome*[91] attempted to explain how irrational behavior by a leader may have tragic consequences for both himself and the nation. His repeated sexual activity in the White House with intern Monica Lewinsky continued to place Clinton in potentially dangerous situations. This author described a variety of therapies to treat this disorder, including psychotherapy, antidepressant drugs, and twelve-step programs. Clinton chose none of these approaches to deal with the underlying causes for the Lewinsky affair, but instead chose spiritual counseling to combat his problem.

Evangelical ministers Tony Campolo and Gordon MacDonald had occasionally given the forty-second president religious counsel since the onset of his presidency. Campolo and MacDonald, motivational speakers and authors of spiritual self-help books, agreed to be Clinton's counselors and his weekly prayer partners as they guided his spiritual recovery. Campolo said that "we will pray with him, study Scripture together and do our best to help him as he searches his heart and soul."[92] The ubiquitous Rev. Jesse Jackson also prayed with Clinton during previous political crises related to his addiction, providing spiritual rather than psychiatric therapy.[93]

Twenty-first-century chief executives Trump and Biden have been challenged with suspicions of dementia, Alzheimer's Disease, and other psychological maladies while president. A full discussion of this matter occurred in Chapter 13.

Several recent American presidents have been selected from the septuagenarian and older age groups, where questions regarding senility, dementia, and Alzheimer's disease are appropriate. The question was provoked when the retired Ronald Reagan, in a thoughtful letter written on November 5, 1994, announced to the nation, "(he) was one of the millions of Americans who will be afflicted with Alzheimer's disease" which was the same affliction that had affected his mother.[94] He was then the oldest U.S. president when he retired in 1989 at nearly seventy-eight years of age. Intense speculation resulted whether the aging Reagan displayed signs of the disease during his two-term presidency. "Most observers, friends, Administration officials, and his physician, Dr. John Hutton, answered: No."[95]

The advice of doctors Norman J. Knorr and Daniel Harrington, in retrospect, is apt: "As an adjunct to the appointment of the president's physician. a Mental Health consultant appointed to assist the White House physician could present opportunities for the president, the first family, and staff to seek advice and counsel regarding psychological matters. The stresses of Watergate and Iran/Contra episode on the president and his staff, and the existence of alcoholism … is good evidence that such a service is needed."[96] Clinton's presidential physician, Connie Mariano, acknowledged that a designated psychiatrist had been named on the approved list of medical consultants to be contacted in case of need. The psychiatrist was a senior staff officer from one of the three Washington area military hospitals. However, these services apparently were not utilized during the tenure of this two-term president.

Psychiatrists at Walter Reed National Military Medical Center remain available for consultation, but have never been consulted.[97] However, the stigma remains.

Chapter 15

The Medical Care of Vice Presidents

In 1875 Henry Wilson, serving as Ulysses Grant's second vice president,[1] returned to Washington "...on November 10th in a weakened condition. He had suffered an acute pain in the back for some days and while in New York during the week had hot irons applied without affect ... he went to the Capitol baths on the morning of the eleventh. After the bath he went to the barber shop and while in the chair he rolled his head in a convulsive manner.... Dr. Baxter, an army man, summoned at Wilson's request, found nothing to indicate brain lesions or paralysis.... Taken to his own room at the Capitol ... there he remained during his last sickness tended by officers of the Senate.... The next few days and nights were restless ones.... On the sixteenth he had a bad night and Dr. Baxter complained that he received too many letters.... Reports claimed that he was gaining, but he lost thirty pounds, and suffered from nervous depression. On the eighteenth he wanted to go out, but the doctors restrained him. On the twenty-second he passed away."[2]

The death of Henry Wilson on November 22, 1875, was the fourth of seven American vice presidents who died in office during the 100-year period of 1812–1912. Fortunately, no vice president has died since then. The narration that follows traces the administration of medical care that was afforded to sitting vice presidents, both before and after President Ronald Reagan, who directed the physicians and staff of the WHMU to extend health care coverage to them after his March 1981 assassination attempt.[3] The seven vice presidents who expired, and an eighth who was disabled by alcoholism, during their tenures, reside among the ranks of the most obscure of American politicians. However, a recounting of their illnesses and a consideration of the doctors whose patients they became may add context to the prior chapters about the White House Medical Unit and the Twenty-fifth Amendment. An examination of the evolution of the WHMU's health monitoring and of the role of consultant doctors in the medical treatment of recent vice presidents G.H. Bush, Dan Quayle, Al Gore, Mike Pence, and, especially, Richard Cheney, conclude this chapter.

The first of the seven near-nonentities had been blessed with a recognizable contemporary surname. George Clinton died from pneumonia on April 12, 1812, in the eighth year of his vice presidency.[4] Clinton served as the perennial governor of New York State almost continuously from the time of the Revolutionary War until his selection and election to replace the nefarious Aaron Burr as Thomas Jefferson's vice president in 1804.[5] His biographers make many references to Clinton's chronic arthritis and ill health, dating as far back as 1779, when his chronic rheumatism is mentioned as a problem to be overcome.[6] Later, in 1795, a biographer recounted, "...there is reason enough to believe that Clinton's health, always uncertain, made it impossible for him to accept another term [as governor of New York]. The governor was so ill at the Greenwich farm that he had to have his message read for him when the legislature met on January 6, 1795, at Poughkeepsie."[7]

Despite his infirmities, and perhaps an indicator of the perceived irrelevancy of the position, Clinton, at age sixty-five, was nominated and elected as Jefferson's vice president in 1804; and four years later, at age sixty-nine, he was renominated and reelected as President James Madison's vice president. In 1808, Dolley Madison, referring to Clinton, wrote, "The Vice-President lies dangerously ill.... His age alone prevented his aspiring to more political honors. He did not carry his [almost] seventy years any too gracefully."[8] His sole constitutional responsibility, presiding officer of the Senate, was handled only intermittently, and, when present, poorly. Federalist New Hampshire senator William Plumer remarked: "He is an old and feeble man—his voice is very weak and feeble." Three years later there was no improvement in Plumer's assessment: "He is old, feeble.... He has no mind ... no memory. He forgets the question."[9]

During the last three years of his life, Clinton was afflicted with various, mostly undefined, ailments which probably were related to arthritis and aging and which prohibited him from carrying out his modest duties. Finally, he was confined to his residence where, after an illness of about four weeks, he was unable "to withstand 'the general decay of Nature and the ravages of pneumonia.'"[10] It is unknown whether he was attended by a physician in addition to his family. During Clinton's Washington career the District of Columbia was in its infancy and professional services were rudimentary. In 1815 there were only nine physicians and two apothecaries in the district.[11] The office of the vice presidency was subsequently vacant for almost a year and the body politic hardly noticed.

Elbridge Gerry, James Madison's second vice president, also died in office in the nation's capital city. The sixty-eight-year-old former Massachusetts congressman, envoy to the French government, and governor was nominated for several reasons, one being that he was too old to challenge James Monroe, the presidential heir apparent in 1816.[12] Surprisingly, the near-septuagenarian Gerry vigorously adapted to his administrative duties and to the capitol's social scene until he suffered a "stroke" in 1813, after which he returned home to Massachusetts.[13] In autumn 1814, Gerry's strength weakened, and in November he became seriously ill. On the morning of November 23, 1814, he awakened with chest pains. Despite this, Gerry attempted to fulfill his sole constitutional duty, to preside over the Senate, but chest pains forced him to retire to his boarding house residence. Gerry's biographer wrote: "He was carried to his room, stretched out on his bed, and died within minutes."[14] Any record of physician attendance at Gerry's deathbed is unknown but his symptoms strongly implicate a heart attack as the cause of his death.[15]

William Rufus King, the third vice-presidential decedent, is so unmemorable that only a single full-length dual biography (with James Buchanan) of his life has been published![16] King, a long-time United States senator from Alabama, had been nominated to run on the same national ticket as the ill-fated Franklin Pierce.[17] During the 1852 national election campaign, King's tuberculosis reduced his activity, although he worked hard regionally to assure Pierce's victory. In September 1852, during the campaign's final weeks, John Martin, in his graduate thesis, recounted: "Tuberculosis ... forced King to restrict his activities during the campaign. He declined to attend a public dinner in his old congressional district in North Carolina because of his infirmity ... he wrote the committee in charge that he had become worn down and expected to spend some time resting."[18] In November, the now vice president-elect developed a worsening cough, lost weight, and began to doubt his recovery. According to Martin, "A month later [King] complained that the cough had worn him to a skeleton."[19] In January 1853, the vice president-elect left Washington for the balmier climate of Cuba with the hope of medical improvement. He departed Key West on the USS *Fulton* and arrived in Havana on February 6.[20] However, King's pulmonary and systemic symptoms did not improve and he realized that he was physically unable to appear in Washington for his March 4 inauguration. He requested, and was granted—for the first and only time in American history—special legislation by Congress to permit his swearing in to occur on foreign soil.[21] At the time of his swearing in to office by William Sharkey, United States Consul to Cuba, the vice president was too feeble to stand.[22]

In April 1853, King despaired of any improvement; he traveled home to Alabama where he succumbed to tuberculosis the day after his arrival.[23] He thus never appeared in the nation's capital to assume his duties as vice president.[24] The onset and the origins of the vice president's tuberculosis are unknown. King engaged in two lengthy diplomatic missions in Europe, to Russia and France, where he feared for his physical well-being.[25] Bailey wrote that King "suspected that he contracted consumption (tuberculosis) during his time as minister to France during 1844–46."[26] Additionally, Martin recorded four episodes when King was prevented from carrying out his political responsibilities because of illness; the most protracted may have been during the winter of 1847–1848, when he became indisposed "because of a severe case of influenza."[27] Tuberculosis is a chronic disease and any of these episodes of illness, especially the spell of "influenza," may have represented its onset. Unfortunately, Martin's thesis and the scattered newspaper accounts of King's health offer no information regarding the identity of his physicians or their treatments, either in Washington or in his home state of Alabama.

Vice President Henry Wilson died during the third year of his tenure as the constitutional successor to President Ulysses Grant. The sixty-one-year-old Wilson, a long time senator from Massachusetts, whose pre-political trade had been that of a cobbler, suffered a cerebrovascular accident (stroke) while in Massachusetts in May 1873, a mere three months into his vice presidency.[28] He was stricken with facial paralysis described by his biographer, "…by which his countenance was slightly altered, and his utterances somewhat impaired."[29] Adopting the habitual response of a politician, Wilson attempted to conceal his illness from the public, but inevitably reports circulated in the press that exaggerated the extent of his disability.[30] That August, Wilson entertained the press in his Natick, Massachusetts, home to clear the air over his illness. One reporter wrote that Wilson "had been attacked with a suspension of muscular action in the right side of his face. He immediately consulted [local physician] Dr. Edward H. Clarke … who enjoined a cessation of all mental labor, and forbade Mr. Wilson to write or read. He has visited his medical advisor once or twice every week since he was attacked, and has been under a course of treatment which has resulted in a slow but sure and steady improvement." However, as a summary to his article, the reporter observed: "The muscles of his forehead and face have been nearly restored to their normal condition, although his speech is still slightly affected."[31] The selection of Dr. Clarke as the treating physician was a most suitable choice. The physician had been professor of *Materia medica* at Harvard Medical School for seventeen years and was described as holding "an enviable position in Boston as consulting physician." In addition, Dr. Clarke maintained professional interest in the areas of otology, and more pertinently, neurology.[32]

Recovering slowly, Wilson finally returned to Washington, hoping to assume the chairing of the Senate's proceedings when it reconvened in December 1873.[33] But, his convalescence continued while he avoided public engagements. He bluntly explained to one inquirer: "It would risk my life."[34] However, in January 1874, continuing "poor health" required him to return to his Massachusetts home where he spent the balance of his vice presidency, out of the public eye, resting and completing a three-volume history of the rise and fall of the slave power.[35] Mark Hatfield, in his tome on American vice presidents, summarized Wilson's vice presidency in the following way: "Wilson's ill health kept him from playing any role of consequence as vice president."[36]

Vice President Wilson suffered a second neurological stroke in Massachusetts in September 1875. He was examined by ex-army surgeon general Dr. William Hammond, who observed the following: severe and generalized agitation associated with more localized complaints of vertigo, slurring of speech, twitching of the facial muscles, difficulty in swallowing, and severe neck pain.[37] Wilson's Boston physician, Dr. E.H. Clarke, had referred his patient to the experienced Hammond. Hammond further noted as part of his examination that the patient had recovered from the hemiplegia (one sided body weakness) suffered in 1873. Disregarding his doctor's advice, an infusion of political ambition compelled Wilson to travel once more to Washington to resume his neglected vice-presidential duties. Unfortunately, on November 10, he suffered his third and ultimately fatal cerebrovascular event while sitting in the Capitol's barber shop. The vice president survived for another twelve days. During the last period of his life, he had lost thirty pounds.[38]

For the first time a confluence occurred between presidential and vice-presidential medical treatment. Army surgeon Dr. Jedediah Baxter, future surgeon general and physician to presidents, presided over the stricken vice president's terminal care.[39] Hammond previously had been Baxter's commanding officer and referred to Baxter as his friend in an article that discussed the decedent's post mortem examination.[40] It is not known whether Hammond had recommended his friend to the vice president to be his doctor while in Washington, but during the Grant administration public officials customarily partook of military medical care, a practice that greatly disturbed the capital city's nonmilitary medical community.[41] The two physicians corresponded regarding Baxter's treatment during Wilson's terminal illness, agreed regarding the diagnosis and treatment, but later expressed dissimilar opinions on the cause of death. The most probable explanation for Wilson's illness was atherosclerosis of the arteries at the base of the brain with a series of subsequent strokes.[42]

Former Indiana senator and governor Thomas A. Hendricks died in 1885 nine months after his inauguration as Grover Cleveland's vice president. In 1880, while vacationing in Hot Springs, Arkansas, Hendricks, like Wilson before him, suffered what was described as "a paralytic stroke," from which he recovered.[43] But the recovery was more complete in his physical than in his psychological well-being. The vice president's physician, a Dr. Thompson, was quoted: "Mr. Hendricks, since his gangrenous attack, four years ago, had been apprehensive of a sudden termination of his life by paralysis.... This fear had grown so strongly upon him in the last few months, that he would not consent for his wife to be separated from him for any prolonged stay ... she has been by his side almost constantly."[44] Two years later he developed erysipelas, an acute inflammation of his toes, a result of his stance while speaking from a podium at numerous political engagements. As a result, lameness developed, requiring six months for recovery.[45] Otherwise the Hoosier appeared to be in good health.

On Tuesday, November 24, 1885, the vice president delayed his departure for Washington, where he was scheduled to preside at the convening of the new session of the Senate, in order to socialize with old friends in Indianapolis. At the reception, he was described as pale and tired; upon returning to his home, he complained of an illness, which was otherwise unspecified. The next morning, complaining of pain in his chest, sides and stomach, Hendricks felt worse and summoned his physician, Dr. Thompson. Simple treatments were administered, consisting of an emetic, bromides, and cupping of the chest. The doctor "apprehended no serious danger," but contradictorily his patient died peacefully later that same day. Dr. Thompson listed as the cause of death "Paralysis of the brain, with a slight complication of heart affection from the same cause."[46]

Presley Rixey, previously identified as the first White House physician,[47] described the responsibilities of that office in a magazine article: "...and it is important that the President keep advised as to the health of his official family, that is, the members of the cabinet and others ... in whom the President might be much interested. Here the President calls in the services of the official White House physician, especially when the illness is serious, as in the case of Vice-President Hobart ... whom I visited at the President's direction."[48] Garret A. Hobart, a little-known attorney and New Jersey state legislator, was elected as William McKinley's vice president in 1896. The McKinleys and the Hobarts bonded both personally and professionally; the president relied upon his vice president for counsel, judgment, social support for his epileptic wife, and even for personal financial advice.[49]

Hobart developed a serious illness as vice president, which both progressively limited his activities and increasingly demanded physician attention. Early in 1899 the symptoms of cardiac disease, most probably secondary to coronary arteriosclerosis, began to significantly affect the vice president.[50] Severe angina pectoris, characterized as "extreme pain" and "severe paroxysms of pain," became debilitating. In addition, his heart began to fail and the effects of congestive heart failure worsened rapidly. Hobart developed shortness of breath, difficulty in sleeping on a flat surface, weakness and a loss of energy. Before his death, it was reported that Hobart "could not take a reclining position without a sense of suffocation, and the only sleep obtained was while he sat on the edge of the bed and leaned forward, resting his head on a table."[51]

Despite his illness, Hobart, to fulfill a commitment to his friend the president, traveled from his New Jersey home to Plattsburgh, New York, where the McKinleys were vacationing. Unfortunately, Hobart's condition deteriorated there. The president abruptly terminated his vacation and the presidential party accompanied the vice president to Hobart's vacation home on the New Jersey shore. Rixey, the presidential physician, traveled with McKinley, and presumably provided medical attention to Hobart.[52] Several months later, McKinley became so concerned that his friend, the vice president, had surrendered to despair, that "he sent a message urging Mr. Hobart to rally his courage and make a new effort, and at the same time sent Dr. Rixey, his official medical attendant, to strengthen the appeal and add his advice."[53]

Hobart, the sixth vice president to die in office, expired on November 21, 1899, in New Jersey, apparently from a heart attack. A newspaper reported that he had suffered two significant attacks of angina pectoris shortly before his death.[54] Present at his bedside was his family physician, Dr. William Newton.[55] Newton's medical interests, in the era prior to the strict delineation of medical specialties, were broad. He practiced as a

New York City coroner, served as the Paterson, New Jersey, public health officer, and was the consulting physician to the Paterson Eye and Ear Infirmary.[56]

The nineteenth and early twentieth-century duties of a vice president were limited and a requisite presence in Washington was at most sporadic. As a consequence, ailing holders of this office, in contrast to the presidents, spent most of their time in their hometowns to be cared for by their local family physicians.

For example, Vice President James S. Sherman, William Howard Taft's vice president (1908–1912) was dying from the chronic renal failure of Bright's disease. As a result, he remained confined to his Utica, New York, home during Taft's 1912 reelection campaign, and was treated there by his family physician, Dr. Fayette H. Peck.[57] Dr. Peck, a graduate of New York University's medical school, engaged in general surgery and public health, in addition to his family practice.[58] Many doctors in the decades prior to the regulation of medical specialties practiced broadly rather than focusing on a limited set of skills and knowledge.

Sherman was the seventh and the last vice president to expire in office. Sherman had contracted Bright's disease in 1904 but the symptoms of kidney failure worsened significantly in 1912.[59] Despite his vice president's apparent illness, President Taft permitted the renomination of Sherman as his running mate. Sherman's ill fortune did not translate into the country's misfortune, since the Taft-Sherman ticket was defeated in the November national election, and the nation was spared the anxiety of yet another lacuna in the constitutional architecture of presidential succession.

The medical travails of the remote and even the relatively recent surviving vice presidents have remained in the shadows, just as the former insignificance of the office has obscured the life histories and reputations of most of its incumbents. However, the addiction of one incumbent, Daniel Tompkins, was so apparent to his peers that, in a modern setting, the intrusive scrutiny of the press would have demanded that he be the recipient of medical or psychological treatment. Tompkins, an effective governor of New York State, was twice elected as James Monroe's vice president (1817–1825). Tompkins initially paid little attention to his vice-presidential duties because ill health arising from a horseback accident had, according to the vice president "increased upon me for several years until finally, for the last six weeks, they have confined me to my house ... and sometimes to my bed." As a consequence, Tompkins gloomily predicted that he would be compelled to "...resign the office of Vice President at the next session, if not sooner, as there is very little hope of my being able to perform its duties hereafter."[60]

Tompkins's riding injury resolved itself, but a far more serious issue, alcoholism, damaged his vice presidency. During the last three years of his first term, it was reported that "he was absent from the Senate nearly three fourths of the time."[61] Instead, he spent much of his first term in New York in an attempt to resolve severe financial problems that were leading to bankruptcy. Despondent over his misfortune, alcohol became his treatment of choice. Referring to Tompkins, the prominent New York politician Dewitt Clinton wrote in September 1819: "Our friend on Staten Island is unfortunately sick in body and mind. His situation upon the whole is deplorable and calculated to excite sympathy."[62] Apprehension over the vice president's alcoholism grew to the point that Martin Van Buren, his political ally, was impelled to inquire of Tompkins's son-in-law whether the vice president was drinking excessively.[63] Van Buren's question was answered in the affirmative.

Both Tompkins's financial woes and his alcoholic response to them continued into his second term. One observer in the Senate noted that Tompkins had never been "perfectly sober during his stay here. He was several times so drunk in the chair that he could with difficulty put the question."[64] Vice presidential duties, albeit minimal, were ignored, his indebtedness and drinking increased, premature aging ensued, and Tompkins returned to New York. He died intestate on June 11, 1825.[65] The extent of medical or psychological support, if any, given to the vice president is not recorded.

It was not until March 1981, that the medical care of a vice president became formalized: Institutionalized coverage by the White House replaced a traditional reliance upon hometown care by the family doctor and the haphazard coverage by the presidential physicians during emergencies in Washington.[66] Reagan physician Burton Smith explained: "After President Reagan was shot, he said that he did not want Vice President Bush having second-class medicine; therefore, he wanted him also to have a doctor assigned anywhere he went."[67] Apparently vice presidential medical coverage also was extended to vice presidential wives. Smith continued: "The President, Vice President Bush, Mrs. Reagan, and Mrs. Bush were my four sole responsibilities. As I say, Vice President Bush was never given a doctor until after the March 1981 shooting."[68]

Since then, White House physicians have been assigned to the vice-presidential family, occasionally on a rotational, but most often on a dedicated, basis, when a single doctor would act as the second family's personal physician. A deviation took place in the case of Vice President Dan Quayle (1989–1993), who was disliked by the Bush presidential physician, Dr. Burton Lee III. Lee decided that Quayle merited coverage only by a physician's assistant, not a physician, during his domestic travel.[69] Quayle's successor, Al Gore (1993–2001), insisted that the vice president's station merited a single doctor to be specifically assigned to vice presidential care, similar to the practice for the president. Air Force physician Dr. Richard Tubb, who later became President George W. Bush's presidential physician, drew this assignment.[70] Subsequent vice presidents Richard Cheney, Joe Biden, and Mike Pence were assigned WHMU physicians Lew Hofmann, Kevin O'Connor, and Jennifer Pena respectively. After a brief hiatus, the practice of WHMU assignment of a specific physician to care for the vice president and family was reinstated. Emergency medicine doctor Josh Simmons is assigned to Vice President Kamala Harris medical care.[71]

Recent vice presidents have undergone annual physical examinations, but, in contrast to the presidents' yearly examinations, the results have been issued quietly and briefly as part of a press release.[72] An exception occurs when an incumbent of the office is considering a future campaign for the presidency.[73] The use of outside medical consultants also may occur. When the wife of the vice president, Tipper Gore, developed a thyroid gland tumor, the benign lesion was surgically removed not at a military hospital but at the Johns Hopkins Hospital in Baltimore, Maryland.[74]

During the past three decades, most vice presidents were healthy and presented no medical emergencies to their WHMU doctors. Vice President Richard Cheney (2001–2009) was a notable exception. Cheney at his inauguration in January 2001 had a history of chronic coronary artery heart disease. He previously survived four heart attacks, the first at age thirty-eight and the most recent shortly before his inauguration during the protracted Bush-Gore Florida recount. Additionally, it was at George Washington Hospital (GWH) that staff cardiac surgeon Dr. Benjamin Aaron performed a quadruple coronary bypass surgery in 1988.[75] A few years earlier, the same Dr. Aaron removed a bullet from the left lung of President Ronald Reagan after his attempted assassination.[76]

Cheney's health was the most precarious of any incumbent since James Sherman's kidneys failed over 100 years previously. As a consequence, prophylaxis became both routine and mandatory for the WHMU as it organized this vice president's day-to-day health coverage. Robust advanced life support capability was always nearby in the form of a WHMU doctor, in addition to a nurse, physician assistant, or medic.[77] The proximity of such coverage proved to be fortuitous when Cheney accidentally sprayed seventy-eight-year-old Harry Whittington, his hunting companion, with birdshot while shooting quail on a Texas ranch.[78] Positioned nearby, the members of Cheney's medical contingent treated Whittington on the spot quickly, competently, and anonymously. The White House Medical Unit was well prepared for this contingency, since it previously had undergone scenario training that consisted of trauma by hunting.[79]

Dick Cheney was entitled to the vice-presidential perquisite of an assigned WHMU doctor for medical care. Lieutenant colonel, later colonel, Lewis (Lew) Hofmann attended Cheney for the entire eight years of his tenure. This vice president was very grateful, writing, "I was extraordinarily fortunate to draw Lew for that assignment. He is a top-notch physician. He was always discrete, worked endless hours, and traveled over a million miles with on Airforce Two.... He played a vital role in dealing with all my health issues during that time. He remains a good friend today and I consult with him from time to time even though we are both civilians. Perhaps Lew's greatest contribution was his ability to adapt to my special requirements."[80]

As therapy, in addition to diet, an exercise regime and various medications, Cheney required a variety of invasive medical procedures, including a four-vessel cardiac bypass surgery, two separate coronary vessel stent procedures, and the placement of an implantable cardioverter defibrillator.[81]

This vice president, who first achieved elective office as the sole U.S. Representative from Wyoming, subsequently held high-level positions in both the Gerald Ford and the G.H.W. Bush administrations. Therefore, as his cardiac health declined, it is unsurprising that he would seek medical care at a major Washington hospital, in his case, George Washington University Hospital (GWH) near the central U.S. government offices.

Cheney's medical care was also provided by GWH physicians, cardiologist Dr. Jonathan Reiner, and internist Dr. Gary Malakoff. Dr. Reiner, a graduate of Georgetown University Medical School is the director of GWH's cardiac catheterization laboratory and a professor of medicine at George Washington University School of Medicine. He holds certification in internal medicine, cardiovascular disease, and interventional cardiology.[82] Richard Cheney has not been ungrateful for his cardiac care. In March 2006, Vice President and Mrs. Cheney donated $2.7 million to GWH to establish the Richard B. and Lynne V. Cheney Cardiovascular Institute at the hospital.[83] Reiner provided cardiac care to the vice president both before and after his tenure and co-authored their medical relationship in "Heart."[84]

Reiner and Hofmann effectively co-managed Cheney's heart issues for eight years, which involved numerous consultations, many heart concerns, arrythmias, and the implantation of an intracardiac defibrillator (ICD).[85]

Cheney's cardiac saga worsened after his vice presidency. Dr. Reiner managed his fifth heart attack in 2010 that was complicated by medically unmanageable congestive heart failure. He became bed ridden while the ejection fraction of his left ventricle fell to a woeful 20 percent (Normal >50%).[86] His life was saved by the introduction of a Left Ventricular Assist Device (LVAD) during a nine-hour surgical intervention July 6–7, 2010 (Heart, 273). On March 23, 2012, the former vice president received a transplanted heart. He remains alive today.[87]

Any consideration of Cheney's doctors illuminates two significant problems that have become increasingly difficult for current medical practitioners. The first relates to the management of relations with the contemporary press corps. Famed Texas cardiac surgeon Dr. Denton Cooley was asked in July 2000, by presidential candidate George Bush, to evaluate the cardiac record of his prospective running mate. In a July 24, 2000, press release, Cooley opined that Cheney "is in good health with normal cardiac function," and that "in my opinion Mr. Cheney's health problems in the past decade should not interfere with a strenuous political campaign."[88] Cooley's statement, meant to be reassuring, was shortly exposed as being glib and superficial. It was soon revealed in the press that his evaluation was based on a ten-minute phone conversation with cardiologist Reiner and did not include a personal physical examination, a review of Cheney's medical records, or any discussion of medications and critical cardiac monitoring data, such as the ejection fraction. Furthermore, Reiner was forced to admit that Cooley had misquoted him in stating that Cheney's cardiac function was normal, when Reiner knew it was decidedly abnormal.[89]

The modern press, increasingly persistent and critical, is apt to question any physician's statements, despite one's prominence or reputation. Burton Lee commented about the Washington press corps after his retirement from the White House. In an interview, Lee complained at length about reporters' behavior: "The press in the White House is obviously a major problem.... Really you cannot do anything in the White House without it getting into the press. Unfortunately, there are scrupulous and unscrupulous press people, just as there are scrupulous and unscrupulous people in everyday life.... I was misquoted recently on a highly controversial subject, and it caused me enormous, paralyzing difficulty.... I would say 5 percent of the press quoted me accurately. The little spin that is put on a statement is the killer."[90]

A second problem concerning doctors was underscored in July 2004 when a spokesman for the vice president announced that Dr. Gary Malakoff had been terminated as Cheney's physician. The announcement was in response to a statement by GWH that Malakoff had been suspended as its director of internal medicine. He was judged to be too impaired to treat patients because of an addiction to prescription drugs. Malakoff, Cheney's internist since 1995, had been in a monitoring and treatment program for prescription drug abuse since 1999.[91] That year the internist had been detected using other doctors' names to prescribe controlled substances for himself. As a consequence, he was placed in a GWH physician-supervised drug monitoring and treatment program, but was permitted to continue treating patients, including Cheney. The vice president was promptly informed about his physician's problem. However, Malakoff's addiction persisted and he was able to deceive the physician monitors of his recovery program. It was discovered that he had placed bulk internet orders of about $50,000 for Stadol, an opiate, fiorinal, a barbiturate, codeine, a narcotic, and other prescription drugs. When these further violations became known, the District's medical society demanded that he discontinue medical practice.[92] Several doctors anonymously interviewed for a newspaper article suggested that GW Medical Center had found itself in a difficult situation over this problem because of GWH's unofficial acknowledgment as "the president's hospital," a relationship that had enhanced its reputation and prestige. One physician continued: "They knew that if they blew the whistle on Gary, it would hurt the center."[93]

Dr. Malakoff is hardly the only prominent physician whose addiction to prescription drugs has received newspaper headlines. A February 2006 headline in the *Des Moines Register* read, "Ex-Iowa health director admits pain killer addiction."[94] Physician misuse of prescription drugs, particularly opiates and benzodiazepines, undetected for the most part in the past, recently has been identified as a significant problem. A review article reported that physicians were five times more likely than matched controls to take sedatives and minor tranquilizers without medical supervision. It further recounted that 11.4 percent of doctors had consumed benzodiazepines in the past year unsupervised and an even higher percentage had engaged in unsupervised use of opioids.[95] High stress professional work, the ability to write prescriptions, and easy access to the aforementioned controlled substances combine to explain the genesis of the problem; computerized tracking of prescriptions and more assertive law enforcement monitoring has unmasked it. Fortunately, physicians generally do well in recovery programs and most return to satisfying professional careers.[96]

WHMU's medical responsibilities have included the care of the vice presidents' spouses. The handling of vice presidential wife Mrs. Karen Pence's illness resulted in both administrative turmoil and personal animus between presidential physician Ronny Jackson and vice-presidential physician Jennifer Pena. Its effects included the sudden departure of one and the eventual departure of the second from both the WHMU and their resignations from the military, an inspector general's investigation into the professional behavior of Dr. Jackson, and probably the derailment of his cabinet nomination.

Jennifer Pena, a board-certified internist, received her medical degree from Yale University, served her internship at Army hospitals William Beaumont and Walter Reed, and completed her internal medicine residency also at Walter Reed. Afterward Pena practiced executive medicine at Fort Belvoir, Virginia. Her service there was of such a high quality that Dr. Ronny Jackson invited her onto the WHMU in 2014 and later proposed her as the vice president's physician in 2016. The initial Pena/Jackson professional relationship was amicable.[97]

But something happened after Karen Pence underwent a still-undisclosed illness at the presidential retreat Camp David Maryland in the Fall of 2017. A heated imbroglio between Pena and Jackson occurred when the patient was transferred to Walter Reed National Military Medical Center in Bethesda, Maryland. The circumstances of her care remain opaque.

However, "according to copies of internal documents obtained by CNN, Pena accused Jackson of overstepping his authority and inappropriately intervening in a medical situation involving the second lady as well as potentially violating federal privacy rights by briefing White House staff and disclosing details to other medical providers—but not appropriate consulting with the vice president's physician."[98] Dr. Pena elaborated on Dr. Jackson in a letter to the author, saying "he has a tendency to inappropriately insert himself in clinical situations in which he is not supposed to intervene."[99] Pena took her concerns about Jackson to Pence's chief of staff, who in turn referred her complaints to President Trump's chief of staff John Kelly. Kelly advised that the proper reporting should have been within her chain of command through the White House Medical Unit.[100]

Dr. Pena was a participant in the presentation of very negative material to the Tester senatorial committee that torpedoed Jackson's nomination for Veterans Affairs Secretary. Was she a leader, as Jackson has written (see previous chapter) or as she alleged merely "the twenty-third person to be interviewed by the Vetting Board.... She was shocked after her name was leaked to the press." That was claimed as the reason for her resignation.[101]

In contrast, Pena claimed that Ronny Jackson's continuing stature in the Trump administration was her real reason to resign.[102]

As the significance of the vice presidency has grown, there has been a corresponding increment in the sum total of official medical attention given to its incumbents. Moreover, the evolution of the type of health care has paralleled that of the president: emphasis is focused upon health maintenance and disease prevention rather than treatment of acute illnesses. Since most recent vice presidents (G.H.W. Bush, Quayle, Gore, Biden, Pence, Harris) have been healthy, their annual examinations and uncommon urgent care have been managed discreetly and with minimal publicity. Vice President Cheney was a notable exception; both his disease prophylaxis and emergent therapy have received intensive public attention. Scrutiny of this vice president's medical ups and downs has been fortuitous, however, for this author, since it provides an opportunity to examine several contemporary medical issues, the most important of which is the problem of physician prescription drug abuse. Richard Cheney was elected with a known chronic health problem, not normative for recent vice presidents, as described above. During earlier administrations, when the vice presidency was viewed as a fatuous responsibility, a number of those elected to this office were widely known to be afflicted with old age (Clinton, Gerry) or by significant illness (Wilson, Sherman) without serious anxiety. Interestingly, as a further mark of this office's previous obscurity, several of these incumbents nursed their medical problems at their homes, far distant from the nation's capital.

Chapter 16

Presidential Physicians After Their Tenures

An opinion piece, titled "The Stain of Torture," appeared on the July 1, 2005, editorial page of *The Washington Post*. Its author, Dr. Burton Lee III, asserted: "Having served as a doctor in the Army Medical Corps early in my career and as presidential physician to George H.W. Bush for four years, I might be expected to bring a skeptical and partisan perspective to allegations of torture and abuse by U.S. forces.... But I cannot do so. It's precisely because of my devotion to country, respect for the military and commitment to the ethics of the medical profession that I speak out against systematic, government-sanctioned torture and excessive abuse of prisoners during our war on terrorism."[1] In this manner the outspoken Dr. Lee reappeared in the public spotlight twelve years after his departure from the White House.

Intermittent glimpses into the careers of former presidential physicians have appeared in previous chapters. Although it is the practice of most recent presidential physicians to avoid public celebrity, professional, academic, public, and personal advantages inevitably accrue as a result of their White House appointment. The biographies of thirteen ex-presidential physicians will be summarized in this, the penultimate chapter, to determine whether they indeed may have an encore after the White House. The post presidential careers of the civilian physicians and their military counterparts will be compared and contrasted. Since the sample sizes are small, any conclusions necessarily will be tentative.

After the formalization of its role in the mid-twentieth century, six civilians (Doctors Sawyer, Travell, Ruge, Smith, Lee, and O'Connor) have been appointed as the physician to the president. Pay limitations and practice constraints have been disincentives for a doctor at a career peak to accept this post; consequently, most of the above were near retirement at the time of their selection. Travell was sixty years of age; Sawyer was sixty-one; Ruge was sixty-three; and Burton Smith was seventy when he joined the White House staff. Dr. Burton Lee was the exception; at age fifty-eight, he arrived in the executive mansion after resigning as chief of the lymphoma service at New York's prestigious Memorial Sloan Kettering Cancer Center. To paraphrase Dr. Lee, "I accepted a demotion to take the job."[2]

Longtime presidential physician navy captain William Lukash concluded that the White House was not a venue conducive to the requirements of a civilian practitioner. Its remuneration in 1988 was $72,000 per year, far below that of a successful practitioner. This opinion was supported by Burton Smith, who explained in his memoir: "I had a successful, six-figure practice in Los Angeles as a surgeon specializing in urology....

I had been building this practice for more than thirty-five years when I gave it up to serve President Reagan for $72,300 a year." Smith emphasized the point by mentioning a friend's consoling words: "He [Smith] was doing so well and now he's just another government doctor with only one patient."[3]

Doctors Willis Hurst and Kenneth H. Cooper chose another option: monitoring their patients' health from a distance, i.e., Atlanta and Dallas respectively, and traveling to Washington to participate in the presidents' annual physical exams or as needed. A prior chapter detailed cardiologist Hurst's decision to remain in his active academic practice rather than to accept Lyndon Johnson's offer of the presidential physician's position.[4] It is unknown whether President George W. Bush offered this post to the famous "Exercise Guru," Dr. Kenneth H. Cooper, who was Bush's personal physician for more than a decade prior to the Bush presidency.[5] Cooper, considered by many to be the father of aerobic exercise, and widely recognized as a leader of the fitness movement, is the founder and head of the well-known Cooper Aerobics Center and the Cooper Institute in North Dallas, Texas, an employer of almost 500.[6] Dr. Cooper had overseen with Dr. Richard Tubb the Bush annual physical examinations in Washington.[7]

The civilian physicians have lived to advanced ages. Homeopathic doctor Charles Sawyer was the exception; he died one year after his presidential patron, Warren Harding, expired in San Francisco, and only four months after his resignation as Calvin Coolidge's White House doctor on June 25, 1924.[8] Sawyer's health had been in decline; moreover, he continued to lose influence over the new president's medical management to the ambitious Dr. Joel Boone. These reasons compelled him to return to his successful medical enterprise, the White Oaks sanatorium, in Marion, Ohio.[9]

In 1895 Dr. Sawyer arrived in Marion to establish the Sawyer Sanatorium for nervous dysfunctions; most of its occupants were treated for mental and psychiatric disorders. Sawyer's practice became so prosperous that, at the turn of the century, it was organized with a capital stock of $450,000. Continual success allowed the sanatorium to relocate to the nearby 103-acre White Oaks Farm. The sanatorium then included a dairy, chicken houses, fruit orchards and vegetable gardens, together with fifteen patient cabins, each containing ten private patient rooms. The cabins were arranged in a cloister configuration; all were connected by an enclosed corridor and faced a large inner courtyard. The courtyard contained larger structures including administrative and treatment facilities. Sawyer's enterprise was so successful that a private railroad spur and train station were constructed in order to accommodate the many patients from afar.[10]

Charles Sawyer dispensed his homeopathic remedies while his son, Dr. Carl Sawyer, an unaccredited but practicing psychiatrist, administered treatments for manic depression, severe depression, paranoia, and other mental disorders.[11] White Oaks sanatorium was left in the capable hands of Carl when the elder Sawyer answered the call to service in Washington: it was to this thriving enterprise that Charles Sawyer returned in 1924.

A frequent visitor to the sanatorium was the senior Dr. Sawyer's most illustrious patient, Florence Harding, before she resided in the nation's capital as the wife of an Ohio Senator and later as the nation's first lady. The sanatorium became Mrs. Harding's temporary residence after her husband's demise; she burned much of the deceased president's personal correspondence in one of its cabins.[12] Florence Harding returned to Washington, where she developed a recrudescence of her chronic kidney disease; she had relied upon the elder Sawyer for its treatment over many years. Subsequently,

Charles and Carl Sawyer prevailed upon the widow to return to their sanatorium for medical care, and it was there that she died from renal failure on November 7, 1924.[13]

Charles Sawyer's post–White House career was brief; he spent his few remaining months immersed in Harding and White Oak affairs, treating Mrs. Harding, and acting as a trustee of the Harding Memorial Foundation. He preceded his patient in death by fewer than six weeks. The proximate dates of the deaths of Warren G. Harding, Florence Harding, and their physician, Charles Sawyer, became the subject of numerous conspiracy theories.[14]

Carl Sawyer lacked the promotional and marketing skills of his father, and failed to either upgrade or improve the White Oaks facility. The enterprise drifted into obsolescence; in 1953 it was converted into a facility for aged care. In the 1960s it was ceded to the city of Marion, which tore it down shortly thereafter.[15]

Doctors Daniel Ruge and Burton Smith retired from the practice of medicine either shortly after or immediately upon their respective White House departures. Ruge departed quietly at the end of Reagan's first term to reassume his position as the director of the Spinal Cord Injury Service at the Washington, D.C., Veterans Administration central office.[16] He retired one year later and moved to Colorado to be near his daughter and grandchildren. His daughter recalled that in his retirement, Ruge was active in his church and spent time fly fishing and cooking.[17] He also volunteered his time to record materials for the blind and dyslexic.[18]

Dr. Ruge did not seek to capitalize upon the prominence of his former position in the form of an autobiography, speeches, or prestigious appointments. He died in Denver at age 88.[19] Ruge publicly emerged from the quiet of his twenty-year retirement only when asked to participate in discussions of the Twenty-fifth Amendment, or to respond to *New York Times* medical reporter Lawrence Altman's inquiries regarding President Reagan's various medical crises.[20]

Dr. Smith retired to his home in Los Angeles. He no longer practiced medicine but remained on the honorary medical staff of the Saint John's Health Center in Santa Monica, where he had been affiliated since 1950. The former presidential physician was described as a "happy retiree" by a long-term colleague on the hospital's medical staff.[21]

Golf surely contributed to the retiree's enjoyment; moreover, it generated an interesting anecdote from Smith regarding ex-president Reagan, a fellow member of the Los Angeles Country Club. Smith, when asked how his former patient was coping with Alzheimer's disease, commented, "They say he plays golf. He does not play 18 holes. He goes over there and plays a few holes, which is very nice.... So physically from the motor side.... [Reagan is] pretty adept."[22]

This observation was the closest that Smith came to the medical care of his ex-patient. The Reagans' medical management was in the care of another set of local doctors that was backed up by the advice of Dr. John Hutton.[23] However, Burton Smith's two years as a presidential physician were not without subsequent advantage. Smith coauthored *White House Doctor*, a memoir of his experience in the White House. Smith acknowledged therein that "A book of this type does not just happen. There must be a unique experience involving engaging personalities, during an interesting period of history. My appointment as Physician to President Ronald Reagan during the Reagan Administration adequately fulfilled these requirements."[24] However, it is striking that Nancy Reagan is mentioned only infrequently in this memoir and the physician's name is missing in the index of her memoir "My Turn." Even more telling was her absence at Dr. and Mrs. Smith's farewell with the president in the Oval Office on January 28, 1987.[25]

Second, at the time of Smith's resignation, President Reagan nominated him to be one of the nine appointed members of the Board of Regents of the Uniformed Services University of the Health Sciences, the medical school for military officers located in Bethesda, Maryland. The Senate approved his nomination a year later.[26] This regent served for over eleven years and on August 2, 1999, was posthumously awarded the university's Distinguished Service Award for his contributions.[27]

Burton Smith also authored a paper that drew upon his White House career. "The Presidential Physician and the Reagan Presidency," is included in the Miller Center's series on the Twenty-fifth Amendment.[28] Burton Smith died from a brain tumor in 1999, at age 84, thirteen years after his retirement as presidential physician.[29]

It is not surprising that Dr. Burton Lee led a colorful and melodramatic life after the White House. Lee's subsequent medical experiences are best defined as eclectic, and the candid doctor continued to voice outspoken views about the medical profession.

Lee did not return to his professional roots at New York's Memorial Hospital in 1993; instead, he embarked upon a geographic and professional journey. His first stop was Greenville, South Carolina; he was hired to oversee the organization, the construction, and the medical care for a cancer center to be built by a local hospital. In an interview, Lee acerbically claimed that, although he successfully generated both medical and community support for the cancer center, the hospital administration reneged on its support for the project. After one year Smith departed for the next location on his sojourn.[30]

His next role was the presidency of Intracel Corporation, a Cambridge, Massachusetts, biotech company. Lee was lured to Intracel by its owner's promise to invest in the development of an AIDS vaccine. Lee's interest was piqued because of his membership on President Reagan's national AIDS commission, an assignment that he considered successful and professionally satisfying. However, this chapter also ended unsuccessfully; Lee recounted with some bitterness his intellectual and economic betrayal by Intracel's chief executive officer. After the doctor's departure, Intracel was taken over by another biotech corporation.[31]

Burton Lee subsequently resided in Florida's Indian River County, where he happily immersed himself in at least three diverse medically related activities. He was elected Commissioner of health for his county's Hospital District. As a consequence, he was able to satisfy his idealism by treating the impoverished at the county's department of health. This position provided Lee with his first opportunity since the White House to treat patients. Ever outspoken, Lee criticized both the state health bureaucracy and the state medical establishment, since both denied willing physician-retirees the opportunity to assist in crowded emergency rooms. It was necessary for Florida governor Jeb Bush, the son of Lee's former White House patient, to intervene on Lee's behalf to secure a limited-practice medical license. Its acquisition has allowed Lee to medically treat the poor.

Dr. Lee's academic interest was satisfied by his membership on the Health Sciences Advisory Council of his alma mater, the Columbia-Presbyterian School of Medicine. He characterized his activities as assisting its dean in various ways, including the raising of money.

The platform for Lee's intense convictions regarding medical ethics is his board membership on the Physicians for Human Rights. From this podium, he again was able to criticize publicly physician behavior in speeches, in *The Washington Post*, and in letters. Describing himself as an "idealistic type doctor," he is "morally appalled" by fellow physicians who participate in or condone what Lee labels as "torture" by Americans in Iraq and Afghanistan.[32] Burton Lee certainly had an encore after his four years as a presidential physician; his thirteen post–White House years have copied his four White House years in being colorful, opinionated, controversial, and resourceful.[33]

He died in November 2016 at his home in Vero Beach, Florida, from the complications of bladder cancer. He was 86.[34]

Janet Travell's professional career in the White House may have been one of considerable turmoil, but her subsequent thirty-year medical practice definitely was one of unqualified success. She practiced, investigated and wrote from her Washington base until 1996, when together with her daughter, she moved to Northampton, Massachusetts, where she died on August 1, 1996, at the age of ninety-five.[35]

Initially, Travell's energy was directed toward writing her autobiography, *Office Hours: Day and Night*, which appeared in November 1968. A major objective of this effort was to present favorably her perspective on President Kennedy's back therapy. The effort was successful since it was only many years later that the success of her treatments were challenged in print.[36] Subsequently, as noted by her daughter, "she never strayed from her primary focus on the diagnosis and management of myofascial pain syndromes due to trigger points."[37] Her research, teachings and clinical observations over many years resulted in the magisterial two-volume *Myofascial Pain and Dysfunction: The Trigger Point Manual*, published in 1983, coauthored with Dr. David Simons.[38] It was reissued as a textbook paperback in 1992, and was reissued in hardcover format after a revision by Simons in 1998.[39]

Dr. Travell first met Simons when she lectured at the School of Aerospace Medicine in San Antonio in the 1960s. Encouraged by Travell, Simons completed a residency in physiatry and subsequently was appointed as director of rehabilitation at the Long Beach Veterans Hospital. He became Travell's professional colleague, disciple and champion; together they coauthored the *Trigger Point Manual*, cowrote a number of clinical papers and consulted on individual patients.[40]

Travell's influence upon osteopathic medicine and massotherapeutist technique has been significant. In 1967 she became president-elect of the North American Academy of Manipulative Medicine at its second annual meeting.[41] Moreover, several authors have noted the similarities of Travell's trigger point therapy to osteopathic treatment.[42] Interestingly, Travell in 1977 authored an article in the major osteopathic journal which localized a trigger point to treat hiccups.[43] In retirement, her interests were protean as evidenced by her editorial correspondence regarding the ozone layer and the proper treatment of the common cold.[44]

While she was Kennedy's physician, Travell joined the staff of George Washington University Hospital and School of Medicine. She taught clinical rehabilitation and physical medicine there and was appointed associate clinical professor of medicine in 1965, emeritus clinical professor of medicine in 1970, and honorary clinical professor of medicine in 1988.[45] She also saw private patients, some of whom were among the political elite, namely Senator Barry Goldwater, Ambassador Chester Bowles and Speaker of the House of Representatives Sam Rayburn.[46]

Janet Travell's professional legacy remains important; she will be remembered far longer for her work on myofascial pain and trigger point therapy than for her selection as John Kennedy's presidential physician. Her papers, consisting of 104 boxes, or 44.5 linear feet of materials, were donated to the Gelman Library of the George Washington School of Medicine and are part of a permanent online exhibit.[47] In 2003 *The Texas Heart Journal* dedicated three retrospectives to her life and work, and her tome on trigger point therapy has been both reissued and revised. Trigger point therapy has become a therapeutic paradigm for which she is greatly responsible. Its significance is such that a recent search of the Barnes and Noble Website discovered 103 titles with the keywords "Trigger Point."[48] Additionally, trigger point theory and methodology are taught in many schools of massage therapy, where Travell remains in high esteem.[49] Finally, and most importantly, the announcement of Travell's death brought forth many letters of appreciation from patients who were helped by her methods.[50]

Since 1960, ten presidential physicians have been drawn from the ranks of the military medical corps. Doctors Burkley, Lukash, Hutton, Mariano, Tubb, Kuhlmann, Jackson, and Conley were serving as White House physicians at the time of their selection; the ninth, Richard Nixon's doctor, Dr. Walter Tkach, had been a member of the WHMU eight years earlier during Nixon's term as vice president. President Biden's physician. Kevin O'Connor had been his WHMU doctor when vice president. O'Connor retired from the military in 2017, but returned as Biden's civilian presidential physician in 2021. In contrast to the civilian selectees, military presidential physicians were in the mid-course of their careers when chosen. All, except Burkley, were fifty-five years or younger; Dr. Mariano was only thirty-eight at the time of her appointment by President Clinton.

Doctors Burkley, Lukash, Mariano, and Kuhlmann retired from military service almost immediately upon the conclusion of their White house tour of duty. However, Tkach and Hutton remained to complete an important command assignment. Walter Tkach was command surgeon for the Air Force Systems Command at Andrews Air Force Base outside Washington, D.C., until he retired in 1979.[51] Tkach's administrative responsibilities as a command surgeon were weighty. His span of responsibility included the budget, personnel, and research for all the medical treatment and research facilities located on this and affiliated bases.[52] He commanded 4,500 medical officers and enlisted men in addition to approximately 1,400 civilians working in the medical field.[53] At the conclusion of President Reagan's two term presidency in January 1989, John Hutton was promoted to brigadier general and to commander of Madigan Army Health Center in Tacoma, Washington. His major responsibility was the oversight of the construction of a new Madigan Hospital.

The post–White House experiences of the military and civilian practitioners likewise have been similarly diverse. Both doctors Tkach and Burkley retired from the practice of medicine to obscurity in California. However, George Burkley, rather than profiting from his White House connection, was disadvantaged by it. He could not escape the aftermath of the Kennedy assassination in Dallas, Texas, in November 1963. He was required to give sworn testimony to two members of the Select Committee on Assassinations in January 1978 and to respond to telephone inquiries into the event by author Henry Hoch in the early 1980s.[54]

On the other hand, doctors Lukash and Hutton continued to practice medicine as civilians, combining teaching with patient care. Lukash worked at the Scripps Clinic and Research Foundation in southern California in the Department of Gastroenterology for nearly ten years.[55] Alzheimer's disease forced his premature retirement and he died at the early age of sixty-six.[56]

John Hutton remained active in medicine for many years after his military retirement. Although he retired from active surgery at the age of seventy, he continued to teach medical students, had written book chapters, and presented lectures.[57] He held many academic appointments with professorships in surgery at the United States Uniformed Health Services School of Medicine, George Washington School of Medicine, and Tulane University School of Medicine.

Hutton formally stopped treating Reagan when he left the White House in 1989, but he would accompany the ex-president and first lady when they traveled to the Mayo Clinic for their annual physical examinations. After the former president announced that he had Alzheimer's disease in 1994, Hutton visited him a number of times, each time for a week or so, to give Nancy Reagan some relief, and he frequently called Mrs. Reagan, the last time a month before the ex-president's death. Dr. Hutton was an honorary pallbearer at his ex-patient's state funeral in June 2004.[58]

Brigadier General Hutton died ten years later on December 19, 2014, at the age of eighty-three with Parkinson's Disease. He is buried in Arlington National Cemetery.[59]

Since her retirement from the navy in 2001, Dr. Connie Mariano has practiced medicine in Arizona, initially as part of the Executive Health Program, in the structured environment of the Mayo Clinic, Phoenix Arizona,[60] and presently in the flexible, independent, and concierge setting of the Center for Executive Medicine, in nearby Scottsdale.[61]

Many features of her presidential physician experience—emphasis on primary care; the ready availability of medical subspecialists if necessary; the promotion of health maintenance and early disease detection; and life style monitoring—are important elements of her practice paradigm.

Additionally, Mariano, like many of her contemporaries, is entrepreneurial; she established her own medical business, the Center for Executive Medicine. Its website prominently displays images of the ex-presidential physician with presidents Clinton, George H.W. Bush and George W. Bush; these associations undoubtedly assist in marketing her medical practice.[62] The website defines the Center for Executive Medicine as a concierge practice: "A concierge practice provides premium-level care and access exclusively to patients enrolled as members."[63] Concierge medicine is an expanding concept of practice management. The Society for Innovative Medical Practice Design recently concluded its third annual conference on concierge medicine; Mariano was a featured speaker.[64]

She authored a memoir, *The White House Doctor*, has organized two monthly podcasts on health matters, and continues her concierge practice of executive medicine.[65]

Richard (Dick) Tubb retired from the military shortly after his eight-year stint as presidential physician. However, he continued to serve as "White House Physician Emeritus" and senior adviser to the Physicians to Presidents Obama and Trump. He also served as a board member to Lexus/Nexis Special Services, and was clinically involved in several national and international health care start-ups.[66]

Jeff Kuhlman retired from both the Navy and the WHMU at the end of President Obama's first term. He had spent thirty years in the Navy, and the combination of his family's desire and the offer of an excellent position attracted him to Florida. He has held numerous clinical and administrative positions with Advent Health.[67]

Ronny Jackson was the natural selection to succeed Kuhlman since he had served as the latter's administrative second. The two respected the other's medical expertise, but they experienced a personal falling out.[68]

Jackson quietly served as Barack Obama's physician during this president's second term. However, as Donald Trump's doctor, chaos and controversy ensued. The apparent media's bias toward this president also engulfed his doctor.

After his unsuccessful cabinet nomination, Jackson returned to the White House as a special assistant to the president, but only briefly. He retired from both the Navy and the White House to run for Congress from the conservative Texas panhandle. He was overwhelmingly elected and reelected to the United States House of Representatives in 2020 and 2022.[69] In the Congress, he is an outspoken foe of Joe Biden's policies and a proponent of the president's cognitive inability to serve as president.[70]

Jackson described his WHMU experience in his 2022 account, *Holding the Line*. He presented his personal version of the controversy over his ill-fated cabinet appointment, the resultant inspector general's investigation into his purported ill-conduct as presidential physician, and the perceived press bias against him. In an unusual breech of the common reticence between White House physicians, Jackson commented harshly upon the behavior of WHMU physicians Jennifer Pena and Kevin O'Connor. This acrimony in the public space was almost unprecedented; it recalled the 1881 Bliss/Baxter imbroglio over the treatment of President Garfield.

He blamed Pena and O'Connor for spreading false information about his performance as presidential physician to Obama and Trump, information that torpedoed his nomination as Secretary of Veterans' Affairs. The rejected nominee alleged that both disliked him since he, in their minds, prevented them from elevation to the president's physician position. Although he was not present when Pena made the allegation, he wrote, "This is not right. I'm taking the fall for all of this! This wasn't even my idea. This was all Kevin O'Connor's idea." Jackson also alleged that "during (my) confirmation process, Kevin O'Connor coordinated with her and a few others and discussed ways to undergo my nomination."[71]

Dr. Pena, in a letter to the author, disputed the accuracy of these allegations and denied any coordinated attempt with O'Connor in the nomination process.[72] Dr. O'Connor when asked to respond to his predecessor's accusations preferred not to respond, first stating that he had not read Jackson's memoir. Further, he added that he agreed with Dr. Mariano's statement in the foreword to this edition, to not speak negatively and publicly about a colleague.[73]

The charges leveled against Jackson precipitated a full investigation into his behavior by the Department of Defense Inspector General. When the Inspector General's tentative conclusions were released, it cited Jackson for creating a toxic work environment in the WHMU, but essentially cleared him of more serious charges. However, in an indication that politics may continue to influence the outcome, on the day of Joe Biden's inauguration, Jackson was informed that his investigation remained open.[74]

In the Acknowledgments of *Holding the Line*, retired captain, presently U.S. Representative Jackson, thanked two previous WHMU presidential physicians, Jeffrey Kuhlman and Richard Tubb. He wrote, "Thank you ... for pushing my early career along and setting me up for success. We did not always see eye to eye, but I would not be here without his early trust in me." "Deep appreciation to my most trusted mentor.... Richard Tubb ... hired me as a junior physician during the George W. Bush administration and later in my career became one of my best friends and biggest supporters."[75]

Sean Conley was promoted to Physician to the President in March 2018 when his predecessor resigned to become a cabinet nominee. At age thirty-eight, Conley became one of the youngest in that post; he had been assigned to the WHMU for barely a year. Conley's near three years as the presidential physician were tumultuous because they coincided with the president's Covid hospitalization. He was happy to leave behind the hostility of the Washington press at the inauguration of Joe Biden and to enter academic medicine at the Uniformed Services University of the Health Sciences in Bethesda, Maryland. His two years in the relative anonymity as professor of Military and Surgical Medicine allowed him to recuperate from the "post-traumatic stress syndrome" of the White House.[76]

After a promotion to director of the emergency medicine department at Walter Reed National Military Medical Center, he was recently promoted once again. He now serves as the emergency medicine consultant for the United States Navy.[77]

In another unfortunate circumstance of Conley's three-year tenure, his rank remained fixed as a Commander in the Navy, an O-5 equivalent to a Lieutenant Colonel in the Army or Air Force. Until 2017, both by tradition and by regulation, the physician to the president was an O-6, a Navy captain or a colonel. However, for apparent budgetary, or suspiciously political, reasons, the rule in his case was suspended and Conley remained a commander during his tenure. He was promoted to captain (USN) two years later.[78]

Chapter 17

Final Thoughts

Future political and scientific developments undoubtedly will affect the present organization and delivery of health care to presidents by the White House Medical Unit. As changes in the social, administrative, professional and educational structure of American medicine accelerate, while the circumstances and complexities of the modern American presidency increase and compound, the responsibilities and structure of the WHMU will necessarily evolve.

Over a span of 235 years the medical care of the American president has shifted from episodic to permanent, informal to formal, civilian to military, and individual to bureaucratic. Emphasis has been redirected from the medical response to an acute illness or a medical emergency toward the maintenance and improvement of the president's baseline health status. Additionally, the responsibilities of the WHMU physicians have proliferated. These include the medical management of the explosive growth of foreign and domestic presidential travel, the continuous care of the vice president and his family, the demands of the Twenty-fifth Amendment, increased public scrutiny and the extraordinary security requirements of the protracted global war on terror. Moreover, the WHMU patient census has burgeoned to include the urgent care of the thousands of military personnel attached to the White House Military Office (WHMO), the members of the presidential staff, and on occasion important domestic and foreign visitors.

One might ask whether the present organization of, and emphasis on, contingency planning by the WHMU has made it a more responsive and effective unit. My answer to this inquiry would be "yes," but a qualified "yes" for the following reasons: first, this medical organization has rarely been politically challenged during the incumbencies of healthy presidents Bill Clinton, George W. Bush and Barack Obama. No medical emergencies arose comparable to those that affected the presidencies of Dwight Eisenhower, John Kennedy, Ronald Reagan, and George H.W. Bush. However, the quiescence was shattered by the Covid hospitalization of President Donald Trump. Moreover, the WHMU effectively responded to the several cardiac crises and one accidental mishap that marked Dick Cheney's vice presidency.

In the previous edition, the author confidently, but incorrectly predicted: "the current media milieu—antagonistic, intrusive and ubiquitous in nature—virtually assures that the finalists in any presidential competition would be free of chronic medical baggage upon entering the White House. As a consequence, there would likely be no Wilson's hypertension, Harding's coronary artery pathology, or Kennedy's Addison's disease. Such an illness would most certainly be common knowledge long before Election Day." But, in a historical anomaly, in the 2016, 2020, and 2024 elections instead of candidates in their fifth to seventh decades competing for the presidency, septuagenarians and octogenarians have vied for the office. Aging has inevitable consequences.

Professional deference had modulated conflicts among the physicians treating an acutely ill president during recent decades. The interprofessional disputes that marked the Garfield, Harding, and Franklin Roosevelt events had been absent with the exception of the O'Connor/Pena/Jackson imbroglio of the recent past. Presently the opinion of the physician to the president prevails more by his or her relationship with the presidential patient, rather than by military rank or professional prestige. But the question remains whether a future medical emergency might unmask the inherent competitiveness and occasional professional arrogance of doctors. The all-military composition until recently of the doctor component of the WHMU encourages a harmony that might be challenged if a future president selects a civilian as his presidential physician. The military chain of command obliges obedience and agreement. In summary, the WHMU has functioned smoothly during the last thirty years due to a confluence of the aforementioned factors. However, its response to a severe medical crisis, although rendered less likely because of better procedures, better health of the incumbent, or by better health maintenance, remains to be judged.

Two issues require further analysis and study. Did the presidents benefit from their lofty position's greater exposure to eminent physicians, as contrasted with the doctor availability extant for their constituents? A second question is whether the changes in the medical care and health delivery afforded the president have in general paralleled the changes in American medicine over the past two centuries.

The president most definitely is a beneficiary of extraordinary medical attention. The American chief executive certainly is advantaged compared to his constituents by a physician's constant attendance, by the ready availability of the most talented medical specialists, and by the continual emphasis on health maintenance and physical fitness. Previously a few medical historians postulated that the heavy responsibilities of the office might outweigh any health premium related to the above. Fortunately, the recent longevity of presidential retirees belies this notion.[1]

Presidents have been treated by doctors whose medical education far surpassed that of most of their contemporaries. Few were graduates of defunct or unaccredited medical schools and, with the exception of Dr. Henry Huntt, no president has been cared for by a non-degreed physician; Huntt served only an apprenticeship. Even the earliest American presidents were treated by medical school graduates. Initially their degrees were obtained from abroad, most notably by the prestigious Edinburgh School of Medicine at a time when American medical schools were either in their infancy or their parturition.

In addition, for over the past hundred years, White House doctors usually acquired advanced training in the form of certification in a medical specialty. At present, board certification is a requirement before selection to the White House Medical Unit.

Over the past century, the principal causes for presidential medical emergencies have been either traumatic (assassination attempts upon McKinley, Kennedy, and Reagan) or cardiovascular (the heart attacks of Harding and Eisenhower and the strokes of Wilson and Franklin Roosevelt). It is likely that a combination of aggressive security arrangements and active health maintenance programs will reduce significantly both of these physical threats. However, other categories of disease should be anticipated. A new infectious agent, e.g., the coronavirus, may infect the president (Trump) before definitive treatment was established. The neurologic nemeses of aging (Alzheimer's Disease,

Chapter 17. Final Thoughts

Parkinsonism, pre dementia) may affect an elderly inhabitant of the oval office, as has been alleged for Joe Biden.

The White House physician experience has been at best only a translucent mirror in reflecting the structural, administrative and educational trends in American medicine over 200 years. It accurately reflects the changes in physician compensation from out-of-pocket reimbursement by the patient to third party payment by insurance companies. Moreover, it has copied accurately the development of postgraduate medical education in the United States—first internship training, then specialization, and finally board certification. As previously stated, all candidates for the White House Medical Unit must be board certified.[2]

Moreover, it has mirrored with precision the allopath-homeopath conflict that came to a boil around 1880 and characterized the emergency care of President James Garfield. The subsequent détente between these two dominant branches of organized medicine was reflected in the significant White House career of the homeopathically trained doctor Joel Boone.

But, in several areas, the White House experience had been unrepresentative. The first president to be hospitalized was Harry Truman, four decades after hospital care in America was judged to be beneficial by the population at large.

Second, at a time when half of the American medical school graduates are female, only two women, doctors Travell and Mariano, had served as White House physicians. The latter incongruity is acknowledged by the WHMU. Attempts to correct the gender disparity were undertaken; however, a previous recruitment of a military cardiologist ended unsuccessfully at the last moment.[3]

The gender disparity has been addressed. During the recent two decades, eight female physicians have joined the WHMU, bringing the historical cumulative White House complement to ten. In addition, Dr. Jennifer Pena served as the doctor to Vice President Pence and family.

In a third area, the mirror has been opaque. Significant numbers of American physicians have been osteopathically trained, but the narrative of osteopathic medicine's involvement with presidential medical care had been written on a nearly blank page. No Doctor of Osteopathy (D.O.) until recently had served as a president's personal physician or as a member of the WHMU. The only entries that were found on this page are those of the notorious Dr. Kenneth Riland, who was a consultant to Richard Nixon, and of navy dermatologist Dr. David W. Corbett. Corbett, on the staff of Bethesda Naval Hospital, removed a precancerous lesion from President Bill Clinton's nose in May 1996, and excised a benign cyst from his neck that September.[4]

This near absence was perplexing, since osteopathic medicine has made significant advances both in numbers and prestige since Dr. Riland's time.[5] The establishment of the Michigan State University College of Osteopathic Medicine in the mid-1990s was a significant event for three reasons. It was the first new school of osteopathic medicine to be founded in several decades; it was the first university-based osteopathic school, thus conferring greater academic prestige; and since it existed side by side with a traditional medical school, it indicated that the two medical professions "were separate but equal."[6] From 1970 to the present, new schools opened in many states, several with state funding, so that the total of osteopathic colleges reached fifteen by 1980 and twenty-one by 2005. Six schools have been established so recently that their charter classes graduated in 2000 or later. A major selling point for the expansion has been the proclivity of osteopathic medical graduates to practice in underserved and rural areas.[7] It has been documented that publicly funded D.O. schools have a stronger record than their respective M.D. schools in state retention of their graduates, especially in the areas of primary care.[8]

The increase in medical schools has produced both an absolute and a relative increase in the numbers of practicing osteopaths. Their numbers have grown from 11,000 in 1962 to 50,532 in active practice and in postdoctoral training by 2005.[9] Osteopathy's proportion of all graduating medical students has risen to 13.9 percent, leading to Gewitz's claim that "osteopathic medicine is now the fastest growing segment of the U.S. physician and surgeon population."[10]

Within the past several decades, osteopathy, determined to maintain an independent medical identity, has reached legal, and possibly also professional, equality with the still predominant M.D. medicine. Its core principles, having been recently restated, emphasize the distinctiveness of its practice and may explain its increasing acceptance. The four core principles are: the body is a unit and a person represents a combination of body, mind and spirit; the body is capable of self-regulation, self-healing and health maintenance; structure and function are reciprocally interrelated; rational treatment is based upon an understanding of body unity, self-regulation, and the interrelationship of structure and function.[11]

In addition to the holistic approach toward patient care articulated above, osteopathic medicine holds the following as additional distinctions from mainstream medicine: the ability to diagnose and treat through their hands; emphasis on the practitioner's interpersonal skills; focus on primary care; and a commitment to serve in underserved areas.[12] During the past two decades, a focus on holistic medicine and the training of primary care physicians have been popular trends; osteopathic medicine's empathy with these goals goes far in explaining its increasing significance. Recent data provided by the American Osteopathic Association determined that almost two thirds of osteopaths self-identify as practicing primary care medicine.[13] Primary care specialties are defined as family medicine, general internal medicine, general pediatrics and obstetrics/gynecology.[14] Therefore it was puzzling that, despite the WHMU's recent emphasis on primary care qualifications, the WHMU continued for so long to be off-limits to D.O.s.

Nor can the absence of an eligible pool of military doctors be postulated to explain this dearth. In 1977 the Association of Military Osteopathic Physicians and Surgeons (AMOPS) was formed to serve and represent osteopathic doctors in the uniformed services of the United States. AMOPS presently claims that there are 2,200 doctors of osteopathy in active service, a number comprising approximately 10 percent of physicians currently in the armed forces.[15]

A recent analysis of U.S. residency programs disclosed that the number of physician-trainees in primary care programs has plateaued, while an increasing proportion has selected subspecialty residencies. The composition of the former increasingly has become represented by osteopaths, women, and graduates of foreign medical schools.[16] Osteopathic medical doctors (DO) have achieved additional prominence since both the presidential physicians (Sean Conley/Kevin O'Connor) of Trump and Biden had the suffix DO attached to their names.

Conversely, international medical graduates (IMGs)—an enlarging portion of the American physician population—are unlikely to serve in the United States military. Consequently, their presence among those who treat a president is at best improbable.

Politically, too, it might be unwise for a president to have a foreign-born doctor. The 2120 Physician Specialty Data Report compiled and published by the American Association of Medical Colleges stated that 24.7 percent of all active U.S. physicians in 2019, or 232,190 doctors were IMGs.[17] However, during the past 100 years, before WHMU's formation, several European physicians, i.e., Dr. Max Jacobson and Dr. Hans Kraus treated President Kennedy. Both were escapees from Nazi Germany.

Professional ethics is a recurrent concern for those doctors who have cared for presidents. A comprehensive examination of the evolution, if any, of behavioral codes remains beyond the scope of this narrative. However, the reader will recall many examples of how White House doctors dealt with the thorny matter of confidentiality. In the main, physicians have been overprotective of the president's privacy, often misleading, denying, and lying, even though the information desired was trivial or not even confidential. Confidentiality has been total, even in selected instances when the president's illness affected national security and foreign policy.[18]

The provision of all relevant information regarding one's illness to the patient by the treating physician, known as informed consent, is a more recent requirement. In retrospect, under this principle Cary Grayson should have informed Wilson of his first wife's terminal kidney disease, Ross McIntire was wrong in prohibiting FDR's treating cardiologist, Howard Bruenn, from discussing with his patient the diagnosis and the prognosis of his heart disease, and did Janet Travell or Max Jacobson ever inform JFK of the ill effects of their unorthodox therapies?[19]

Medical ethical codes also address consultation and second opinions. Travell's reluctance to seek one was problematical, but perhaps not unethical. However, Hans Kraus was very careful to avoid any professional conflict with Travell when he was approached by a third physician to intervene in the case of President Kennedy. Dr. D.W. Bliss undoubtedly violated professional rules when he aggressively intervened in the case of James Garfield and banished the president's personal physician from any association with the case.[20]

In this author's numerous personal, telephone, and electronic communications, not once has any of these White House Physicians violated the rules of patient confidentiality.

Several recent presidential physicians[21] commented whether the responsibilities of the first family's medical care ought to be discrete from the multiple administrative and clinical functions of the WHMU, which include the advance planning for trips, staffing the outpatient clinic, Camp David, the care of the vice president and selected VIPs and other miscellaneous activities. Earlier these responsibilities were combined in a single person—the presidential physician was also the WHMU director. The unified model was employed by Dr. Mariano, and in the main by Drs. Tubb and Jackson.

However, present consensus supports separate lines of authority. The presidential physician is a political appointee who reports directly to the president; the WHMU director is a military and medical appointee who now is usually a non-physician but a nurse or a physician's assistant, who reports directly to the WHMO. A dotted line of cooperation and communication between the presidential physician and the director must be maintained for the arrangement to function.

The medical care of the first family has become extremely time consuming and increasingly complex. Moreover, the merged lines of authority had become confusing[22] and uncommonly very fractious.[23]

This narrative has not attempted to analyze in detail the strictly medical aspects of presidential illness or to judge the efficacy of the treatments by the presidential physicians. It also generally avoided any discussion of the advances in medical diagnosis and treatment over the preceding two centuries. It has attempted to restrict consideration to the presidents' tenure in office rather than detailing their health either before or after their presidencies.

We leave it to future studies to examine whether the medical care of presidents compared with both the customary and the best practice level of diagnosis and treatment generally available at the time. A future analysis might also consider other models for the optimal structure and organization of the White House Medical Unit and whether additional responsibilities may be appropriate, as, for example, the medical care of ex-presidents and whether the conflicts and intimate relationship with the patient rules out the presidential physician from a role in application of the Twenty-fifth Amendment.

Chapter Notes

Introduction

1. Robert F. Gilbert, ed., *Managing Crisis: Presidential Disability and the 25th Amendment* (New York: Fordham University Press, 2000), 26–29; Michael P. Riccards, "The Presidency in Sickness and in Health," *Presidential Studies Quarterly* (Summer 1977): 215–231. Both of these present excellent synopses of the significant medical problems that affected sitting presidents.

2. Rudolph Marx, M.D., *The Health of the Presidents* (New York: G.P. Putnam's Sons, 1960). This remains as the most comprehensive and well written book in this genre. It covers all the presidents from George Washington to Franklin Roosevelt. However, a major deficiency is an absence of notes and bibliography. Robert F. Gilbert's *Mortal Presidency: Illness and Anguish in the White House* (New York: Basic Books, 1992), while not as comprehensive, provides new information on presidents Dwight Eisenhower, John F. Kennedy and Ronald Reagan. Lesser works include Warren G. Harding II and Mark Stewart, *Mere Mortals: The Lives and Health Histories of American Presidents* (Worthington, OH: Renaissance Publications, 1992), and John R. Bumgarner, M.D., *The Health of the Presidents: The 41 United States Presidents through 1993 from a Physician's Point of View* (Jefferson, NC: McFarland, 1994).

3. Kenneth R. Crispell and Carlos F. Gomez, *Hidden Illness in the White House* (Durham: Duke University Press, 1988). Bert Edward Park, M.D., *The Impact of Illness on World Leaders* (Philadelphia: University of Pennsylvania Press, 1986) foreshadowed Crispell and Gomez but dealt with world figures in general, of which several were U.S. presidents. A follow-up book by Park, *Aging, Ailing, Addicted: Studies of Compromised Leadership* (Lexington: University Press of Kentucky, 1994), explores the cover-ups of Woodrow Wilson and John F. Kennedy. Robert H. Ferrell, *Ill-Advised: Presidential Health and Public Trust* (Columbia: University of Missouri Press, 1992) is an excellent book that provides new information, especially regarding Dwight Eisenhower. An earlier study is Edward B. MacMahon, M.D., and Leonard Curry, *Medical Cover-Ups in the White House* (Washington, D.C.: Farragut, 1987).

4. Edwin A. Weinstein, *Woodrow Wilson: A Medical and Psychological Biography* (Princeton: Princeton University Press, 1981). This is one of the first and most useful of these monographs. Doctor Weinstein is a neurologist-psychiatrist. Other worthy sources are: James C. Clark, *The Murder of James A. Garfield: The President's Last Days and the Trial and Execution of His Assassin* (Jefferson, NC: McFarland, 1993); Robert H. Ferrell, *The Strange Deaths of President Harding* (Columbia: University of Missouri Press, 1996); Robert H. Ferrell, *The Dying President: Franklin Roosevelt 1944–1945* (Columbia: University of Missouri Press, 1998); Clarence G. Lasby, *Eisenhower's Heart Attack: How Ike Beat Heart Disease and Held On to the Presidency* (Lawrence: University Press of Kansas, 1997).

5. Rear Admiral Cary T. Grayson, *Woodrow Wilson: An Intimate Portrait* (Washington: Potomac Books, 1960).

6. Vice Admiral Ross T. McIntire, *White House Physician* (New York: G.P. Putnam's Sons, 1946).

7. Janet Travell, *Office Hours Day and Night: The Autobiography of Janet Travell, M.D.* (New York: World Publishing, 1968).

8. T. Burton Smith, M.D., *White House Doctor* (Lanham, MD: Madison Books, 1992).

9. These generally have been more interesting and candid, since the authors have somewhat less reason to be defensive in their narratives, even though a few were written by the subjects' relatives. They include: Charles S. Foltz, *Surgeon of the Seas: The Adventurous Life of Surgeon General Jonathan M. Foltz in the Days of Wooden Ships* (Indianapolis: Bobbs-Merrill, 1931); Rear Admiral William C. Braisted and Captain William H. Bell, *The Life Story of Presley Marion Rixey* (Strasburg, VA: Shenandoah Publishing, 1930); Milton F. Heller, Jr., *The Presidents' Doctor: An Insider's View of Three First Families* (New York: Vantage Press, 2000); Susan E.B. Schwartz, *Into the Unknown: The Remarkable Life of Hans Kraus* (New York: iUniverse, 2005).

10. J. Brett Langstaff, *Dr. Bard of Hyde Park* (New York: E.P. Dutton, 1942).

11. E. Connie Mariano, M.D., interview by the author, Scottsdale, Arizona, 18 July 2003.

12. Paul Starr, *The Social Transformation of*

American Medicine (New York: Basic Books, 1982), 41.

13. Ibid., 42–43.

14. Ibid., 118–121.

15. John D. Thompson and Grace Goldin, *The Hospital: A Social and Architectural History* (New Haven, CT: Yale University Press, 1974), 97.

16. Charles E. Rosenberg, *The Care of Strangers: The Rise of America's Hospital System* (New York: Basic Books, 1987).

17. David McCullough, *Truman* (New York: Simon & Schuster, 1992), 902.

Chapter 1

1. J. Brett Langstaff, *Doctor Bard of Hyde Park* (New York: E.P. Dutton, 1942), 167.

2. William A. DeGregorio, *The Complete Book of Presidents*, 4th ed. (New York: Wings Books, 1993), 8.

3. Langstaff, 168.

4. George Washington, letter, to James McHenry, July 3, 1789, *The Writings of George Washington from the Original Manuscript Sources, 1745–1786*, ed. John C. Fitzpatrick, vol. 30, *The George Washington Papers of the Library of Congress, 1741–1799*.

5. Langstaff, 167–8.

6. "The Medical History of George Washington (1732–1799) I," *Staff Proceedings of the Mayo Clinic* (February 11, 1942): 82–96; "The Medical History of George Washington (1732–1799) II," *Staff Proceedings of the Mayo Clinic* (February 18, 1942): 107–112; and "The Medical History of George Washington (1732–1799) III," *Staff Proceedings of the Mayo Clinic* (February 25, 1942): 116–123, is an excellent three-part review of Washington's health. Many compilations of the first president's illnesses have been written, and a second excellent treatment is Abraham Blinderman, "George Washington's Health in Peace and War," *New York State Journal of Medicine* (January 1975): 122–132.

7. R. Walton Moore, address: "Dr. James Craik. Chief Physician and Surgeon of the Continental Army," delivered in Alexandria, VA, printed in the Congressional Record (February 22, 1929): 1–8. There is a discrepancy between the dates of departure from Edinburgh. Moore records 1750, while Martin Kaufman, Stuart Galishoff and Todd Savitt, eds., *Dictionary of American Medical Biography*, vol. 1 (Westport, CT: Greenwood Press), 164–165, state that he departed in 1758. Howard A. Kelly and Walter L. Burrage, *Dictionary of American Medical Biography* (New York: D. Appleton, 1928), 265, present parallel biographical material, but add the information on Craik's honorary doctorate.

8. The following periodization is used: Colonial, to 1775; Early National, 1775 to 1800; National, 1800 to 1830; Ante Bellum, 1830 to 1861.

9. Rosemary Stevens, *American Medicine and the Public Interest: A History of Specialization*, updated ed. (Berkeley: University of California Press, 1998), 18–19.

10. J.B. Morrell, *Medicine and Science in the Eighteenth Century*, in *Four Centuries: Edinburgh University Life 1583–1983*, ed. Gordon Donaldson (Edinburgh: University of Edinburgh Press, 1983), 47.

11. The Edinburgh Medical School, http://www.mvm.ed.ac.uk/history/index/htm (accessed December 16, 2004).

12. D.H. Horn, *A Short History of the University of Edinburgh, 1556–1889* (Edinburgh: University of Edinburgh Press, 1967), 41–42.

13. There are several excellent narratives of the history of the University of Edinburgh and its medical college. The sources referenced here include The Foundation of the Faculty of Medicine; http://www.mvm.ed.ac.uk/history2.htm (accessed 12/16/2004); John Harrison, *Oure Tounis College: Sketches of the History of the Old College of Edinburgh* (Edinburgh: William Blackwood and Sons, 1884), 90–91, 94–95; D.H. Horn, *A Short History of the University of Edinburgh, 1556–1889* (Edinburgh: Edinburgh University Press, 1967), 42–43; J.B. Morrell, *Medicine and Science in the Eighteenth Century*, in *Four Centuries: Edinburgh University Life, 1583–1983*, ed. Gordon Donaldson (Edinburgh: Edinburgh University Press, 1983), 38–39.

14. Leiden University Medical Center History; http://145.88.210.153/englishj/general/history.html (accessed December 18, 2004).

15. Harrison, 100.

16. Horn, 46.

17. Alyn Brodsky, *Benjamin Rush: Patriot and Physician* (New York: St. Martin's, 2004), 45, is the source for Edinburgh's population.

18. "Edinburgh and Medical Schools in North America," http://www.mvm.ed.ac.uk/history/note11.tmm (accessed December 16, 2004). Whitfield J. Bell, Jr., "Some American Students of 'That Shining Light of Physic,' Dr. William Cullen of Edinburgh, 1755–1766," in *Proceedings of the American Philosophical Society* 94(3) (June 1950): 275–281. Bell lists the dates of attendance of the American students of William Cullen in Edinburgh. Alyn Brodsky, *Benjamin Rush Patriot and Physician* (New York: St. Martin's, 2004), 89, contains material on Shippen's career. Kuhn's career is found in "Penn in the 18th Century," http://www.archives.upenn.eduhisty/features/1700s/people/kuhn_adam html (accessed April 17, 2006).

19. James Monroe, letter, to Thomas Jefferson, June 28, 1813, 271–272, in *The Writings of James Monroe*, ed. Stanislaus Hamilton (New York: G.P. Putnam's Sons, 1901) contains the scant details of Dr. Tucker's attendance to Madison. Bell and http://www.bioguide.congress.gov/scripts/biodisplay.pl?index=T000403 are sources for Tucker's career.

20. Charles A. Roos, "Physicians to the Presidents, and Their Patients: A Bibliography," *Bulletin of the Medical Library Association* 49 (1961): 310–311.

21. Howard A. Kelly and Walter L. Barrage, *American Medical Biographies* (Baltimore: Norman, Remington Company, 1920), 1196–1197.

22. Bell is the source for the date of Brown's Edinburgh graduation. Brown's association with the medical and chirurgical faculty of Maryland is derived from the following sources: John Tilden Howard, "The Doctors Gustavus Brown, Father and Son, of Charles County, Maryland," *Annals of Medical History* 9 (1937): 437–448; John French, *Celebration of the Sesquicentennial of the Medical and Chirurgical Faculty of Maryland, 1799–1949* (Baltimore: Waverly Press, 1949), 9–13. Brown's participation in the treatment of the moribund Washington is well depicted in the following: David M. Morens, "Death of a President," *New England Journal of Medicine* 341(4) (December 9, 1999): 1845–1849; D. Pelisati and G. Sperati, "George Washington," *Acta Otorhinolaryngology Ital* 25 (2005): 55–58; F.A. Willis and T.E. Keys, "The Medical History of George Washington III," *Staff Meetings of the Mayo Clinic* (February 25, 1942): 116–121.

23. "Mitchill, Samuel Latham," in *Samuel Latham Mitchill Papers, William L. Clements Library, The University of Michigan*, http://www.clements.umich.edu/Webguides/M/Mitchill.html (accessed January 20, 2006).

24. J. Brett Langstaff, *Dr. Bard of Hyde Park* (New York: E.P. Dutton, 1942), 51.

25. *Ibid.*, 57–58.

26. *Ibid.*, 84–85.

27. "Samuel Bard (1742–1821) Colonial Physician," editorial, *Journal of the American Medical Association* 205 (8) (August 19, 1968): 114–5. This is a very succinct summary of Samuel Bard's illustrious career. Langstaff's *Doctor Bard of Hyde Park* referenced above gives the same information in much greater detail.

28. Langstaff, 119.

29. *Ibid.*, 121.

30. *Ibid.*, 122.

31. *Ibid.*, 132–4.

32. *Ibid.*, 136.

33. *Ibid.*, 147–9.

34. *Ibid.*, 168; Blinderman, 128, specifies that Bard's reputation was so great that Washington overlooked his previous Loyalist sympathies.

35. Douglas Southall Freeman, *Washington* (New York: Simon & Schuster, 1992), 571.

36. Blinderman, 128.

37. Many narratives of this episode exist. The most useful has been Langstaff, 168–175, and Blinderman, 128.

38. Stephen Decatur, Jr., *Private Affairs of George Washington from the Records and Accounts of Tobias Lear, Esquire, His Secretary* (Boston: Houghton Mifflin, 1933), 68.

39. Arthur L. Bowley, *Wages in the United Kingdom in the Nineteenth Century* (Cambridge, MA: The University Press, 1900), 64, 82.

40. Decatur, 133.

41. Freeman, 582.

42. "John Jones (1729–1791), Physician to Washington and Franklin," editorial, *Journal of the American Medical Association* 202(1) (October 2, 1967): 152–3.

43. Freeman, 582.

44. Donald Jackson and Dorothy Twohig, eds., *The Diaries of George Washington*, vol. 6 (Charlottesville: University Press of Virginia, 1979), 76–7.

45. John D. Thompson and Grace Goldin, *The Hospital: A Social and Architectural History* (New Haven, CT: Yale University Press, 1974), 97.

46. James J. Walsh, *History of Medicine in New York: Three Centuries of Medical Progress*, vol. 3, *Medical Institutions* (New York: National Americana Society, 1919), 748–753.

47. *Ibid.*, 748.

48. Langstaff, 179–198.

49. Decatur, 255, "Penn in the 18th Century."//

50. James Thomas Flexner, *George Washington: Anguish and Farewell, 1793–1799* (Boston: Little, Brown, 1972), 46.

51. *Ibid.*, 149.

52. *Ibid.*, 146–7.

53. John M. Holmes, *Thomas Jefferson Treats Himself* (Fort Valley, Virginia: Loft Press, 1997), 18. This is an excellent compilation of Jefferson's health practices.

54. *Ibid.*, 21

55. *Ibid.*, 18–19.

56. See Chapter 2.

57. See Chapter 13.

58. Brodsky, 335–336, 352–355, 365–366.

Chapter 2

1. History of the Medical Society of the District of Columbia (Washington, D.C.: The Medical Society of the District of Columbia, 1909), 5–7.

2. *Ibid.*, 426.

3. *Ibid.*, 433.

4. *Ibid.*, 55.

5. Roos, 305–326. These pages cover the Madison-Lincoln period. This invaluable source not only contains a listing of the presidential physicians and brief synopses of each president's health but also provides important citations from primary sources.

6. As defined in Chapter 1, 1800–1865.

7. Paul E. Kopperman, "Venerate the Lancet: Benjamin Rush's Yellow Fever Therapy in Context," *Bulletin of the History of Medicine* 78 (2004): 539–574. There are two useful recent biographies of Benjamin Rush: David Barton, *Benjamin Rush: Signer of the Declaration of Independence* (Aledo, TX: Wall builder Press, 1999) and Alyn Brodsky, *Benjamin Rush: Patriot and Physician* (New York: St. Martin's, 2004).

8. Samuel C. Busey, *Personal Reminiscences and Recollections of the Medical Society of Forty-six Years Membership in the Medical Society of the District of Columbia* (Philadelphia: Dornan, printer, 1895), 148–9.

9. Two significant sources for the history of the District of Columbia Medical Society and the biographies of its physician members are *History of the Medical Society of the District of Columbia, 1817-1890* (Washington, D.C.: The Medical Society of the District of Columbia, 1909) and Samuel C. Busey, *Personal Reminiscences and Recollections of Forty-six Years Membership in the Medical Society of the District of Columbia* (Philadelphia: Dornan, printer, 1895).

10. Rudolph Marx, *The Health of Presidents* (New York: G.P. Putnam's Sons, 1960), 85–6.

11. Allan Nevins, ed., *The Diary of John Quincy Adams, 1794-1845* (New York: Charles Scribner's Sons, 1951), 299.

12. Wyndham B. Blanton, *Medicine in Virginia in the Eighteenth Century* (Richmond: Garrett & Massie, 1931), 82. Everett's required dissertation was on the function of menstruation, which is verified in http://www.franklin.library.upenn.edu/cgi-bin/Pwebrecon.cgi?Search_Arg=Everett%2C+Ch (accessed on February 4, 2005).

13. W.P. Cresson, *James Monroe* (Chapel Hill: University of North Carolina Press; 1946), 248.

14. James Monroe has been the subject of many biographies. Only a few have been useful in charting his medical history. In addition to Cresson above, two others have been helpful, especially with regard to his 1818 illness: Harry Ammon, *James Monroe: The Quest for National Identity* (New York: McGraw-Hill, 1971), 420–421, and Arthur Styron, *The Last of the Cocked Hats; James Monroe & the Virginia Dynasty* (Norman: University of Oklahoma Press; 1845), 350.

15. Lyon G. Tyler, *Tyler's Historical Quarterly and Genealogical Magazine* 5 (1924): 18, 21, 22, 23.

16. *Ibid.*, 18.

17. Roos, 307.

18. Tyler, 21–2.

19. Roos, 307.

20. Busey, 174, and *The History of the Medical Society of the District of Columbia*, 214, 238, are encyclopedic with information of this era. Thomas Miller's accomplishments were recorded in an address by his daughter, Virginia Miller, to the May 1, 1899, meeting of the Columbia Historical Society, *Records of the Columbia Historical Society* 3 (1900): 303–323. *Transactions of the American Medical Association*, 32 (1881): 506–513, contains a lengthy obituary of James C. Hall.

21. *History of the Medical Society of the District of Columbia*, 239; *Transactions of the American Medical Association* 32 (1881): 506–513; J.K. Crellin, "Robert King Stone, M.D., Physician to Abraham Lincoln," *Illinois Medical Journal* (February 1979): 97–99 was helpful in corroborating and expanding Stone's academic credentials.

22. *Transactions of the American Medical Association* 32; *Records of the Columbia Historical Society*, "A Biographical Sketch of the Late Henry Huntt, M.D.," *The Medical Examiner* 1 (1838): 363–5; *The History of the Medical Society of the District of Columbia*, 149.

23. *Transactions of the American Medical Association* 32.

24. "The Late Dr. Hall," *The Boston Medical and Surgical Journal* 102 (1880): 621–2.

25. Ludwig M. Deppisch, "Andrew Jackson and American Medical Practice: Old Hickory and His Physicians," *Tennessee Historical Quarterly* 62(9) (Summer 2003): 130–151.

26. *Ibid.*

27. *History of the Medical Society of the District of Columbia, 1807-1909* (Washington, D.C.: The Medical Society of the District of Columbia, 1909), 214, and Thomas Miller, "A Biographical Sketch of the Professional Life and Character of the Late Henry Huntt, M.D., of Washington, D.C.," *The Medical Examiner* 1 (1838): 363–365 both allude to Huntt's lack of an M.D. other than an honorary one. Deppisch, 130–151, summarizes what is known of May's and Esselman's training.

28. Paul Starr, *The Social Transformation of American Medicine* (New York: Basic Books, 1982), 40.

29. Starr, 63–64.

30. Many references agree upon the predominance and historical period of apprenticeship and include Abraham Flexner, *Medical Education in the United States and Canada: A Report to the Carnegie Foundation for the Advancement of Teaching, 1910*, Bulletin 4 (Boston: D.B. Updike, Merrymount Press, 1960), 3; Wyndham B. Blanton, *Medicine in Virginia in the Eighteenth Century* (Richmond: Garrett & Massie, 1931), 76; Richard H. Shryock, *Medical Licensing in America, 1650-1965* (Baltimore: Johns Hopkins Press, 1967), 3; William G. Rothstein, *American Physicians in the 19th Century: From Sects to Science* (Baltimore: Johns Hopkins University Press, 1985), 85; Robert C. Derbyshire, *Medical Licensure and Discipline in the United States* (Westport, CT.: Greenwood Press, 1978), 3. Derbyshire commented upon the exclusion of women from the medical apprentice system.

31. Blanton, in his review of Virginia medicine of this period, discussed both the age of entry and a duration that could reach seven years. Rothstein, 87, and Starr, 40, agreed that the usual time span was three years. Flexner and Rothstein, 87, discussed the qualities of the physician preceptor.

32. Starr, 40; Rothstein, 85; Blanton, 76. Blanton is responsible for the Mount Vernon anecdote.

33. Starr, 40.

34. Blanton, 76, quotes the stricture placed upon the apprentice's behavior. Flexner, 3, and Starr, 40, provided general information regarding the apprentice's duties.

35. Flexner, 3; Blanton, 76; Rothstein, 86–87; Starr, 40, are in agreement in their assessment of the quality of apprenticeships. The macabre anecdote regarding anatomical study is from Blanton.

36. Blanton, 76; Derbyshire, 3; Rothstein, 85; Starr, 40.

37. Shryock, 27.

38. "Report on Hall, James Crowdhill, M.D.,"

Transactions of the American Medical Association 33 (1881): 506–513.

39. Virginia Miller, "Dr. Thomas Miller and His Times," *Records of the Columbia Historical Society* 3 (1900): 303–323.

40. Derbyshire, 6.

41. James Parton, *The Life of Andrew Jackson in Three Volumes,* vol. 3 (New York: Mason Brothers, 1860), 608. Additional information regarding Sim was obtained in a personal communication from David R. Hoth, assistant editor of the "Papers of Andrew Jackson," September 8, 1998.

42. Library of Congress, *Andrew Jackson Correspondence,* March 27, 1833; January 1, 1836; January 2, 1836; January 3, 1837.

43. Library of Congress, *Andrew Jackson Correspondence,* January 1, 1832; January 9, 1832; September 14, 1833; June 9, 1834; April 6, 1835.

44. Andrew Donelson to Emily Donelson, June 24, 1833, *Donelson Papers.*

45. Fielding H. Garrison, *An Introduction to the History of Medicine,* 4th ed. (Philadelphia: W.B. Saunders Co., 1963), 499–500.

46. Deppisch, 142.

47. Deppisch, 140.

48. Rudolph Marx, *The Health of the Presidents* (New York: G.P. Putnam's Sons, 1960), 127–131.

49. Miller, *Records of the Columbia Historical Society,* 311-2.

50. Irving Brant, *James Madison: Commander in Chief* (Indianapolis: Bobbs-Merrill, 1961), 187.

51. Miller, 312; Roos, 313.

52. Thomas Miller, "Case of the Late William H. Harrison, President of the United States," *The Boston Medical and Surgical Journal* 24 (June 2, 1841): 267.

53. *Niles National Register,* March 27, 1841.

54. Miller, "Case of the Late William H. Harrison," 261-7.

55. Statute I, Chapter II of the Acts of the Twenty-seventh Congress of the United States, passed on June 30, 1841. The Act for the relief of Mrs. Harrison, widow of the late president of the United States, stipulated a payment of $25,000 minus any sum of money previously paid to the personal representatives of the deceased president. This same congress (House of Representatives, 27th Congress, 1st session, document #55) on August 16, 1841, provided $3,088.09 for expenses for the funeral of William Henry Harrison.

56. Starr, 42–43; Flexner, 6.

57. Starr, 42–43.; Flexner, 6–7.

58. Daniel Drake, *Practical Essays on Medical education and the Medical Profession in the United States, 1832* (Baltimore: Johns Hopkins Press, 1953), 45

59. Starr, 42–43; Flexner, 7; Drake, 47.

60. Roos, 316.

61. *Ibid.,* 324–5.

62. Samuel X. Radbill, "The Autobiographical Ana of Robley Dunglison, M.D.," *Transactions of the American Philosophical Society* 53(8) (December 1963): 26. Dunglison recounts a comment by ex-president Jefferson, in the presence of Dr. Charles Everett, "that whenever he saw three physicians together, he looked up to discover whether there was not a turkey buzzard in the neighborhood." Everett apparently was not amused by Jefferson's remark.

63. *History of the Medical Society of the District of Columbia,* 228.

64. "The Late Dr. Hall," *Boston Medical and Surgical Journal* 102 (January-June 1880): 621–622.

65. Blockley, "The Memory Lingers On," http://www.uchs.net/Rosenthal/Blockley.html (accessed January 12, 2005); "Old Blockley," Philadelphia General Hospital, http://www.phila.gov/health/history/parts/part_5.html (accessed January 12, 2005).

66. J.R. Crellin, "Robert King Stone, M.D., Physician to Abraham Lincoln," *Illinois Medical Journal* (February 1979): 97–9.

67. Miller, 63–65.

68. Crellin, 97–99; *History of the Medical Society of the District of Columbia,* 238–239.

69. Rosemary Stevens, *American Medicine and the Public Interest: A History of Specialization* (Berkeley: University of California Press, 1998), 100–101.

70. Roos, 321-6.

Chapter 3

1. Charles S. Foltz, *Surgeon of the Seas: The Life of Surgeon General Jonathan M. Foltz* (Indianapolis: Bobbs-Merrill, 1931), 132–133.

2. Ludwig M. Deppisch, "President Cleveland's Secret Operation: The Effect of the Office Upon the Care of the President," *Pharos* 58(3) (Summer, 1995): 11–16.

3. Roos' bibliography continued as a significant source in researching this chapter. An important primary source was the military records of army and navy officers on file in the National Archives. Biographies of the presidents of the period and of navy admiral Jonathan Foltz were helpful secondary sources.

4. Lisa Odum (Associate Librarian, Mount Vernon Ladies' Association), in a telephone interview with the author, 1 July 2002.

5. *History of the Medical Society of the District of Columbia, 1817–1909* (Washington, D.C.: Medical Society of the District of Columbia, 1909), 222, 433.

6. *Ibid.,* 2.

7. *Ibid.,* 222; "Obituary of Bailey Washington," *JAMA:* 28 (1897): 431.

8. Rudolph Marx, *The Health of Presidents* (New York: G.P. Putnam's Sons; 1960), 86; John R Bumgarner, *The Health of the Presidents* (Jefferson, NC: McFarland, 1994), 34.

9. Allan Nevins, ed., *The Diary of John Quincy Adams, 1794–1845* (New York: Charles Scribner's Sons, 1951): 299.

10. "History of the Washington Navy Yard," http://www.history.navy.mil/faqs/faq52-1.htm (accessed February 11,2005); "Old Naval Hospital Building," http://www.nlm.nih.gov/hmd/medtour/oldnavy.html (accessed February 19, 2005).

11. Leon G. Tyler, ed., *Tyler's Quarterly Historical and Genealogical Magazine*, 5 (1921): 21-2.

12. Harold D. Langley, *A History of Medicine in the Early U.S. Navy* (Baltimore: Johns Hopkins University Press, 1995), 298-300.

13. Robert V. Remini, *Andrew Jackson*, vol. 1, *The Course of American Empire* (Baltimore: Johns Hopkins University Press, 1977), 181-6.

14. *The Washington Globe*, 14 January 1832.

15. Robert V. Remini, *Andrew Jackson*, vol. 2, *The Course of American Freedom* (Baltimore: Johns Hopkins University Press, 1981), 346; *The Washington Globe*, 14 January 1832.

16. Louis Roddis, "Thomas Harris, M.D.: Naval Surgeon and Founder of the First School of Naval Medicine in the New World," *Journal of the History of Medicine* (Summer 1950): 236-250.

17. John S. Bassett, ed., *Correspondence of Andrew Jackson*, 7 vols. (Washington, D.C.: Carnegie Institute of Washington, 1926-35).

18. Bumgarner, 72-6; Marx, 148-55.

19. Samuel W. Francis, "Biographical Sketch of General R.C. Wood," *The Medical and Surgical Reporter* 20 (April 10, 1869): 275-6.; Holman Hamilton, *Zachary Taylor: Soldier in the White House* (Indianapolis: Bobbs-Merrill, 1951): 38-9, 47, 140, 199, 216.

20. Roger D. Hunt and Jack R. Brown, *Brevet Brigadier Generals in Blue* (Gaithersburg, MD: Lode Soldier Books, 1990), 689.

21. R.C. Wood, letter, to Brigadier General Thomas Lawson, August 1, 1849, *Robert C. Wood's Medical Officer's files*, National Archives and Records Administration.

22. Hamilton, 224-6.

23. K. Jack Bauer, *Zachary Taylor: Soldier, Planter, Statesman of the Old Southwest* (Baton Rouge: Louisiana State University Press, 1985), 314-6; Hamilton, 386-93.

24. Charles A. Roos, "Physicians to the Presidents, and Their Patients: A Bibliography," *Bulletin of the Medical Library Association* 49 (1961): 315-6; A.S. Wotherspoon, "Some Cases of a Rare Form of Exanthem," *American Periodical Series* II(ii) (1844): 203-217 describes investigative work by Wotherspoon performed during his stay at the New York Hospital.

25. Roos, 315-16; Wotherspoon, 203-217; Bauer, 314-6; *History of the Medical Society of the District of Columbia*, 250-1.

26. Robert C. Wood to Brigadier General Thomas Lawson, October 17, November 25, December 10, 1850, March 10, 1851; *Robert C. Wood's Medical Officer's Files*, National Archives and Records Administration.

27. Francis B. Heitman, *Historical Register and Dictionary of the United States Army* (Washington: Government Printing Office, 1903), 1061.

28. Howard A. Kelly & Walter L. Burrage, *Dictionary of American Medical Biography* (New York: D. Appleton, 1928), 963.

29. Charles S. Foltz, *Surgeon of the Seas: The Life of Surgeon General Jonathan M. Foltz* (Indianapolis: Bobbs-Merrill, 1931), 19.

30. J.H. Kidder, "Foltz, Jonathan Messersmith," *Transactions of the American Medical Association* 33 (1882): 555-8.

31. Foltz, 15-16; Francis, 275.

32. Foltz, 132-3.

33. Mile Milton Quaife, ed., *The Diary of James K. Polk During His Presidency, 1845 to 1849* (Chicago: A.C. McClurg, 1910), 85-103.

34. Foltz, 130-1.

35. *Ibid.*, 131.

36. Franklin & Marshall College Collection of Jonathan Messersmith Foltz Papers, January 30, 1856, February 23, 1857, July 18, 1857.

37. Foltz, 180-1; "National Hotel Disease," as found in http://www.everything2.com/index.pl?node=National%20Hotel1%disease (accessed August 22, 2005).

38. *Ibid.*, 183.

39. George T. Curtis, *Life of James Buchanan: Fifteenth President of the United States* (Freeport, NY: Books for Libraries Press, 1883), 188.

40. Foltz, 184.

41. Ross T. McIntire, *White House Physician* (New York: G.P. Putnam's Sons, 1946), 58-9.

42. Foltz, 185-6.

43. *Ibid.*, 186.

44. *Ibid.*

45. Franklin and Marshall College: Special Collection of Jonathan Messersmith Foltz Papers, notation for December 15, 1857.

46. Foltz, 191.

47. *Ibid.*, 339.

48. Jonathan Messersmith Foltz to A.J. Steinman, June 16, 1868.

49. *Ibid.*

50. Foltz, 337. The Naval Appropriations Act of 3 March 1871, Section 5173, added the title of Surgeon General to the Chief of the Bureau of Medicine and Surgery. Henceforth Surgeon General will be the term used for this position.

51. Paul Starr, *The Social Transformation of American Medicine* (New York: Basic Books, 1982), 150; Charles E. Rosenberg, *The Care of Strangers: The Rise of America's Hospital System* (New York: Basic Books, 1987), 4-5.

52. Samuel C. Busey, *Personal Reminiscences and Recollections of Forty-Six Years Membership in the Medical Society of the District of Columbia* (Washington, D.C., 1895), 212.

53. *Ibid.*; *History of the Medical Society of the District of Columbia 1817-1909* (Washington, D.C.: The Medical Society of the District of Columbia, 1909), 33.

54. *History of the Medical Society of the District of Columbia*, 34.

55. Starr, 149-151.

56. Rosenberg, 4.

57. *History of the Medical Society of the District of Columbia*, 33-37; Busey, 224-229. Additional information on Providence Hospital was found at http://www.provhosp.org/history_&_mission.htm (accessed on May 23, 2004).

58. Julie A. Stanish, personal correspondence with the author, 25 February 2005.

Chapter 4

1. James C. Clark, The Murder of James A. Garfield: The President's Last Days and the Trial and Execution of His Assassin (Jefferson, NC: McFarland, 1993), 76.

2. *Ibid.*

3. *Ibid.*

4. Charles A. Roos, "Physicians to the Presidents, and Their Patients: A Bibliography," *Bulletin of the Medical Library Association* 49 (1961): 322-3.

5. Harvey C. Browne, *The Medical Department of the United States Army from 1775 to 187*, Part III, *From the Revolution of the Corps in 1821 to the Declaration of War Against Mexico* (Washington, D.C.: Surgeon General's Office, 1873), 139-140; Mary C. Gillett, *The Army Medical Department, 1865-1917* (Washington, D.C.: U.S. Government Printing Office, 1994), 11.

6. Roos, 321-2.

7. *Ibid.*, 321-5.

8. James Evelyn Pilcher, *The Surgeon General of the Army of the United States* (Carlisle, Pennsylvania: Association of Military Surgeons, 1905), 60-63; William B. Atkinson, ed., *A Biographical Dictionary of Contemporary American Physicians and Surgeons* (Philadelphia: D.G. Brinton, 1880), 459-460; "Joseph K. Barnes," in *Museum of History*, http://www.virtualmuseumofhistory.com/josephkbarnes (accessed May 27, 2001); Roos, 323.

9. Roos, 326.

10. Monthly duty reports, Basil Norris to Surgeon Generals of the Army, 1863-1884.

11. Atkinson, 106.

12. Roos, 326-7.

13. Frank Cowan, *Andrew Johnson, President of the United States: Reminiscences of His Private Life and Character* (Greenesburgh, PA: Oliver Publishing, 1894), 7.

14. Lately Thomas, *The First President Johnson: The Three Lives of the Seventeenth President of the United States of America* (New York: Morrow; 1968), 349-350; Hans L. Trefousse, *Andrew Johnson: A Biography* (New York: W.W. Norton, 1989), 229.

15. Trefousse, 285.

16. Thomas, 350.

17. Letter from ex-president Johnson to Norris, July 12, 1870; Telegram from Mary Stover, Johnson's daughter, to Norris, March 24, 1869. Both from Basil Norris Military Records.

18. Rudolph Marx, *The Health of the Presidents* (New York: G.P. Putnam's Sons, 1960), 216-7.

19. U.S. Grant to Basil Norris, surgeon, USA, August 15, 1877, Basal Norris Military Records. In this letter, which Grant signed "Your Friend," the ex-president also wrote, "It seems more like a breaking up of a family to part from you, who have been a welcome visitor for so many years, than a mere separation from Government officials."

20. *History of the Medical Society of the District of Columbia* (Washington, D.C.: The District of Columbia Medical Society, 1909), 31-2.

21. Samuel C. Busey, *Personal Reminiscences and Recollections of Forty-Six Years Membership in the Medical Society of the District of Columbia* (Washington, D.C.: Dornan, printer, 1895), 105.

22. *Ibid.*, 305.

23. *Ibid.*

24. *Ibid.*, 309.

25. *Ibid.*, 312.

26. Harold D. Langley, *A History of Medicine in the Early U.S. Navy* (Baltimore: Johns Hopkins University Press, 1995), 338.

27. Bureau of Medicine and Surgery Administration Activities, http://www.navymedicine.med.navy.mil/burned/index.cfmocid=10259 (accessed February ,11, 2005).

28. Basil Norris to Assistant Surgeon General Joseph R. Smith, January 4, 1863; Basil Norris military records.

29. Joseph B. Moore to Secretary of War McCreary, September 25, 1878. A previous letter by Moore to the Secretary of War with the same complaint was written April 10, 1876. Basil Norris military records.

30. Gillett, 56.

31. Pilcher, 74-8; T. Harry Williams, ed., *Hayes: The Diary of a President, 1875-1881* (New York: David McKay, 1964), 259, 266.

32. Busey, 306-8.

33. Pilcher, 76.

34. Pilcher, 74-78; "Jedediah Hyde Baxter," http://www,arlingtoncemetary.com/jhbaxter.htm (accessed June 8, 2001).

35. Williams, 259.

36. Tom Culbertson, Spiegel Grove curator, personal correspondence with the author, 7 June 2001.

37. Kenneth E. Davison, *The Presidency of Rutherford B. Hayes* (Westport, CT: Greenwood Press, 1972), 78.

38. Harry James Brown and Frederick D. Williams, eds., *The Diary of James A. Garfield*, vol. 2, *1872-1874* (Lansing: Michigan State University Press, 1967), 275, 287-8, 387.

39. Harry James Brown and Frederick D. Williams, eds., *The Diary of James A. Garfield*, vol. 4, *1878-1881* (Lansing: Michigan State University Press, 1981), 36, 41, 406.

40. *Ibid.*, 406.

41. *Ibid.*, 418-9.

42. James C. Clark, *The Murder of James A. Garfield: The President's Last Days and the Trial and Execution of His Assassin* (Jefferson, NC: McFarland, 1993), 42.

43. Howard A. Kelly and Walter L. Burrage, *American Medical Biographies* (Baltimore: Norman, Remington, 1920): 75-6.

44. Martin Kaufman, *Homeopathy in America: The Rise and Fall of a Medical Heresy* (Baltimore: Johns Hopkins Press, 1971), 27. Hahnemann stated that orthodox doctors prescribed medicinals not on the basis of "contraria" (opposite in reaction to the symptoms) or "similia" (like the symptoms, a basic tenet of homeopathy) but rather "allos," other basis for prescription.

45. Roos, 330–337.

46. Clark, 61.

47. *Ibid.*, 76–7.

48. See Chapter 4.

49. Kaufman, 88–90.

50. *Ibid.*, 52–53.

51. James C. Whorton, *Nature Cure: The History of Alternative Medicine in America* (New York: Oxford University Press, 2002), 68–69.

52. Clark, 75.

53. Clark, 74–5, and Kaufman, 86–87, detail the circumstances of Barnes' consultation with Verdi. Verdi's interesting biography is documented in http://www.famousamericans.net/tulliosuzzaraverdi; http://www.hoemeoint.org/history/cleave/v/verdits.htm; and http://www.hoemoint.org/photo/uv/verfdits.htm (accessed September 15, 2005). The *History of the Medical Society of the District of Columbia*, 110–112, details the Society's fulminations over the board of health matter.

54. Busey, 274.

55. Ludwig M. Deppisch, "Homeopathic Medicine and Presidential Health: Homeopathic Influences upon Two Ohio Presidents," *Pharos* 60(4) (Fall, 1997): 5–10.

56. Busey, 290; Kaufman, 88–90.

57. Kaufman, 23–27.

58. Deppisch, 5.

59. Clark, 99; Roos, 330.

60. Editorial, "A Violation of Medical Ethics," *Walsh's Retrospect: A Quarterly Compendium of American Medicine and Surgery* (1881): 457–9.

61. Deppisch, 5–10.

62. Allan Peskin, *Garfield* (Kent, OH: Kent State University Press, 1978), 9.

63. H.J. Brown and F.D. Williams, eds., *The Diary of James A. Garfield*, vol. 1, *1848–1871*, and vol. 4, *1878–1881*(East Lansing: Michigan State University Press, 1967, 1981).

64. W.H. King, ed., *History of Homeopathy and Its Institutions in America*, vol. 3 (New York: Lewis, 1905).

65. H.J. Brown, *The Diary of James A. Garfield*.

66. *Ibid.*, 590.

67. Clark, 42–43.

68. D.G. Swainn to Silas A. Boynton, July 4, 1881, James A. Garfield Papers, Western Reserve Historical Library, Cleveland, OH. Originals in the Manuscript Division, Library of Congress.

69. Deaths: Susan A. Edson, M.D., *Transactions of the 54th Session of the American Institute of Homeopathy* (New York: Troy Directory, Printing and Bookbinding, 1899).

70. R.S-B. Feis, *Mollie Garfield in the White House* (Chicago: Rand McNally, 1963), 70.

71. James S. Brown to Susan A. Edson, July 1, 1881, James A. Garfield Papers, Western Reserve Historical Library, Cleveland, OH. Originals in the Manuscript Division, Library of Congress.

72. M. Leech and H.J. Brown, *The Garfield Orbit* (New York: Harper & Row, 1978).

73. Deppisch.

74. Deppisch; Robert Reyburn, "Clinical history of the case of President James Abram Garfield," *JAMA* 22 (1894): 411–417, 440–464, 578–582, 621–624, 664–669; S.M. Brooks, *Our Murdered President: The Medical Story* (New York: Frederick Fell, 1966), 80.

75. Deppisch; Clark, 110–112.

76. D.W. Bliss, "Report of the Case of President Garfield," *The Medical Record* 20(15) (October 8, 1881): 393–402.

77. Richard W. Pritchard and A.L. Herring, "The Problem of the President's Bullet," *Surgery, Gynecology and Obstetrics* 92 (1951): 631.

78. "Expenses of President Garfield's Illness and Death," Miscellaneous Document #14, House of Representatives, 47th Congress, 2d session (December 11, 1882):1–12.

79. Anne Taylor Kirschmann, *A Vital Force: Women in Homeopathy* (New Brunswick, NJ: Rutgers University Press, 2004), 5.

80. *Ibid.*, 35.

81. *Ibid.*, 56, 46.

82. *Ibid.*, 74, 83.

83. "Susan Edson, MD," *Homeopathy Today* 17(9) (October 17, 1997): 1.

84. Homer E. Socolofsky and Allan B. Spetter, *The Presidency of Benjamin Harrison* (Lawrence: University of Kansas Press, 1987), 164–180.

85. Deppisch.

86. Pilcher, 77.

87. Harry J. Sievers, *Benjamin Harrison, Hoosier President* (Newton, CT: American Political Biography Press, 1996), 207n, 218–219, 241–243, provides information on Caroline Harrison's illness and death. Information regarding Franklin Gardner is obtained from Roos, 341, and Dana Ullman Homeopathic (Educational Services), personal correspondence with the author, June 2, 2006. Gardner was a participant in the end-of-the-century truce between the two major sects of American medicine; he became a member of the American Medical Association at that time.

88. "Robert Maitland O'Reilly," http://www.armymediicne.army.mil/history/tsgs/O'Reilly.htm (accessed May 31, 2001).

89. *Ibid.*

90. A. Scott Earle, ed., *Surgery in America: From the Colonial Era to the Twentieth Century,* 2nd ed. (New York: Praeger Scientific, 1965), 343.

91. http://www.armymedicine.army.mil/history/tsgs/O'Reilly.htm; Correspondence from Surgeon R. O'Reilly to Surgeon General U.S. Army, Washington, D.C., September 1, 1888; Military Officer Records, National Archives.

92. Marx, 265.

93. http://www.armymedicine.army.mil/history/tsgs/O'Reilly.htm.
94. Pilcher, 90.
95. Military Officers Records, Robert O'Reilly, National Archives, August 1894, March 1895, June 1895, December 1896, January 1896, June 1896.
96. Allan Nevins, *Grover Cleveland: A Study in Courage* (New York: Dodd, Mead, 1948), 528; Ludwig M. Deppisch, "President Cleveland's Secret Operation: The Effect of the Office Upon the Care of the President," *Pharos* 58(3) (1995): 11–16.
97. Earle, 343; Marx, 255.
98. Nevins, 529.
99. Deppisch, "Grover Cleveland," 12–3.
100. Joseph D. Bryant, "A History of Two Hundred and Fifty Cases of Excision of the Superior Maxilla," *Transactions of the Medical Society of the State of New York* (1890): 63–76.
101. Deppisch, "Grover Cleveland," 13.
102. Grover Cleveland Papers, the Library of Congress, April 8, 1885; April 14, 1885.
103. *Ibid.*, April 24, 1887: April 30, 1887.
104. *Ibid.*, February 16, 1886; September 6, 1887; June 7, 1888.
105. *Ibid.*, November 4, 1887.
106. *Ibid.*, September 26, 1887.
107. *Ibid.*, June 7, 1888; July 19, 1888; May 16, 1892.
108. *Ibid.*, December 18, 1890; December 31, 1892.
109. *Ibid.*, June 12, 1890.
110. Richard D. Welch, Jr., *The Presidencies of Grover Cleveland* (Lawrence: University Press of Kansas Press; 1988), 100.
111. Deppisch, "Grover Cleveland," 11–16.
112. Nevins, 529; Deppisch, "Grover Cleveland," 13.
113. C.L. Moreels, Jr., "New Historical Information on the Cleveland Operations," *Surgery* 62 (1967): 542–551.
114. Deppisch, "Grover Cleveland."
115. http://www.armymediicne.army.mil/history/tsgs/O'Reilly.htm.
116. Mary Gillett on page 96 reports that in the 1890s a small staff of six medical officers worked in the surgeon general's office to coordinate the efforts of all the army surgeons in the field; Personnel: Bureau of Medicine and Surgery Office of the Historian: http://www.nsvymedicine.med.navy.mil/burned//index.cfm?docid=10258 (accessed February 11, 2005) indicated that until the Civil War, the navy surgeon's staff consisted of the chief, an assistant surgeon, two clerks, and a messenger.
117. Mary Gillett, 96, 150.
118. Harold D. Langley, *A History of Medicine in the Early U.S. Navy* (Baltimore: Johns Hopkins University Press, 1995), 351–360.
119. K. Jack Bauer, *Zachary Taylor: Soldier, Planter, Statesman of the Old Southwest* (Baton Rouge: Louisiana State University Press, 1985), 314–316.
120. Robert V. Remini, *Andrew Jackson*, vol. 2, *The Course of American Freedom* (Baltimore: Johns Hopkins University Press, 1981) 346; *The Washington Globe*, 14 January 1832.
121. The dates of Harris' tenure as surgeon general as stated in "Chiefs of the Bureau of Medicine and Surgeons General of the Navy Medical Department," http://www.navymediicne.med.navy.mil/bumed/index.cfm?docid=10328 (accessed February 11, 2005).
122. "The Surgeon Generals of the U.S. Army and Their Predecessors, 1775–2000," http://history.amedd.army.mil.tsgs/defaylt.htm (accessed February 11, 2005).
123. Mary A. Gillett, *The Army Medical Department, 1865–1917* (Washington, D.C.: Center of Military History, 1994) 9.
124. P.M. Ashburn, *A History of the Medical Department of the United States Army* (Boston: Houghton Mifflin, 1929), 143.
125. http://www.history.amedd.army.mil/tsgs/default.htm.
126. Gillett, 314–315, and Ashburn, 283, disagree whether O'Reilly had received preferential treatment in his promotion. Gillett claimed that Colonel O'Reilly was appointed over the heads of several medical officers who had more time in service. Ashburn countered by claiming that O'Reilly was then the senior medical officer and would be able to serve a full four year term before reaching the mandatory retirement age of sixty four years.
127. Charles S. Foltz, *Surgeon of the Seas: The Adventurous Life of Surgeon General Jonathan M. Foltz in the Days of Wooden Ships* (Indianapolis: Bobbs-Merrill, 1931), 337.
128. It is the opinion of John T. Greenwood, Ph.D., Chief, Office of Medical History, Office of the Army Surgeon General (personal communication, February 4, 2005) that Wood was passed over in 1861 because he was too old, and in 1854 because of the political influence of Joseph Barnes; Louis C. Duncan, "The Days Gone By—The Strange Case of Surgeon Hammond," *Military Surgeon* 64(1) (January 1929): 98–100, and 64(2) (February 1929): 252–262 discusses the cashiering of then Surgeon General Louis Hammond and his replacement by Barnes; Ashburn, 773.
129. Clark, 76–77.
130. Mary C. Gillett, *The Army Medical Department, 1865–1917* (Washington, D.C.: Center of Military History United States Army, 1994), 7.
131. See chapters 5 and 7.
132. See Chapter 6.

Chapter 5

1. William C. Braisted and William H. Bell, The Life Story of Presley Marion Rixey (Strasburg, VA: Shenandoah Publishing, 1930). The quotation is found on page 30. Rixey's connection with the Long family is found on pp. 19, 21 and 27. Rixey's elite Washington practice is noted on page 27.
2. James Evelyn Pilcher, *The Surgeon Generals of*

the Army of the United States of America (Carlisle, PA: Association of Military Surgeons, 1905), 77.

3. Braisted and Bell. This most useful source is in two parts, the first of which is a biography of Rixey written by two admiring colleagues. The second and somewhat longer part of the book consists of Rixey's previously unpublished autobiography that contains many interesting primary source documents.

4. *Ibid.*, 7. Rixey sought a commission in the United States Navy after graduation from medical school because "it was absolutely necessary for him to make a decision of how to make a living."

5. Abraham Flexner, *Medical Education in the United States and Canada: A Report to the Carnegie Foundation for the Advancement of Teaching*, Bulletin Number Four (Boston: D.B. Updike, Merrymount Press, 1910).

6. Braisted and Bell, 1–10; "Editorial Expression," *The Military Surgeon* 23(5) (November 1908): 406–8.

7. Braisted and Bell, 11–22.

8. *Ibid.*, 19.

9. *Ibid.*, 19–21.

10. *Ibid.*, 27.

11. Navy Bureau of Medicine and Surgery—History, http:/www./navymedicine.med.navy.mil/bumed/index.cfm?docid=10259 (accessed February 11, 2005).

12. Braisted & Bell, 30–31.

13. Margaret Leech, *In the Days of McKinley* (New York: Harper, 1959), 17.

14. John DeToledo, Brian DeToledo, and Meredith Lowe, "The Epilepsy of First Lady Ida Saxton," *Southern Medical Journal* 93(3) (March 2000): 267–271.

15. "Mrs. McKinley Dies in Canton Cottage," *New York Times*, 26 May 1907. See Chapter 6 Florence Harding.

16. Braisted & Bell, 31.

17. *Ibid.*, 32–3.

18. *Ibid.*, 30, 84, 239.

19. *Ibid.*, 239.

20. Leech, 459.

21. Braisted & Bell, 37, 47.

22. *Ibid.*, 37.

23. Leech, 567.

24. Braisted & Bell, 27.

25. See Chapter 4.

26. Selig Adler, "The Operation on President McKinley," *Scientific American* 208(3) (March 1963): 118–130. The report on the autopsy of the president is included in "The Official Report on the Case of President McKinley," *JAMA* 37 (1901): 1029–1036 asserted, "The extensive necrosis of the pancreas would seem to be an important factor in the cause of death...." However, the report confused the issue by concluding that "changes in the heart ... indicate that the condition of this organ was an important factor in the extensive brown atrophy and diffuse fatty degeneration of the muscle, but especially the extent to which the pericardial fat had invaded the atrophic muscle fibers of the right ventricular wall, to sufficiently explain the rapid pulse and lack of response of this organ to stimulation during life." Subsequent pathologic doctrine has shown that this conclusion is erroneous.

27. Roswell Park, "Emergency Hospital at the Pan-American Exposition," *Buffalo Medical Journal* (1901): 701–704.

28. James E. King, "In Memoriam: Matthew Derbyshire Mann," *Transactions of the American Gynecological Society* 46 (1921): 386–389; Adler.

29. The operative and postoperative course of McKinley's assassination has been the subject of several publications. The official report was by P.M. Rixey, Matthew D. Mann, Herman Mynter et al., "The Official Report on the Case of President McKinley," *JAMA* 37 (October 19, 1901): 1029–1036. This was reprinted as "Report of the Medical Staff Attending the Late President William McKinley," *New York Medical Journal* 74 (1901): 732–743. An overview of the case with commentary appeared as "Death of President McKinley," *JAMA* 37 (September 21, 1901): 779–787. Additionally, there were two further eyewitness accounts: John Parmenter, "The Surgery in President McKinley's Case: An Account of the Operation by One of the Surgeons," *Buffalo Medical Journal* 41 (1901): 205–206, and Nelson W. Wilson, "Details of President McKinley's Case, Narrated by the Recorder at the Operation," *Buffalo Medical Journal* 41 (1901): 207–225.

30. P.M. Rixey et al., *JAMA*, 1030.

31. Michael L. Palmer, Robert J. Weiss, and Lilli Sentz, "Dr. Roswell Park and the McKinley Assassination," in *Medical History in Buffalo, 1846-1996, Collected Essays*, ed. Lilli Sentz (Buffalo: 1996), 183.

32. *Ibid.*, 187–188.

33. "Death of President McKinley," *JAMA* 37 (September 21, 1901): 782.

34. Rudolph Marx, *The Health of the Presidents* (New York: G.P. Putnam's Sons, 1960), 276–7.

35. Michael L. Palmer, Robert J. Weiss and Lilli Sentz, 180.

36. Braisted and Bell, 49.

37. Rixey et al., *JAMA*.; Palmer, 186.

38. Roswell Park, "Report of the Medical Department of the Pan-American Exposition, Buffalo, 1901," *Buffalo Medical Journal* (December 1901), http://www.panam1901.bfn.org/medical/parkreport.html (accessed June 5, 2004); Adele Pillitteri, "OR Nursing 100 Years Ago: Nursing Care of President McKinley," *Today's OR Nurse* 12(12) (December 1991): 19–24.

39. Pillitteri.

40. *Ibid.*

41. See Chapter 4.

42. James J. Walsh, *History of Medicine in New York: Three Centuries of Medical Progress*, vol. 3, *Medical Institutions* (New York: National Americana Society, 1919). The Bellevue quote is lifted from pages 725–726, and the historical references to the other listed hospitals are found in pages 748–767.

43. John E. Lynaugh, "From Respectable Domesticity to Medical Efficiency: The Changing Kansas City Hospital, 1875-1920," in *The American General Hospital: Communities and Social Contexts*, Diane Elizabeth Long and Janet Golden, eds. (Ithaca, NY: Cornell University Press, 1989), 24.
44. Charles E. Rosenberg, *The Care of Strangers: The Rise of America's Hospital System* (New York: Basic Books, 1987), 4-5.
45. Paul Starr, *The Social Transformation of American Medicine* (New York: Basic Books, 1982), 154-157; Rosenberg, 148-149; Lynaugh, 29-31.
46. Braisted and Bell, 101.
47. *Ibid.*, 83.
48. *Ibid.*, 102.
49. *Ibid.*
50. Record of Service of Surgeon Presley M. Rixey, Naval Service Records, St. Louis, Missouri.
51. Braisted & Bell, 102.
52. *Ibid.*, 45.
53. *Ibid.*, 92-3.
54. *Ibid.*, 106.
55. *Ibid.*, 101-2.
56. Edmund Morris, *Theodore Rex* (New York: Random House, 2001), 150.
57. *Ibid.*, 376.
58. James L. Mooney, *Dictionary of American Naval Fighting Ships*, vol. 6 (Washington: Navy Dept., Office of the Chief of Naval Operation, 1976).
59. Braisted and Bell, 7.
60. Rosenberg, 67.
61. *Ibid.*
62. See Chapter 3.
63. Rosemary Stevens, *In Sickness and in Wealth: American Hospitals in the Twentieth Century* (Baltimore: Johns Hopkins University Press, 1999), 65-67.
64. *Ibid.*
65. *History of the Medical Society of the District of Columbia, 1817-1909* (Washington, D.C.: The Medical Society of the District of Columbia, 1909), 250-251.
66. Joseph K. Barnes, http://www.history.amedd.army.mil/tsgs/Barnes.htm (accessed April 3, 2005).
67. Jedediah Hyde Baxter, http://www.arlingtoncemetery.net/jhbaxter.htm (accessed April 3, 2005).
68. Janeway's career is documented in Martin Kaufmann, Stuart Galishoff, Todd L. Savitt, eds., *Dictionary of American Medical Biography* (Westport, CT: Greenwood Press, 1984), 391. The dates and venues for Roswell Park's early medical career in Chicago are somewhat confusing. "Obituary, Roswell Park, M.D., LL.D.," *The Lancet* (March 14, 1914): 780 mentions an internship in two of the largest hospitals in Chicago, lasting for two- and one-half years. Kelly and Burrage, 881, state that Park served as an intern at Cook County Hospital, starting in 1876. Finally, an obituary in the *British Medical Journal* 69(8) (March 1914) states that he was a demonstrator of anatomy at the Women's Medical College in Chicago from 1877-1979. Erdmann's resume is specific: Loyd Thompson and Winfield S. Downs, eds., *Who's Who in American Medicine* (New York: Who's Who Publications, 1925), 464.
69. Bliss' and Reyburn's curricula vitae appear in the *History of the Medical Society of the District of Columbia, 1817-1909* on pages 277 and 281-282 respectively; Robert O'Reilly, http://www.armymedicine.army.mil/history/tsgs/O'Reilly.htm (accessed May 31, 2001); William Sternberg, http://www.arlingtoncemetray.com/gmsternb.htm (accessed July 2, 2001).
70. James E. King, "In Memoriam: Matthew Derbyshire Mann, A.B., A.M., M.D., F.A.C.S.," *Transactions of the American Gynecological Society*, 46 (1921): 386-389; Kaufman, 406-407.
71. Thomas N. Bonner, *American Doctors and German Universities: A Chapter in International Intellectual Relations, 1870-1914* (Lincoln: University of Nebraska Press, 1963), 23.
72. *Ibid.*, 3.
73. *Ibid.*, 75.
74. Abraham Flexner, *Medical Education in the United States and Canada: A Report to the Carnegie Foundation for the Advancement of Teaching* (New York: Carnegie Foundation Bulletin Number Four, 1910, reproduced in 1960).
75. Paul Starr, *The Social Transformation of American Medicine* (New York: Basic Books, 1982), 118-121. In 1906 the number of American medical schools was 162; the complement declined to 131 in 1910 when the report was published, and further fell to 81 in 1922. The number of medical graduates in 1922 was 2,529. Thomas N. Bonner (see note 76) says that in the first decade of the twentieth century 25,000 students were enrolled in American medical schools.
76. Thomas N. Bonner, *Iconoclast: Abraham Flexner and a Life in Learning* (Baltimore: Johns Hopkins University Press, 2002), 63, 67, 68, 69, 71.
77. Flexner, 6.
78. *Ibid.*, 151-154.
79. Harold J. Abrahams, *Extinct Medical Schools of Nineteenth-Century Philadelphia* (Philadelphia: University of Pennsylvania Press, 1966), 111-160.
80. Heidi Syler (Reference Librarian, Sewanee University), personal correspondence with the author, 2 August 2004 and 16 August 2004.
81. Flexner, 292.

Chapter 6

1. Milton F. Heller, *The President's Doctor: An Inside View of Three First Families* (New York: Vantage Press, 2000), 127.
2. *Ibid.* Milton Heller married Dr. Boone's only child, Suzanne. In this book's preface, Heller cites as his source material the voluminous documents, notes and newspaper clippings kept by its subject. Additionally, Dr. Boone had organized this

mass of material as an autobiographical account that emphasized his dealings with the three first families.

3. *Ibid.*, 5.
4. *Ibid.*, 26–7.
5. *Ibid.*, 39.
6. *Ibid.*, 127–9.
7. *Ibid.*, 129.
8. *Ibid.*, 131–3.
9. *Ibid.*, 124–125.
10. An Act Allowing the rank, pay, and allowances of a colonel, Medical Corps, United States Army, or of a captain, Medical Corps, United States Navy, to any medical officer below such rank assigned to duty as physician to the White House, Public, No. 89, Chapter 104 (April 4, 1930).
11. An Act Allowing the rank, pay, and allowances of a colonel, Medical Corps, United States Army, to the medical officer assigned to duty as personal physician to the President, Public, No. 393, Chapter 573 (May 16, 1928).
12. Heller, 110.
13. *Ibid.*, 124–5.
14. Physician to White House: assignment: grade, Title 10, 70A Stat. 34, Chapter 1041 (August 10, 1956).
15. Heller, 5.
16. *Ibid.*, 5–7; Charles A. Roos, "Physicians to the Presidents, and Their Patients: A Bibliography," *Bulletin of the Medical Library Association* 49 (1961): 353.
17. Ludwig M. Deppisch, " Homeopathic Medicine and Presidential Health: Homeopathic Influences Upon Two Ohio Presidents," *Pharos* 60(4) (1997): 5–10.
18. Three reference works containing excellent histories of American homeopathy are available. In no particular order of importance they are James Whorton, *Nature Cures: The History of Alternative Medicine in America* (New York: Oxford University Press, 2002); William G. Rothstein, *American Physicians in the 19th Century. From Sects to Science* (Baltimore: Johns Hopkins University Press, 1972); Martin Kaufman, *Homeopathy in America: The Rise and Fall of a Medical Heresy* (Baltimore: Johns Hopkins Press, 1971). The specific references here are Whorton, 222, 272–276, and Rothstein, 235–240.
19. Rothstein, 307; Kaufman, 141–142.
20. Flexner, 157.
21. Flexner, 158–159, reported that of the fifteen existing schools none required more than a high school graduation for admission and the majority required even less.
22. *Ibid.*, 159–161.
23. Whorton, 222.
24. Whorton, 272–276; Rothstein, 236–246; Kaufman, 124, 183.
25. Heller, 7–16.
26. *Ibid.*, 26–7.
27. *Ibid.*, 29–31.
28. *Ibid.*, 32–3.
29. *Ibid.*, 35.
30. *Ibid.*, 36–7.
31. *Ibid.*, 39–44.
32. *Ibid.*, 73.
33. *Ibid.*, 78–80.
34. *Ibid.*, 81.
35. *Ibid.*, 39, 84–5.
36. Heller, 113, 115; Robert F. Gilbert, *The Tormented President: Calvin Coolidge, Death, and Clinical Depression* (Westport, CT: Praeger, 2003), 219–220. Gilbert's work is one of the first to document Coolidge's debilitating depression after the death of his son. This book also provides many details of the Coolidges' personal life and interpersonal relationships.
37. Gilbert, 223–5; Ishbel Ross, *Grace Coolidge and Her Era* (New York: Dodd, Mead, 1962), 159; Edmund M. Starling, *Starling of the White House* (Chicago: People's Book Club, 1946), 238.
38. Heller, 139.
39. *Ibid.*, 35; Robert H. Ferrell, *The Strange Deaths of President Harding* (Columbia: University of Missouri Press, 1996), 7.
40. Heller, 47.
41. *Ibid.*, 138.
42. *Ibid.*, 108–9.
43. *Ibid.*, 35–9.
44. Gilbert, 169.
45. Gilbert, 151–6; Heller, 84–5.
46. Ross, 135, 244.
47. Ross, 342; Gilbert, 169; Heller 84–5.
48. Robert H. Ferrell, *The Presidency of Calvin Coolidge* (Lawrence: University of Kansas Press, 1998), 21; Ross, 68.
49. Heller, 151.
50. *Ibid.*, 135.
51. Anne Beiser Allen, *An Independent Woman: The Life of Lou Henry Hoover* (Westport, CT: Greenwood Press, 2000), 141.
52. *Ibid.*, 161.
53. Jerrold M. Post and Robert S. Robins, *When Illness Strikes the Leader: The Dilemma of the Captive King* (New Haven, CT: Yale University Press, 1993), 78–120.
54. *Ibid.*, 161.
55. Heller, 79.
56. Deppisch, 9.
57. Eugene P. Trani and David Wilson, *The Presidency of Warren G. Harding* (Lawrence: University of Kansas Press, 1977), 45.
58. Deppisch, 8–9.
59. Francis Russell, *The Shadow of Blooming Grove: Warren G. Harding in His Times* (New York: McGraw-Hill, 1968), 100–101.
60. *Ibid.*, 101.
61. "Obituary: Dr. Charles E. Sawyer,"*J. Am. Inst. Homeopathy* 17 (1924): 1020–1023.
62. Russell, 162.
63. Warren G. Harding to Charles E. Sawyer, January 11, 1916; Warren G. Harding Papers, Ohio Historical Society, Columbus.
64. Russell, 438.
65. *Ibid.*, 549–550.
66. Sawyer to Harding, February 4, 1916, Warren G. Harding Papers.

67. Harding to Sawyer, July 17, 1919, Warren G. Harding Papers.
68. Harding to Sawyer, August 29, 1922, Warren G. Harding Papers.
69. Sawyer to Harding, April 25, 1923, Warren G. Harding Papers.
70. Heller, 58–61.
71. *Ibid.*, 73.
72. Trani and Wilson, 177.
73. Charles A. Roos, "Physicians to the Presidents, and Their Patients: A Bibliography," *Bulletin of the Medical Library Association* 49 (1961), 291–360.
74. "Obituary of James Francis Coupal, M.A., M.D.," *Bulletin of the International Society of Medical Museums*: 14 (March 1935): 114–116; Roos, 354.
75. Heller, 124.
76. Gilbert, 151–6.
77. Calvin Coolidge Papers, Library of Congress Manuscript Division (Washington: Library of Congress, 1965) 3632.
78. Calvin Coolidge Papers, 3632: Calvin Coolidge to Dwight Davis, May 16, 1928; Davis to Coolidge, May 18, 1938.
79. Calvin Coolidge Papers, 3632: Coolidge to Davis, February 21, 1929; Davis to Coolidge, February 26, 1929.
80. "Obituary of James Francis Coupal, M.A., M.D."
81. Heller, 157.
82. *Ibid.*, 160–5.
83. Milton Heller, *Joel Thompson Boone: The Maverick Physician*, http://www.joeltboone.com/ (accessed January 20, 2003).
84. Milton Heller, "The USS Boone," http://www/joeltboone.com/uss_boone.htm (accessed November 20, 2002). Andre Sobocinski, personal correspondence, January 2022
85. Janet Travell, *Office Hours Day and Night: The Autobiography of Janet Travell, M.D.* (New York: Word Publishing, 1968), 390.
86. E. Connie Mariano, *The Evolution of the White House Medical Unit in Managing Crisis: Presidential Disability and the Twenty-fifth Amendment*, ed. Robert E. Gilbert (New York: Fordham University Press, 2000), 84.

Chapter 7

1. Jim Bishop, *FDR's Last Year* (New York: William Morrow, 1974), 18–19.
2. Edwin A. Weinstein, *Woodrow Wilson: A Medical and Psychological Biography* (Princeton: Princeton University Press, 1981), 279. Weinstein's volume was perhaps the first and may remain the best of the longitudinal studies of a disease process that affected a president. Edith Bolling Galt Wilson, *My Memoir* (Indianapolis: Bobbs-Merrill, 1939), 59, 75–8. Presidential wives have been authors and subjects of many volumes. The process of self-recognition definitely did not commence with Hillary Clinton.
3. Robert H. Ferrell, *Ill-Advised: Presidential Health and Public Trust* (Columbia: University of Missouri Press, 1992), 16–7. The energetic Professor Ferrell has written a series of fact-filled monographs that discuss the illnesses of presidents of the early and mid-twentieth century.
4. Ross McIntire, *White House Physician* (New York: G.P. Putnam's Sons, 1946), 215.
5. Ferrell, 118–133.
6. Weinstein, 99.
7. Kenneth R. Crispell and Carlos F. Gomez, *Hidden Illness in the White House* (Durham: Duke University Press, 1988), 49.
8. Weinstein, 256.
9. Howard G. Bruenn, "Clinical Notes on the Illness and Death of President Franklin D. Roosevelt," *Annals of Internal Medicine* 72 (1970): 579–591. This report by the treating physician affords the best insight into FDR's final illness.
10. Jim Bishop, *FDR's Last Year: April 1944–April 1945* (New York: William Morrow: New York, 1974), 37.
11. *Ibid.*, 268.
12. Clarence G. Lasby, *Eisenhower's Heart Attack: How Ike Beat Heart Disease and Held on to the Presidency* (Lawrence: University Press of Kansas, 1997), 207.
13. William Braisted and William H. Bell, *The Life Story of Presley Marion Rixey* (Strasburg, VA: Shenandoah Publishing, 1930), 390.
14. Robert H. Ferrell, *The Dying President: Franklin D. Roosevelt 1944–1945* (Columbia: University of Missouri Press, 1998), 140.
15. *Ibid.*, 8.
16. Ferrell, *Ill-Advised*, 62–3.
17. *Ibid.*, 66.
18. Cary T. Grayson, *Woodrow Wilson: An Intimate Memoir* (Washington: Potomac, 1960, 1977).
19. Ross McIntire, *White House Physician* (New York: G.P. Putnam's Sons, 1946).
20. Ferrell, *Ill-Advised*, 66.
21. Milton F. Heller, Jr., *The Presidents' Doctor. An Insider's View of Three First Families* (New York: Vantage Press, 2000), 155.
22. Thompson, Loyd and Winfield Scott Downs, *Who's Who in American Medicine 1925* (New York: Who's Who Publications, 1925), 594; "Deaths," *Journal of the American Medical Association* 110 (January–March 1938).
23. Thompson and Downs, 594; "Deaths," *Journal of the American Medical Association* 110 (January–March 1938).
24. *Ibid.*; *Who Was Who in America*, vol. 1, 1897–1942 (Chicago: Marquis, 1966), 480.
25. Braisted and Bell, 391.
26. *Ibid.*
27. Weinstein, 249–50.
28. Braisted and Bell, 132–4.
29. Weinstein, 250.
30. Grayson, 1–2.
31. Edith Wilson, 144.
32. Stockton Axson and Arthur S. Link, "Brother Woodrow": *A Memoir of Woodrow*

Wilson (Princeton: Princeton University Press, 1993), 208.

33. Grayson, v–vii.
34. *Ibid.*, ix.
35. *Ibid.*, x.
36. Edmund W. Starling, *Starling of the White House* (Chicago: People's Book Club, 1946), 86, 88.
37. *Ibid.*, 34.
38. Edith Wilson, 51.
39. *Ibid.*, 59.
40. *Ibid.*, 75–8.
41. Arthur S. Link and James R. Carroll, *The Real Woodrow Wilson: An Interview with Arthur S. Link, the Editor of the Wilson Papers* (Bennington, VT: Images from the Past, 2001), 36.
42. Axson and Link, 228.
43. Braisted and Bell, 390.
44. *Ibid.*, 392.
45. Starling, 137.
46. *Ibid.*, 148–9.
47. Edith Wilson, 86, 144.
48. Weinstein, 305.
49. Rudolph Marx, *The Health of the Presidents* (New York: G.P. Putnam's Sons, 1960), 318–22; Weinstein, 355–70; Crispell and Gomez, 67–74.
50. Crispell and Gomez, 72.
51. Herbert Hoover, *The Ordeal of Woodrow Wilson* (New York: McGraw Hill, 1958), 272–3; Edith Wilson, 288; Grayson, 100.
52. James Hendrie Lloyd, "Obituary of Francis X. Dercum," *Archives of Neurology and Psychiatry* 25 (1931): 1333–35.
53. Edward Jackson, "Obituary of George E. de Schweinitz," *American Journal of Ophthalmology* 21(3) (1938): 1285–7.
54. "Obituary of Charles H. Mayo," *Journal of the American Medical Association* 112 (April–June 1939): 2342.
55. Miley B. Wesson, "Hugh Hampton Young," *The Journal of Urology* 57 (1957): 203–8.
56. Weinstein, 320.
57. Braisted and Bell, 389–93.
58. *Cary Travers Grayson*, http://www.1upinfo.com/encyclopedia/E/E-GraysonC.html (accessed July 7, 2003).
59. Ferrell, *The Dying President*, 8.
60. Bert E. Park, *Ailing, Aging, Addicted: Studies of Compromised Leadership* (Lexington: University Press of Kentucky, 1993), 198–200.
61. William J. Stewart, "McIntire, Ross," in *Dictionary of American Biography*, Supplement 6 (1956–1960): 413–4, 1980; Ferrell: *The Dying President*, 8.
62. McIntire, 55–6.
63. McIntire, 55–6; Ferrell, *The Dying President*, 8.
64. Patricia Socha (American Board of Medical Specialties), personal correspondence with the author, 15 November 2004. Rosemary Stevens, *American Medicine and the Public Interest: A History of Specialization* (Berkeley: University of California Press, 1971, 1998), 158–159, notes that traditionally the study and carte of diseases of the ears, nose and throat (ENT) had been conflated with diseases of the eye. However, in 1920 the leading academic ophthalmology society severed its ENT connection, and in 1924 the National Board of Examiners in Otolaryngology was formed, becoming either the second or the third American medical specialty board. Many of its early diplomats were grandfathered in without examination. The mechanism of McIntire's certification is unknown.
65. McIntire, 57.
66. Frank Friedel, *Franklin Roosevelt: A Rendezvous with Destiny* (Boston: Little, Brown, 1990), 512.
67. Bishop, 292.
68. *Ibid.*, 450.
69. McIntire, 64.
70. Bishop, 15.
71. *Ibid.*, 101, 138, 206, 237.
72. Doris Kearns Goodwin, *No Ordinary Time* (New York: Simon and Schuster, 1994), 216, 222; Jeanne Nienaber Clarke, *Roosevelt's Warrior: Harold L. Ickes and the New Deal* (Baltimore: Johns Hopkins University Press, 1996), 153, 248, 349.
73. Goodwin, 113.
74. Bishop, 283, 333.
75. McIntire, 67.
76. Bruenn.
77. Bruenn; Ferrell, *The Dying President*, 27; Bert E. Park, *The Impact of Illness on World Leaders* (Philadelphia: University of Pennsylvania Press, 1986), 225–6.
78. Bruenn.
79. Bruenn; Ferrell, *The Dying President*, 39–40.
80. *Ibid.*
81. Bruenn.
82. Ferrell, *The Dying President*, 69.
83. *Ibid.*, 140.
84. Bishop, 19.
85. Goodwin, 497.
86. *Ibid.*, 545.
87. Bishop, 268.
88. *Ibid.*, 487.
89. Goodwin, 579.
90. Catherine Grace Katz, *The Daughters of Yalta* (New York: Houghton Mifflin Harcourt, 2020), 40–49, 201–7; Howard Bruenn oral history.
91. Bishop, 534.
92. Stewart.
93. "Federal Health Service Obituaries: Major General Howard McCrum Snyder, USA (Ret.)," *Military Medicine* (1970): 1180–1.
94. *Ibid.*; Clarence G. Lasby, *Eisenhower's Heart Attack: How Ike Beat Heart Disease and Held on to the Presidency* (Lawrence: University of Kansas Press, 1997), 29; Robert H. Ferrell, *Ill-Advised*, 62–3.
95. Lasby, 29–30.
96. *Ibid.*, 29.
97. Ferrell, *Ill-Advised*, 60.
98. Lasby, 59.
99. Ferrell, *Ill-Advised*, 108–9.

100. T. Burton Smith, "The Presidential Physician and the Reagan Presidency," 85, in *Papers on Presidential Disability and the Twenty-fifth Amendment*, vol. 2, ed. Kenneth W. Thompson (Lanham: University Press of America, 1991).
101. Lasby, 59–60.
102. Stephen E. Ambrose, *Eisenhower: The President* (New York: Simon and Schuster, 1984), 529.
103. *Ibid.*, 221.
104. Lasby, 60.
105. *Ibid.*, 250
106. Ferrell, *Ill-Advised*, 81–2.
107. Lasby, 80–3.
108. More complete discussions of the decision to invite Paul White may be found in Lasby, 78: Ferrell, 82; Paul Dudley White, *My Life and Medicine* (Boston: Gambit, 1971), 176–179; Paul Oglesby, *Take Heart: The Life and Prescription for Living of Dr. Paul Dudley White* (Boston: Harvard University Press, 1986), 157–158.
109. Ferrell, *Ill-Advised*, 109.
110. Lasby, 141–2, 164–70, 204, 206, 251–2.
111. *Ibid.*, 137. See also Ferrell, 106–107.
112. Ferrell, 125.
113. Anthony Leviero, "Truman in Hospital for Health Check," *New York Times*, 17 July 1952.
114. For discussion of the hospital admissions of Ronald Reagan and George H.W. Bush. Richard Nixon's hospitalization at Bethesda Naval Hospital with viral pneumonia in July 1973 is recorded in John R. Bumgarner, *The Health of the Presidents: The 41 United States Presidents Through 1993 from a Physician's Point of View* (Jefferson, NC: McFarland, 1994), 265, and in Jonathan Aitken, *Nixon: A Life* (London: Weidenfeld and Nicolson, 1993), 498–499. Bumgarner, 256, and Irwin Unger and Debi Unger, *LBJ: A Life* (New York: John Wiley & Sons, 1999), 379–380 discuss Lyndon Johnson's stay at Bethesda Naval Hospital where his gall bladder was removed on October 8, 1965.
115. Robert H. Ferrell, *The Dying President: Franklin D. Roosevelt, 1944–1945* (Columbia: University of Missouri Press, 1998), 86–88.
116. Charles E. Rosenberg, *The Care of Strangers: The Rise of America's Hospital System* (New York: Basic Books, 1987), 114–115.
117. Joan E. Lynaugh, "From Respectable Domesticity to Medical Efficiency: The Changing Kansas City Hospital, 1875–1920," in *The American General Hospital: Communities and Social Contexts*, ed. Diana Long and Janet Golden (Ithaca: Cornell University Press, 1989), 29–31.
118. Paul Starr, *The Social Transformation of American Medicine* (Basic Books, 1982), 167.
119. Ferrell *Ill-Advised*, 122.
120. *Ibid.*, 123.
121. *Ibid.*, 128–30.
122. *Ibid.*, 75–80.
123. Lasby, 207.
124. *Ibid.*, 244.
125. Lasby, 207.
126. *Ibid.*, 244.
127. Ferrell, *Ill-Advised*, 123.
128. *Ibid.*, 96–9.
129. *Ibid.*, 106–7, 125.
130. *Ibid.*, 66.
131. Robert B. McLean, "Leonard Heaton—Military Surgeon," *Military Medicine* 147 (September 1982): 717–727.
132. Rosemary Stevens, *American Medicine and the Public Interest: A History of Specialization* (Berkeley: University of California Press, 1998), 325.
133. *Ibid.*
134. Clarence G. Lasby, *Eisenhower's Heart Attack: How Ike Beat Heart Disease and Held on to the Presidency* (Lawrence: University Press of Kansas, 1997), 250.
135. McLean, 722.
136. McLean.
137. "Surgeon Generals of the U.S. Army and Their Predecessors, 1775–2000," http://www.history.amedd.army.mil/tsgs/defau;t.htm; 2/11/2005. See also "Heaton New Army Surgeon General," *New York Times*, 8 April 1959.
138. "Heaton and 3 Nominated for Lieutenant General," *New York Times*, 8 August 1959.
139. McLean, 723.
140. Leonard D. Heaton, interview by Colonel Robert B. McLean, Senior Officer Oral History Program of the United States Army War College, October, November and December 1978.
141. Paul Dudley White, *My Life and Medicine: An Autobiographical Memoir* (Boston: Gambit, 1971), 184.
142. Carl Jackson, personal correspondence with the author, 15 September 2004, regarding review of the Paul Dudley White file at the Countway Medical Library, Boston.
143. Edwin L. Dale, Jr., "President to Pay $23.10 to Hospital," *New York Times*, 1 July 1956.
144. Wallace H. Graham, oral history interview by Neil M. Johnson, March 30, 1989; Truman Presidential Museum and Library; http://www.trumanlibrary.org/oralhist/grahamw.htm (accessed May 25, 2005).
145. *Ibid.*
146. Margaret Truman, *Harry S. Truman* (New York: William Morrow, 1973), 332–333.
147. *New York Times*, 14 March 1952; 22 March 1952.
148. David McCullough, *Truman* (New York: Simon and Schuster, 1992), 487–488, 510–511.
149. Oral history interview with Wallace H. Graham.
150. *Ibid.*
151. Margaret Truman, 363.
152. Wallace H. Graham, oral history interview.
153. Harry Truman to Ethel Noland, September 24, 1950, in *Off the Record: The Private Papers of Harry S. Truman*, ed. Robert H. Ferrell (New York: Harper & Row, 1980), 194.
154. Wallace H. Graham, oral history interview. Jimmy Byrnes was Truman's secretary of state and Lord Edward Wood Halifax was the British ambassador to the United States.

155. Harry Truman to Bess Truman, September 1, 1951, in *Off the Record*, 216–217; Wallace H. Graham, oral history interview.
156. Wallace H. Graham, oral history interview.
157. Margaret Truman, 281; Wallace H. Graham, oral history interview.
158. *Ibid.*; Wallace H. Graham, oral history interview.
159. Wallace H. Graham, oral history interview.
160. McCullough, 944, 981, 987; Wallace H. Graham, oral history interview.
161. *New York Times*, 14–19 July 1952.
162. *New York Times*, 12 May 1949; Wallace H. Graham, oral history interview.
163. See *New York Times*, 29 December 1947; 2 January, 6 January, 13 January, 17 January 1948; McCullough, 594. Graham's explanation is found in oral history interview with Wallace H. Graham.
164. Ward O. Griffen, Jr., *The American Board of Surgery in the Twentieth Century—Then and Now*, unpublished (Chicago: The American Board of Surgery, 2004), 35. Subsequently the American Board of Surgery made an exception for military surgeons by allowing one year of postgraduate credit for military service. It is unknown whether this partial exemption had any bearing upon Graham's application.
165. Frank Lewis, M.D. (Executive Director of the American Board of Surgery), personal correspondence with author, 7 September 2004.
166. Wallace H. Graham, oral history interview.
167. Rosemary Stevens, *American Medicine and the Public Interest: A History of Specialization* (Berkeley: University of California Press, 1998), 325.
168. *Ibid.*, 318.
169. Wallace H. Graham, oral history interview.
170. Wallace H. Graham, oral history interview, 1989; Truman Library, 69.
171. Wallace H. Graham, *Wallace H. Graham, The Man Who Became President Truman's Physician* (Columbia, MO: Compass Flower Press, 2019). ED: Main file did not have a superscript #171, I added at end to use this note. LR

Chapter 8

1. Miller Center of Public Affairs, Dwight Eisenhower: Administration of the White House, http://www.americanpresident.org/history/dwighteisenhower/staffadvisors/adminsitrtaionoft (accessed August 8, 2005); Oglesby Paul, Take Heart: The Life and Prescription for Living of Dr. Paul Dudley White (Cambridge, MA: Harvard University Press, 1986), 151.
2. See Chapter 7.
3. Clarence G. Lasby, *Eisenhower's Heart Attack: How Ike Beat Heart Disease and Held on to the Presidency* (Lawrence: University Press of Kansas, 1977), 209.
4. "Walter Tkach, 72; Served as the Doctor to Three Presidents," *New York Times*, 9 November 1989; Major General Walter Robert Tkach, http://www.af.mil/bios/bio.asp?bioID=7401 (accessed August 8, 2005).
5. "Citation to Accompany the Award of the Bronze Star Medal to Walter R. Tkach," National Archives and Records Administration.
6. Walter Tkach, *New York Times*.
7. W.J. Weatherby, "Obituary of Walter Tkach," *The Guardian* (London), 11 November 1989.
8. Janet Travell, *Office Hours Day and Night* (Cleveland, OH: World Publishing, 1968), 369.
9. *Ibid.*, 369–370.
10. See Chapter 7.
11. Richard Reeves, *Alone in the White House* (New York: Simon & Schuster, 2001), 290–291.
12. H.R. Haldeman, *The Haldeman Diaries: Inside the Nixon White House* (New York: G.P. Putnam's Sons, 1994), 227.
13. John Hebers, "Ford Aides Silent on Link of Pardon and Nixon Health," *New York Times*, 14 September 1974; "Doctor Says Nixon Feared Hospital Stay," *New York Times*, 15 August 1974.
14. Lawrence K. Altman, *New York Times*, 16 September 1974.
15. "Unhealthy Trifling," editorial, *New York Times*, 17 September 1974.
16. *New York Times*, 13 December 1973, 29 December 1973
17. *New York Times*, 11 February 1970, 11 February 1972.
18. "Citation to Accompany the Award of the Distinguished Service Medal to Walter R. Tkach," National Archives and Records Administration. The accompanying citation read in part: "General Tkach distinguished himself as the Physician to the President of the United States from 20 January 1969 to 9 August 1974. In this important assignment, General Tkach served with eminence and rendered the highest degree of professional attention to the President, the First Family and the Nixon Administration Cabinet members. The singularly distinctive accomplishments of General Tkach in this position were remarkably substantial and of paramount importance to the President and to the Nation."
19. Patricia Socha (American Board of Medical Specialists), personal correspondence with the author, 10 August 2005.
20. Blaine Taylor, "An Exclusive Interview with William Lukash, M.D., Personal Physician to the President of the United States," *MD State Medical Journal* (November 1977): 35–71.
21. Patricia Socha (American Board of Medical Specialties), personal correspondence with the author, 15 November 2004.
22. Taylor.
23. *Ibid.*
24. Taylor; Louis Estrada, "William Lukash Dies at 66, Chief Presidential Physician," *Washington Post*, 7 February 1998; Wolfgang Saxon, "William Lukash, Doctor Who Watched Over Presidents," *New York Times*, 7 February 1998.
25. See chapters 5 and 9.

26. Saxon.
27. Estrada.
28. "Lukash, WM" (Author), as found in http://www.pubmed.gov (accessed January 10, 2006). Pub Med is a service of the National Library of Medicine and the National Institutes of Health. It lists many, but not all, of an author's medical articles.
29. *New York Times*, 15 February Note 1974:
30. Comments of Dr. Joseph Schanno in Blaine Taylor, "The Aftermath of the Wallace Shooting: A Maryland Medical Success Story," *MD State Medical Journal* (May 1976): 35–50.
31. John C. Lungren and John C. Lungren, Jr., *Healing Richard Nixon: A Doctor's Memoir* (Lexington: University Press of Kentucky, 2003), 13–17.
32. *Ibid.*, 22–23.
33. *Ibid.*, 83–125.
34. *Ibid.*, 114–115.
35. *New York Times*, 23 September 1974, 28 October 1974.
36. Jimmy Carter, "Opening Address, January 26, 1995," in *Presidential Disability: Papers, Discussions and Recommendations on the Twenty-fifth Amendment*, ed. James F. Toole and Robert J. Joynt (Rochester NY: University of Rochester Press, 2001), 19–20.
37. J. Willis Hurst and James C. Cain, *LBJ: To Know Him Better* (Austin, TX: LBJ Foundation, 1995).
38. *Ibid.*, 1.
39. Megan Woolhouse, "Hurst: The Heart of Emory," *Atlanta Business Chronicle*, 17 May 2004.
40. Hurst and Cain, 1. Janet Travell had heard rumors that television pictured Johnson holding his left arm as he boarded *Air Force One* for its return trip to Washington from Dallas. Travell feared that the new president had suffered an angina attack. The rumor was unfounded.
41. "Johnson's Doctor Says Heart 'Is Doing Fine,'" *New York Times*, 4 December 1963.
42. Charles Mohr, "President's Health Is Rated Excellent," *New York Times*, 29 December 1964; *New York Times*, 6 October 1965; John W. Finney, "Johnson Enters Naval Hospital; Surgery Is Today," *New York Times*, 16 November 1966; Harold M. Schmeck, Jr., "Physicians Doubt Ailments, Return," *New York Times*, 17 November 1966.
43. "President Attends Church with His Heart Specialist," *New York Times*, 28 July 1968.
44. J. Willis Hurst, personal correspondence with the author, 25 June 2004.
45. Hurst and Cain, 1.
46. *Ibid.*, 5.
47. *Ibid.*, 9–10.
48. J. Willis Hurst, personal correspondence with the author.
49. *New York Times*, 12 April 1972.
50. *New York Times*, 11 April 1973.
51. Norman Gevitz, *The DOs: Osteopathic Medicine in America*, 2nd ed. (Baltimore: Johns Hopkins University Press, 2004), 15–19. Still's early career and his disillusion with orthodox medicine are also well presented in James C. Whorton, *Nature Cures: The History of Alternative Medicine in America* (New York: Oxford University Press, 2002), 141–149.
52. Whorton, 149.
53. Gevitz, 20–22.
54. *Ibid.*, 21.
55. *Ibid.*, 69–70, 75–76.
56. *Ibid.*, 77–84.
57. *Ibid.*, 108.
58. Abraham Flexner, *Medical Education in the United States and Canada: A Report to the Carnegie Foundation for the Advancement of Teaching* (Boston: D.B. Updike, Merrymount Press, 1910), 163–166.
59. *Ibid.*, 172.
60. Gevitz, 93.
61. *Ibid.*, 115–134.
62. *Ibid.*, 143–144.
63. *Ibid.*, 143.
64. *Ibid.*, 109.
65. *Ibid.*, 174.
66. *Ibid.*, 98.
67. *Ibid.*
68. U.S. Colleges of Osteopathic Medicine, www.aacom.org, accessed 19 June 2022.
69. Osteopathic Medical Professional Report, American Osteopathic Association: osteopathic.org/about/aoa/statistics; U.S. Medical Schools 2022 total graduates: www.aamc.org/data/reports, accessed 19 June 2022.
70. "Dr. W.K. Riland, 76, Osteopath," *New York Times*, 15 March 1989; *New York Times*, 16 March 1974.
71. "Dr. W.K. Riland, 76, Osteopath," *New York Times*, 15 March 1989.
72. Emanuel Perlmutter, *New York Times*, 6 March 1974; *New York Times*, 5 May 1973.
73. Edith Evans Asbury, *New York Times*, 11 May 1974.

Chapter 9

1. Susan E.B. Schwartz, *Into the Unknown: The Remarkable Life of Hans Kraus* (New York: iUniverse, 2005), 184. This biographer knew Dr. Kraus personally and had unlimited access to his personal papers and to his family. Her initial interest in the doctor was through their shared passion for rock climbing.
2. Daniel Ruge was certified by the American Board of Neurological Surgery and Burton Lee III was certified by the American Board of Internal Medicine but did not have subspecialty certification in oncology (American Board of Medical Specialties), http://www.abms.org (accessed June 11, 2005). Burton Smith was certified by the American Board of Urology (personal correspondence with Patricia Socha, ABMS, 15 November 2004). John Hutton, who succeeded Burton Smith as personal physician to Ronald Reagan, had been certified by the American Board of Surgery (personal

correspondence with Dr. Frank Lewis, September 7, 2004).

3. Burton J. Lee III, "The Role of the Presidential Physician," in *Papers on Presidential Disability and the Twenty-fifth Amendment*, vol. 3, ed. Kenneth W. Thompson (Lanham, MD: University Press of America, 1996), 32.

4. Bradley Peterson, oral interview with Daniel Ruge, M.D., obtained October 11, 1986.

5. Janet Travell, *Office Hours Day and Night: The Autobiography of Janet Travell, M.D.* (New York: World Publishing, 1968), 119.

6. See Chapter 4.

7. See Chapter 9.

8. Thomas N. Bonner, *To the Ends of the Earth: Women Search for Education in Medicine* (Cambridge, MA: Harvard University Press, 1992), 29, 121, and 130.

9. Mary R. Walsh, *"Doctors Wanted, No Women Need Apply": Sexual Barriers in the Medical Profession, 1835–1975* (New Haven, CT: Yale University Press, 1977), 179–183; Paul Starr, *The Social Transformation of American Medicine* (New York: Basic Books, 1982), 117.

10. Starr, 117.

11. Bonner, 15.

12. *Ibid.*, 16.

13. See Chapter 4.

14. Walsh, 31–35, 179–183.

15. Bonner, 140–141.

16. Walsh, 176–177; Bonner, 149–152; Starr, 117. A comprehensive discussion of this gift is present in A. McGehee Harvey, Gert H. Brieger, Susan L. Abrams and Victor A. McKusick; *A Model of Its Kind*, vol. 1, *A Centennial History of Medicine at Johns Hopkins* (Baltimore: Johns Hopkins University Press, 1989), 27–28.

17. Walsh, 176–177.

18. Bonner, 167.

19. Ellen S. More, *Restoring the Balance: Women Physicians and the Profession of Medicine* (Cambridge, MA: Harvard University Press, 199),109.

20. Walsh, 241; More, 97; Starr, 124.

21. Starr, 124.

22. Walsh, 224. See also More, pages 95–109, for the difficulties in obtaining internships.

23. More, 221.

24. Barbara Barzansky and Sylvia I. Etzel, "Educational Programs in U.S. Medical Schools, 2003–2004," *JAMA* 293(9) (September 1, 2004): 1025–1031.

25. 2022 Application and matriculation data, AAMC.org, accessed June 20, 2023.

26. *Ibid.*, 192–8.

27. *Ibid.*, 249.

28. *Ibid.*, 285–9.

29. Janet G. Travell and David G. Simons, *Myofascial Pain and Dysfunction: The Trigger Point Manual*, 2 vols. (New York: Lippincott, 1983).

30. David G. Simons, Lois S. Simons, Janet G. Travell, *Travell and Simons Myofascial Pain and Dysfunction*, 2 vols. (New York: Lippincott Williams & Wilkins, 1999).

31. Travell, *Office Hours*, 5–7.

32. Thomas C. Reeves, *A Question of Character: A Life of John F. Kennedy* (New York: Free Press, 1991); Seymour M. Hersh, *The Dark Side of Camelot* (Boston: Little, Brown, 1997).

33. Travell, 305, 320, 341.

34. *Ibid.*, 327.

35. *Ibid.*, 319.

36. *Ibid.*, 327–8.

37. *Ibid.*, 331.

38. Kenneth R. Crispell and Carlos F. Gomez, *Hidden Illness in the White House* (Durham: Duke University Press, 1988), 103–4.

39. George D. Lundberg, "Closing the Case in JAMA on the John F. Kennedy Autopsy," *Journal of the American Medical Association* 268(13) (October 7, 1992): 1736–8.

40. Crispell and Gomez; Robert H. Ferrell, *Ill-Advised: Presidential Health and Public Trust* (Columbia: University of Missouri Press, 1992), 154.

41. Travell, 358.

42. Reference Archivist, John F. Kennedy Library, personal correspondence with the author, July 27, 2004. In a sample pay period (10/14–10/27/1962) Travell received a base pay of $769.60, or roughly $20,000 per year.

43. Travell, 370.

44. George G. Burkley, oral history interview conducted October 17, 1967, http:///www.geocities.com/jfkinf03/testimony/burkley.htm (accessed August 7, 2003).

45. Travell., 388–9.

46. *Ibid.*

47. *Ibid.*, 408.

48. *Ibid.*, 369. Medicare, federal government health insurance for seniors, did not become law until 1965, during the presidency of Kennedy's successor, Lyndon Johnson.

49. Notable exceptions to this discretion have been Wallace Graham, who commented upon his patient Harry Truman's support for national health insurance (see Chapter 7), and Burton Lee, who was very quotable on many topics when he served as George Bush's physician (see Chapter 10).

50. Travell, 369.

51. Robert Dallek, *An Unfinished Life: John F. Kennedy* (Boston: Little, Brown, 2003), 581.

52. Travell, 370.

53. George G. Burkley, oral interview.

54. Richard Reeves, *President Kennedy: A Profile of Power* (New York: Simon & Schuster, 1993), 36.

55. *Ibid.*, 15.

56. Procaine, as found on the Internet, http://www.en.wikipedia.org/wiki/Procaine (accessed November 2, 2005). Procaine, first synthesized in 1905, was the first injectable man-made local anesthetic. It is rarely used today because more effective alternatives exist.

57. Travell, 260.

58. Susan E.B. Schwartz, *Into the Unknown: The Remarkable Life of Hans Kraus* (New York: iUniverse, 2005), 170–1.

59. Parmet, 122; Dallek, 472; R. Reeves, 242, reported that the injections totaled up to five or six times a day.
60. Dallek, 472-3; R. Reeves, 242-3.
61. Schwartz, 164-166, 176.
62. Burkley.
63. Dallek, 472-3; R. Reeves, 242-3. According to Schwartz, 176, Burkley and Cohen issued an ultimatum to Travell that either she requests a second opinion from Kraus or the former two physicians would directly inform the president that Travell was inept and should be fired.
64. Patricia Socha (American Board of Medical Specialties), personal correspondence with the author, 15 November 2004.
65. American Board of Physical Medicine and Rehabilitation; http://www.abpmr.org/about/ (accessed June 10, 2005).
66. Dallek, 473; R. Reeves, 243.
67. Schwartz, 177-179.
68. Hersh, 581.
69. Schwartz, 177-179.
70. Schwartz, *Into the Unknown*, 6-7. Schwartz, a rock climber like her subject, had access to the Kraus family and to Hans Kraus' records of Kennedy's treatments.
71. Schwartz, 48-55.
72. *Ibid.*, 64-116.
73. *New York Times,* March 7, 1996; Jane Ogle, "Contrast in Exercise," *New York Times,* 7 March 1982; "Say Goodbye to Back Pain Biographies," http://www.saygoodbyetobackpain.com/biographies (accessed November 16, 2005). According to Pat Socha (American Board of Medical Specialties) in personal correspondence with the author, Dr. Hans Kraus received a lifetime certification by the American Board of Physical Medicine and Rehabilitation in 1949. An interesting literary anecdote was reported in Smallwood, *The Guardian* (London), January 4, 1992: the author James Joyce taught Kraus English as a boy in Trieste and Zurich, Switzerland. Also see Schwartz, 116-123.
74. "Kennedy Exercising Daily to Help Back," *New York Times,* 21 October 1961; "President's Back Reported Better," *New York Times,* 13 December 1961; "Doctor Examines President's Back," *New York Times,* 25 November 1962.
75. Dallek, 472-3.
76. Schwartz, 177-179.
77. *Ibid.*, 188.
78. Patricia Socha (American Board of Medical Specialties), personal correspondence with the author, 23 November 2005.
79. Obituaries, *New York Times,* 17 and 18 January 1999; Travell, 315, 326, 332, 352.
80. Travell, *Office Hours Day and Night*, 388.
81. Schwartz, 183-185.
82. R. Reeves, 243.
83. Herbert S. Parmet, *JFK: The Presidency of John F. Kennedy* (New York: Dial Press, 1983), 123. Parmet wrote that presidential aide Kenneth O'Donnell had asked for her resignation at the end of 1962. "White House Denies Physician Has Quit," *New York Times,* 19 July 1963, reported that although Travell had not yet resigned her departure was expected shortly.
84. Dallek, 581.
85. Parmet, 124.
86. *Ibid.*, 581-2.
87. Burkley.
88. Travell, 388.
89. Schwartz, 198.
90. *Ibid.*, 191, 197-198.
91. *Ibid.*, 179-180.
92. Seymour Hersh, *The Dark Side of Camelot* (Boston: Little, Brown, 1997), 234.
93. Boyce Rensberger, "Amphetamines Used by a Physician to Lift Moods of Famous Patients," *New York Times,* 4 December 1972. According to Richard Reeves, 739a, Jacobson practiced medicine in Berlin and lived there from 1920 to 1934.
94. R. Reeves, 146-7; Lawrence Leamer, *The Kennedy Men, 1901-1963: The Laws of the Father* (New York: William Morrow, 2001), 543, records that Dr. Jacobson billed the president for incidental expenses and travel, but not for his professional services, in 1961.
95. Hersh, 235.
96. The abundant JFK literature is rich with material on this pairing. Sources include Robert Dallek, *An Unfinished Life* (Boston: Little, Brown, 2003); Seymour M. Hersh, *The Dark Side of Camelot* (Little, Brown, 1997); C. David Heymann, *A Woman Named Jackie* (London: Heinemann, 1989); Lawrence Leamer, *The Kennedy Men, 1901-1963: The Laws of the Father* (New York: William Morrow, 2001); Herbert S. Parmet, *JFK: The Presidency of John F. Kennedy* (New York: Dial Press, 1983); Richard Reeves, *President Kennedy: Profile of Power* (New York: Simon & Schuster, 1993); and Thomas C. Reeves, *A Question of Character: A Life of John F. Kennedy* (New York: Free Press, 1991).
97. Leamer, 525.
98. Hersh, 234.
99. R. Reeves, 364.
100. *Ibid.*
101. Hersh, 236-7.
102. R. Reeves 146-7.
103. Heymann, 312.
104. Heymann, 319. Heymann also notes that Jacobson never once requested or received a single penny above or beyond immediate expenses.
105. R. Reeves, 146-7, 158-9, 243, 698-9n.
106. Travell, *Office Hours Day and Night*.
107. Leamer, 544.
108. Boyce Rensberger, "Amphetamines Used by a Physician to Lift Moods of Famous Patients," *New York Times,* 4 December 1972.
109. *New York Times,* 25 April 28 April, 25 June 1975; Hersh, 234.
110. Travell, 430.
111. *Ibid.*, 454.
112. *Ibid.*, 452.
113. *Ibid.*, 406.
114. David Stout, "Janet Travell, Pain Specialist

and Kennedy's Personal Doctor," *New York Times*, 2 August 1997.
115. "George Gregory Burkley," Arlington National Cemetery Website, http://www.arlingtoncemetary.net/ggburklle.htm (accessed August 7, 2003).

Chapter 10

1. See Chapter 12 for further discussion of the misapplication of the amendment.
2. Herbert L. Abrams, *The President Has Been Shot: Confusion, Disability, and the 25th Amendment in the Aftermath of the Attempted Assassination of Ronald Reagan* (New York: W.W. Norton, 1992), 203. The test letter read: "Following up on my letter to you of this date, please be advised I am able to resume the discharge of the Constitutional powers and duties of the President of the United States. I have informed the Vice President of my determination and my resumption of those powers and duties."
3. *Ibid.*, 200–204.
4. Abrams, 232–3.
5. T. Burton Smith, *White House Doctor* (Lanham, MD: Madison Books, 1992), 5.
6. Hugh Smith, M.D. (a former student of Ruge at Northwestern School of Medicine), personal interview with the author, 5 September 2005.
7. Bradley H. Patterson, *The White House Staff. Inside the West Wing and Beyond* (Washington: Brookings Institution Press, 2000).
8. *Ibid.*
9. *Ibid.*
10. Lawrence Altman, "Unique Problems for a Physician Who Makes House Calls," *New York Times*, 21 February 1989.
11. *Ibid.*
12. Ann Devroy, "Interview with Dan Ruge," *USA Today*, 29 March 1984.
13. Altman.
14. *Ibid.*
15. Patterson; Smith, 5.
16. Altman
17. Smith, 5.
18. Patterson.
19. Abrams, 59.
20. *Ibid.*, 182.
21. Abrams, 192; Kenneth Crispell, Carlos Gomez and Kenneth W. Thompson, *Papers on Presidential Disability and the Twenty-fifth Amendment*, vol. 4 (Lanham, MD: University Press of America, 1997), 106–7.
22. Abrams, 146.
23. *Ibid.*, 144.
24. Smith, 15–16.
25. *Ibid.*, 4–5.
26. *Ibid.*
27. *Ibid.*
28. *Ibid.*, 7, 17.
29. *Ibid.*, 10.
30. Press Release, "Appointment of T. Burton Smith as Physician to the President," Administration of Ronald Reagan, January 4, 1985; Patricia Socha (American Board of Medical Specialties), personal correspondence with the author, November 15, 2004.
31. Smith, 19.
32. *Ibid.*, 19–20.
33. *Ibid.*, 54–5.
34. *Ibid.*, 75.
35. *Ibid.*, 21.
36. *Ibid.*, 123.
37. *Ibid.*, 86–7.
38. *Ibid.*, 168; T. Burton Smith, "The Presidential Physician and the Reagan Presidency," in *Papers on Presidential Disability and the Twenty-fifth Amendment*, vol. 2, ed. Kenneth W. Thompson (Lanham, MD: University Press of America, 1991), 65–87.
39. Smith, *White House Doctor*, 159.
40. Smith, *The Presidential Physician*, 65–87.
41. *Ibid.*, 77.
42. *Ibid.*
43. Smith, *The Presidential Papers*, 86–87; Larry Speakes and Robert Pack, *Speaking Out: The Reagan Presidency from Inside the White House* (New York: Charles Scribner's Sons, 1988), 190. Therein Speakes quotes Smith as saying, "The anesthetic will have no more effect on the President than drinking a couple of martinis." In the former 1991 publication, Dr. Smith responded to Speakes' criticism by explaining that by saying "It's like having a martini" he had attempted to give an explanation of what sedation was like to a layman. The number of imbibed martinis that Smith had in mind in his explanation remains open to question.
44. Abrams, 199; Speakes, 190.
45. Speakes, 190.
46. Smith, *The Presidential Physician*, 86–7.
47. Speakes, 195–201.
48. Nancy Reagan, *My Turn: The Memoirs of Nancy Reagan* (New York: Random House, 1989), 245, 253, 255–6, 272, 276–7, 289, 294, 296, 301, 303, 310–11, 368–9.
49. T. Burton Smith, "The Presidential Physician and the Reagan Presidency," in *Papers on Presidential Disability and the Twenty-fifth Amendment*, vol. 2, ed. Kenneth Thompson (Lanham, MD: University Press of America, 1996), 67. Smith explained: "I would have gone four years. I anticipated staying there four years, but I had a younger brother who was a surgeon dying of cancer, and my mother was dying. My brother was to take care of my mother; he was no longer able to take care of her, so I had to go home. I think it's proper that I did."
50. "Reagan Physician Chosen," Associated Press, 12 December 1986; Frank Lewis, M.D. (American Board of Surgery), personal correspondence with the author, 7 September 2004.
51. Bill McAllister, "The Precarious Role of the President's Physician," in *Papers on Presidential Disability and the Twenty-fifth Amendment*, vol. 4, ed. Kenneth Thompson (Lanham MD: University Press of America, 1997), 121.

52. *New York Times*, 5 January 1987; 7 January 1987; 2 August 1987; 16 January 1988; 23 April 1988; 9 December 1988; 4 January 1989.
53. Karen Tumulty, *The Triumph of Nancy Reagan* (New York: Simon & Schuster, 2021), 546.
54. McAllister; Oliver H. Baehrs, "The Medical History of President Ronald Reagan," *Journal of the American College of Surgeons* 178 (January 1994): 86–96.
55. Baehrs; Lawrence K. Altman, "President Is Well After Operation to Ease Prostate," *New York Times*, 6 January 1987.
56. Altman, "The President Is Well after Operation to Ease Prostate."
57. See Chapter 11.
58. Philip M. Boffey, "Cancer Is Removed from Reagan's Nose," *New York Times*, 1 August 1987; "Dr. Diane Colgan Elected to Suburban Hospital Board of Trustees," http://www.suburbanhospital.org/publications/pr052605.html (accessed April 5, 2006).
59. Philip M. Boffey, "Mrs. Reagan's Skin Cancer Removed," *New York Times*, 22 December 1982.
60. Barbara Bush, *Barbara Bush: A Memoir* (New York: Charles Scribner's Sons, 1994), 282; Robert Pear, "A Blunt-Speaking Doctor (Bush's Own) Leads Team Treating President," *New York Times*, 5 May 1989.
61. Walter Bogdanovich, "Role of President's Doctor Scrutinized as Concern over Bush's Health Persists," *Wall Street Journal*, 1991.
62. Pear; Lawrence Altman, "Every Time Bush Says 'Ah,' Second Guessers of His Doctor Cry 'Aha,'" *New York Times*, 18 February 1992.
63. Altman; Pear.
64. Smith, *White House Doctor*, 22; Pear.
65. Pear.
66. Smith, *White House Doctor*, 22; Burton J. Lee III, "The Bush Presidency and Presidential Disability," in *Papers on Presidential Disability and the Twenty-fifth Amendment*, vol. 3, ed. Kenneth W. Thompson (Lanham, MD: University Press of America, 1996), 188–9.
67. Altman.
68. Lawrence K. Altman, "The Doctor's World: A Clinician Reflects on 30 Years of Change," *New York Times*, 1989.
69. Dennis Breo, "Tough Talk from the President's Physician," *Journal of the American Medical Association* 262(9) (November 17, 1989): 2742–5.
70. Ibid.
71. Altman, "Every Time."
72. Lawrence K. Altman, "The Doctor's World: Unique Problems for a Physician Who Make (White) House Calls," *New York Times*, 21 February 1989.
73. See Chapter 7.
74. Altman, "Every Time."
75. Breo.
76. Ibid.
77. Ibid.
78. Lee, "The Role of the Presidential Physician," 34.
79. Ibid., 32.
80. Ibid., 37.
81. Lee, "The Bush Presidency," 185–9.
82. Lawrence K. Altman, "Doctor in the White House Is Dismissed," *New York Times*, 29 January 1993.
83. E. Connie Mariano, correspondence with the author, 8 September 2003.
84. Louie Estrada, "William Lukash Dies at 66," *Washington Post*, 7 February 1998.

Chapter 11

1. Richard Tubb, personal interview by author, 16 December 2021.
2. Ibid.
3. Ibid.
4. The White House Office of the Press Secretary, "Summary of the President's Physical Examination," 4 August 2001, https.//georgewbushwhitehouse.archives.gov//news/releases/2001/08/04, accessed 25 June 2021.
5. Richard Tubb, personal interview by author, 16 December 2021.
6. David Jackson, "George W. Bush has heart surgery for blocked artery," *USA Today*, 6 August 2013; Richard Tubb, personal conversation with author, 12 December 2023.
7. The White House Office of the Press Secretary, "Summary of President Barack Obama's Physical Examination," 12 June 2014.
8. Jeffrey Kuhlman, personal interview with author, 25 February 2022.
9. Ibid. His prime achievement as the Obamas' presidential physician was "persuading the president to quit smoking and keeping him safe."
10. Ibid.; Kuhlman, Transform Healthcare: https://jeffreykuhlman.com/about, accessed 24 November 2020.
11. Had an unfavorable opinion of Jackson, but not clinically. Possessed a different personality than his successor, and "would have handled events differently." Jeffrey Kuhlman, personal interview by the author, 25 February 2022.
12. Ronny Jackson, *Holding the Line: A Lifetime of Defending Democracy and American Values* (New York: Post Hill Press, 2022) 15–17.
13. Ibid.; 23–4. "I was really excited when I finally got accepted at my number one choice at the University of Texas Medical Branch in Galveston," "I got out of med school and had money in the bank."
14. Ibid.; 51–55.
15. Ibid.: 73: "The family, was good to me, and the president wrote me excellent evaluations. He even promoted me to rear admiral."
16. Ibid.: 80–81.
17. Richard Tubb, personal interview by author, 16 December 2021.
18. Ibid.
19. Ibid.
20. The White House Office of the Press

Secretary, "Summary of the President's Physical Examination," 4 August 2001, https. //georgewbush-whitehouse archives.gov//news/releases/2001/08/04, accessed 25 June 2001.

21. Richard Tubb, personal interview by author, 16 December 2021.

22. Press briefing by D. Connie Mariano on the occasion of the president's annual checkup, 12 January 2001; Lawrence K. Altman, "Months of Healing Will Accompany Healing," *New York Times*, 15 March 1997; Mariano, personal interview by author; Romero P. Marquez, "In the Line of Fire," http://www.filipinasmag.com/magazine/issues/nov2000, accessed 12 May 2001; Frank L. Murray, "White House Doctor Promoted to Admiral," *Washington Times*, 31 July 2000.

23. David Jackson, "George W. Bush has heart surgery for blocked artery," *USA Today*, 6 August 2013.

24. The White House Office of the Press Secretary, "Summary of President Barak Obama's Physical Examination," 12 June 2014.

25. Jeffrey Kuhlman, personal interview with author, 25 February 2022.

26. *Ibid.* His prime achievement as the Obamas' presidential physician was "persuading the president to quit smoking and keeping him safe."

27. *Ibid.*; Kuhlman, Transform Healthcare, https://jeffreykuhlman.com/about, accessed November 24, 2020.

28. Had an unfavorable opinion of Jackson, but not clinically. Possessed a different personality than his successor, and "would have handled events differently." Jeffrey Kuhlman, personal interview with author, 25 February 2022.

29. Ronny Jackson, *Holding the Line: A Lifetime of Defending Democracy and American Values* (New York: Post Hill Press, 2022) 15–17.

30. *Ibid.*; 23–4. "I was really excited when I finally got accepted at my number one choice at the University of Texas Medical Branch in Galveston," "I got out of med school and had money in the bank."

31. *Ibid.*; 51–55.

32. *Ibid.*: 73: "The family, was good to me, and the president wrote me excellent evaluations. He even promoted me to rear admiral."

33. United States Code.1994 Edition: Containing the General and Permanent Laws of the United States in Force on January 3, 1995. Volume Three. Chapter 104: "That the officer of the Medical Corps, United States Army, or of the Medical Corps, United States Navy, below the rank of colonel or captain respectively, who is now, or hereafter may be assigned to duty as physician to the White House, shall have the temporary rank and the pay and allowances of a colonel, Medical Corps, United States Army, or of a captain, United States Navy, while serving; Sobocinski, Andre, personal interview with author. Communication with Director of Medical Corps, 20 April 2021.

34. Sean Conley, personal interview by the author, 2021; "Sean Conley," Wikipedia, https://en.wikipedia.org/wiki/Sean_Conley, accessed 30 March 2021.

35. "Sean Conley," Wikipedia, https: en.wikipedia.org/wiki/Sean Conley, accessed 31 May 2022.

36. "Transcript: President Trump's Doctors Provide Saturday Update on His Health," NPR playlist as viewed on YouTube, 3 October 2020.

37. Mark Meadows, *The Chief's Chief* (St. Petersburg: All Seasons Press, 2021), 200–201.

38. *Ibid.*, 147–187.

39. Remdesivir: https://www.drugs.com/mtm/remdesivir.html.

40. "FDA authorizes REGEN-COV antibody therapy for post-exposure prophylaxis (prevention) for Covid-19," www.fda.drugs, 10 August 2021.

41. Meadows, 198.

42. *Ibid.*, 199.

43. "Biden removes Dr. Sean Conley, Trump physician accused of misleading the public about Trump's Covid-19 diagnosis," Yahoo News, 27 January 2021, https://yahoo.com/biden/removes-dr-sean-conley-003458829.html, accessed 3 May 2022.

44. Jeremy Herb and Kevin Liptak, "Trump's White House doctor facing fresh scrutiny over Covid test timeline," CNN Politics, 3 February 2021.

45. Sean Conley, personal interview, 2021.

46. *Ibid.*

47. Jackson, *Holding the Line*.

48. "Joe Biden," https://www.brittanica.com.biography/Joe-Biden, accessed 11 July 2023.

49. Randall Chase, "Vice President's son Beau Biden dies of brain cancer."

50. Richard Harris, "Joe Biden Is 'Healthy' and 'Vigorous,'" NPR, 7 December 2019; Joe Biden, *Promises to Keep* (New York: Random House, 2008) 213–232.

51. For Biden's personal recall of the operations for cerebral aneurysms.

52. "Kevin O'Connor Biography," www.gw/docs.com/find-a-doctor/kevin-ocnnor, accessed 20 November 2020.

53. Jill Sedersttum, "FP Reflects on Service on Front Lines of Family Medicine," AAFP, June 2019, https://www.aafp.org/news/family-doc-focus/20190603fdf-oconnor-html, accessed 9 November 2019; Kevin O'Connor, personal interview, 15 December 2023.

54. Richard Tubb, personal interview, 23 November 2020.

55. *Ibid.*; "Kevin O'Connor Biography."

56. YouTube interview before Federation of State Medical Boards Spotlight: https://www.youtube.com/watch?v=eCBTPuQGZlA) accessed 31 January 2021; O'Connor personal interview, 15 December 2023, 28 December 2023.

57. Brandon Holveck, "Joe Biden suffers hairline fractures after twisting his ankle playing with his dog, his doctor says," *USA Today*, 29 November 2020.

58. Christian Datoc, *Washington Examiner*, 19 November 2021.

59. "Polyp in Biden's colon was benign, potentially pre-cancerous," AP Politics, 25 November 2021.

60. Andrew Restuccia, Catherine Lucey and Ken Thomas, "President Biden Tests Positive for Covid-19," *Wall Street Journal*, 21 July 2022.

61. "Biden tests positive for Covid -19 again," www.foxnews.com/politics/biden-tests-positive, accessed 3 August 22; Cristina Laila, "Quadruple Vaxxed Joe Biden Tests Positive Again for Covid Again This Morning," www-thegatewaypundit.com/2022/08quadruple-vaxxed; accessed 1 August 2022.

62. Steven Nelson, "Biden using CPAP machine for sleep apnea, White House admits, after strap lines appear on prez's face," 30 June 2023.

63. Kevin Tober, "OUCH! Doocy, Portnoy Torch WH Over Biden's Doctor Hiding from Press," 25 July 2022; Katie Pavlich, "White House Won't Make Biden's Doctor Available for Questioning," Town Hall, 21 July 2022, townhall.com/tipsheet/katiepavlich/2022/07/21/white-house, accessed 21 July 2022; Kevin O'Connor, text to author, 2 November 2023.

64. Kevin O'Connor, personal interview with the author, 15 December 2023.

65. Steven Nelson, "Biden gets two-day root canal after report president eats 'like a child,'" *New York Post*, June 12, 2023.

Chapter 12

1. John M. Broder and Don Van Natta, Jr., "Clinton and Starr, a mutual admonition society," *New York Times* News Service, 19 September 1998.

2. "Richard Tubb, White House Physician," *Washington Post*, 9 February 2003.

3. Jackson, *Holding the Line*, 69–70.

4. E. Connie Mariano, "In Sickness and in Health: Medical Care of the President of the United States," in *Managing Crisis*, ed. Robert E. Gilbert (New York: Fordham University Press, 2000), 83. Mariano states that the medical presence in the White House was formally given the name White House Medical Unit by Congress in the 1920s. However, this term did not receive wide usage until the 1990s.

5. Romero P. Marquez, "In the Line of Fire," http://www.filipinasmag.com/magazine/issues/nov2000/eature.html (accessed May 12, 2001).

6. Kate Molan, National Archives and Records Administration, personal communication with the author, 26 October 2022; Law Library of Congress, personal communication with the author, 7 October 2022. Neither the National Archives nor the Library of Congress has any record of a law or regulation establishing the White House Medical Unit; Connie Mariano, personal communication with the author, 10 October 2022: "I don't think WHMU was established by law or admin fiat.... We formalized it when I became director in 1994."

7. Bradley Patterson, *The White House Staff*, 163–173.

8. Connie Mariano, personal communication.

9. Ronny Jackson, personal interview, 12 December 2020.

10. E. Connie Mariano, interview by the author, Scottsdale, Arizona, 18 July 2003; Mariano, "In Sickness and in Health," 83–96.

11. Mariano, interview by the author.

12. Mariano, interview by the author.

13. Gerald R. Cox, interview by the author, 16 June 2006. Dr. Cox described a group interview, chaired by Dr. Richard Tubb, then senior White House physician. The interview occurred at the time of the Senate trial of Bill Clinton. Tubb insisted that Cox respond when asked whether he, as a senator, would vote to convict President Clinton of impeachable offenses. Cox's third answer, "yes," did not disqualify him from receiving the position; rather it indicated that grace under pressure and a working knowledge of current events were prerequisites for the job.

14. Mariano, "In Sickness and in Health," 91–2.

15. Louis Estrada, "William Lukash Dies at 66: Chief Presidential Physician," *Washington Post*, February 1998.

16. Thomas Kaplan, "Biden Names His Personal Doctor, Kevin O'Connor, to Be His White House Physician," *New York Times*, January 25, 2021.

17. Mariano, interview by the author. Primary care specialties have been differentiated from subspecialties for purposes of determining present and future physician needs. Examples of subspecialties are surgery and all the surgical subspecialties, e.g., urology, plastic surgery, ophthalmology, pathology, radiology, etc. In distinction, the primary care specialties are the following: family medicine, internal medicine, obstetrics/gynecology and pediatrics. Only the first two specialties are relevant to the WHMU's normal function.

18. "About ABMS," http://www.abms.org/about.asp (accessed December 7, 2005).

19. American Board of Medical Genetics, http://www.abmg.org/genetics/abmg/general.htm (accessed December 7, 2005).

20. American Board of Emergency Medicine, http://www.abem.org/rainbow/portal/alias (accessed December 5, 2005). At the present time (2007) no emergency room physician serves as a member of the WHMU.

21. Patricia Socha (American Board of Medical Specialties), telephone interview with the author, 29 June 2005.

22. Mariano, personal correspondence with the author, 1 May 2006.

23. Mariano, interview by the author.

24. Mariano, interview by the author, Tempe, AZ, 27 August 2005.

25. See Chapter 15 for a complete discussion of the vice presidents' health care.

26. George F. Fuller, "White House Medical Support," http://www.afip.org/Departments/

legalmed/legmed2003?Fuller.pdf (accessed July 30, 2004).
    27. *Ibid.*
    28. Mariano interview, August 27, 2005.
    29. Mariano, "In Sickness and in Health," 87.
    30. Peter Baker, "In Morocco, a Diplomatic Hillary Clinton Emerges," *Washington Post*, 1 April 1999, page A17.
    31. Hillary Rodham Clinton, *Living History* (New York: Scribner, 2003). Page references to her travels are too numerous to enumerate in this autobiography *cum* travelogue.
    32. Navy captain Dr. Robert Darling traveled extensively with Mrs. Clinton on her overseas journeys. He specifically mentioned her trips to the Central Asian republics and to the nations of sub-Saharan Africa. The rationale was that, in these primitive countries, Darling, an ER boarded physician, would be able to keep this first lady alive until more comprehensive medical resources would arrive. Robert Darling, personal interview with the author, 29 December 2005.
    33. "Which First Lady Flies Highest? Michelle vs. Laura," 9 July 2013 https://www.ntu.org/publications/detail/which-first-lady-flies-highest-michelle-vs-laura; accessed 26 February 2023.
    34. Bradley H. Patterson, *The White House Staff: Inside the West Wing and Beyond* (Washington: Brookings Institution Press, 2000), 362.
    35. Robert Darling, telephone interview with the author, 29 December 2005.
    36. Mariano, personal correspondence with the author, 1 May 2006.
    37. "Man Sets Himself Ablaze at White House," http://www.foxnews.som/story/0,2933,138621,00.html (accessed November 15, 2004).
    38. "Cheney calls in personal physician to help ailing supporter," The Associated Press, 16 July 2004. For a more recent example of the fortuitous presence of Vice President Cheney's WHMU, see Chapter 15.
    39. Jackson, *Holding the Line*, 69.
    40. Mariano correspondence with the author, 19 March 2004; "Ashcroft hospitalized with pancreas condition," The Associated Press, 6 March 2004.
    41. *Ibid.*; "Attorney General Is Hospitalized," *Seattle Times*, 6 March 2004.
    42. Mariano, correspondence with the author, 19 March 2004.
    43. Mariano, interview by the author.
    44. Mike Allen, "A Dog's Life Remembered: Spot Is Dead at Age 14," *Washington Post*, 22 February 2004; "Bushes' 'loyal, loving companion' Spot dies," *Ottawa Citizen*, 22 February 2004.
    45. Jackson, *Holding the Line*, 66.
    46. Alben W. Barkley, *That Reminds Me* (Garden City, NY: Doubleday, 1954), 230. Vice President Barkley recounted a July 1952 White House political session attended by Truman and his close political observers. Barkley wrote: "Among then was Dr. Wallace Graham, the President's physician. I never did quite understand what the good doctor was there for, unless it was to look me over covertly and render a professional opinion as to whether I would survive a campaign. Anyhow, he never took his stethoscope out."
    47. "Taft Again Refuses to Pardon Morse," *New York Times*, 25 December 1911. Morse's wife had been very active in campaigning for her banker husband's pardon on the grounds of ill health. She had importuned half the members of the U.S. House of Representatives to sign her petition for a pardon. See Chapter 7 for Dr. Graham's politically motivated problems with the Senate and the AMA.
    48. Fuller.
    49. Allen; Fuller.
    50. T. Burton Smith, *White House Doctor* (Lanham, MD: Madison Books, 1992), 88.
    51. Mariano, interview by the author
    52. "Tipper Gore and Thyroid Problems," in *Johns Hopkins Medicine Patient Care*, http://www.hopkins.med.jhu.edu/news/thyroid/ (accessed May 11, 2001).
    53. Lawrence K. Altman, "Checkup Finds Bush Fit and Healthy," *New York Times*, 4 August 2001. See this chapter regarding medical consultants.
    54. Mariano, interview by the author; see Chapter 7 (White) and Chapter 9 (Jacobson, Kraus). See Chapter 8 (Hurst).
    55. "Clinton's Knee Bill," *Pittsburgh Post-Gazette*, 3 June 1997.
    56. Mariano, Connie, *The White House Doctor* (New York: St. Martin's Press, 2010) 282. "My work in the military and my life in the kill zone for nine years widened the distance between us."
    57. Mariano, interview by the author.
    58. Frank J. Murray, "White House Doctor Promoted to Admiral," *Washington Times*, 31 July 2000.
    59. Mariano, interview by the author.
    60. Rebecca L. Sutphin, "Nurse Practitioner vs Physician Assistant: What's the Difference?" Nurse Journal, 13 February 2023; trend is physician practices nationwide.
    61. Ronny Jackson, interview with the author, 12 December 2020.
    62. Denise Whitfield, interviews with the author, 15 May, 8 November 2023; Francesco Cimino, interview with the author, 5 June 2023.
    63. Sean Conley, interview with the author, 24 March 2021.

Chapter 13

    1. John D. Feerick, *The Twenty-Fifth Amendment: Its Complete History and Applications* 3d edition (New York: MJF Books, 2014), 125.
    2. Connie Mariano, "In Sickness and in Health: Medical Care for the President of the United States," 902, in *Managing Crisis: Presidential Disability and the 25th Amendment,* ed. Robert E. Gilbert (New York: Fordham University Press, 2000).
    3. Kenneth W. Thompson, ed., *Papers on*

Presidential Disability and the Twenty-fifth Amendment, vols. 1, 2, 3, 4 (Lanham, MD: University Press of America, 1988, 1991, 1996, 1997). These four volumes contain significant and important discussions of these issues. The discussants were medical historians, medical, legal and political authorities, and several White House physicians.

4. James F. Toole and Robert J. Joynt, eds., *Presidential Disability: Papers, Discussions and Recommendations on the Twenty-fifth Amendment and Issues of Inability and Disability in Presidents of the United States* (Rochester: University of Rochester Press; 2001). This is a comprehensive accounting of all the pertinent issues. The participants were ever greater in number and in prestige than the Miller Conference attendees. Several White House physicians were active participants, and both presidents Gerald Ford and Jimmy Carter gave presentations. This discussion is useful in that the experts gave recommendations to resolve the ambiguities, dilemmas, and conflicts of the amendment.

5. Robert E. Gilbert, ed., *Managing Crisis: Presidential Disability and the 25th Amendment* (New York: Fordham University Press, 2000).

6. Feerick, *The Twenty-Fifth Amendment*, 2014.

7. Brian C. Kalt, *Unable* (New York: Oxford University Press, 2019).

8. William A. DeGregorio, *The Complete Book of U.S. Presidents from George Washington to Bill Clinton*, 4th ed. (New York: Wings Books, 1993).

9. Herbert L. Abrams, *"The President Has Been Shot": Confusion, Disability and the 25th Amendment in the Aftermath of the Attempted Assassination of Ronald Reagan* (New York: W.W. Norton, 1992), 269–271. An excellent discussion of the misuse of this amendment during President Reagan's two health crises.

10. Toole and Joynt, xiii.

11. Ibid.

12. Abrams, 178.

13. *New York Times*, 21 August ,10 October, 16 November, 19 November, 5 December 1974.

14. Toole and Joynt, xiii.

15. T. Burton Smith, *White House Doctor* (Lanham, MD: Madison Books, 1992), 106.

16. Ibid., 112. Smith believes that the president did indeed set precedent by being the first to implement section three.

17. Abrams (201) correctly disagreed, stating that the section had not been invoked; Kalt, 69.

18. Smith, 116; Abrams, 203–5, 261. An example of the concern over Vice President Dan Quayle's competence to fulfill the responsibilities of acting president, albeit on a very temporary basis, is exemplified in Jules Witcover, *Crapshoot: Rolling the Dice on the Vice Presidency* (New York: Crown, 1992): 4–8, 394–5.

19. E. Connie Mariano, "In Sickness and in Health: Medical Care for the President of the United States," in *Managing Crisis*, ed. Robert Gilbert (New York: Fordham University Press, 2000), 86; "Surgeons to Repair Torn Tendon," *Youngstown Vindicator*, 14 March 1997; Mariano, 93.

20. "Propofol," Wikipedia https://en.wikipedia.og//wiki//Propofol, 10 July 2022.

21. Richard Tubb, letter to the author, 14 December 2023.

22. Richard Tubb, interview with the author, 16 December 2021; Feerick, 202.

23. Richard Tubb, interview with the author,16 December 2021, Feerick, 203.

24. Ashley Parker, Matt Viser and John Wagner, "Biden deemed fit after routine physical," *Washington Post*, 20 November 2021.

25. Jimmy Carter, Message, xv and "Opening Address," in Toole and Joynt, 15–21.

26. Toole and Joynt, xiii; John Calvin Batchelor, *Father's Day* (New York: St. Martin's Paperbacks, 1994); Frederick Forsyth, *The Negotiator* (New York: Bantam Books, 1989); Mario Puzo, *The Fourth K* (New York: Ballantine Books, 1990); William Safire, *Full Disclosure* (New York: Ballantine Books, 1977); Robert Serling, *The President's Plane Is Missing* (London: Cassell and Co., 1968); Brad Thor, *The Lions of Lucerne* (New York: Pocket Star Books, 2002).

27. Jerrold M. Post and Robert S. Robins, *When Illness Strikes the Leader* (New Haven, CT: Yale University Press, 1993), 96.

28. Toole and Joynt, 119.

29. Ibid., 213.

30. W.T. Reich, ed., *Encyclopedia of Bioethics* (New York: MacMillan, 1995), 2632.

31. Harold Brody, *The Physician Patient Relationship*, in *Medical Ethics,* 2nd ed., ed. Robert M. Veatch (Sudbury, MA: Jones and Bartlett, 1997), 89–90.

32. K. Coblens et al., "American College of Physicians Ethics Manual," *Annals of Internal Medicine,* 3rd ed., 117 (1992): 947–60.

33. Toole and Joynt, 211.

34. Thompson, vol. 2, 93–104.

35. Toole and Joynt, 266.

36. Thompson, vol. 3, 183.

37. Mariano, 92.

38. Ibid., 93.

39. Bandy Lee, editor, *The Dangerous Case of Donald Trump* (New York: St. Martin's Press, 2017).

40. "Dr. Bandy Lee warned five years ago that Trump was dangerous," *Independent*, www.independent.co.uk/news/world/Americanbandy,-less-trump; accessed 8 February 2023.

41. Nick Givas, "New book claims Rod Rosenstein thought John Kelly and Jeff Sessions would back use of 25th Amendment against Trump," Fox News, 8 October 2019; Hoft, Jim: "Deep State Rod Rosenstein Now Admits He Talked with Andrew McCabe About Recording President Trump—After Lying During Senate Testimony," *The Gateway Pundit*, 6 March 2021; Andrew McCarthy, "McCabe, Rosenstein and the real truth about the 25th Amendment coup attempt," *Fox News*, 16 February 2019.

42. John Martin-Joy, *Donald Trump and the 25th Amendment*, "Errors of judgement and lack

of popularity do not constitute an inability"; "How Would It Work," *Psychology Today*, https://psychologytoday/.com/us/blog/politics, accessed 4 April 2021.

43. Ted Rall, "Joe Biden Obviously Has Dementia and Should Withdraw, Political Commentary, Rasmussen Reports," 14 March 2020; Caitlin Johnstone, "Stop Calling It a Stutter: Dozens of Examples Show Biden's Dementia Symptoms," *Consortium News*, 6 March 2020; Alana Goodman, "Not The Same Joe Biden: White House Stenographer Says Former VP's Mental Acuity Has Deteriorated," *Washington Free Beacon*, 8 September 2020.

44. "Is Joe Biden Mentally Fit for the Presidency? No, and These 10 Gaffes Show Why." https://genzconservative.com/is-joe-biden-mentally-fit-for-the-presidency, accessed 16 December 2020; Cheryl Crumley, "Biden's cognitive dysfunction takes front and center," *Washington Times*, 27 July 2021.

45. *Fox News*, https://www//breitbart.com/politics/2021/09/20/49-percent/think-joe-biden-is-mentally-stable-enough-to-be-president; accessed 20 September 2021; Snejana Farberov, "How Concerned Are You About President Biden's Mental Health," *New York Post*, 11 August 2022.

46. "Ronny Jackson, House Republicans Call For Joe Biden's Cognitive Assessment," *Breitbart*, 18 June 2021; Samuel Chamberlain, "GOP lawmakers led by ex-White House doc ask Biden to take cognitive test," *New York Post*, 17 August 2021.

Chapter 14

1. Bob Woodward and Carl Bernstein, *The Final Days* (New York: Simon and Schuster, 1976), 395.

2. Roy Franklin Nichols, *Franklin Pierce: Young Hickory of the Granite Hills* (Philadelphia: Pennsylvania University Press, 1931, 1969), 233.

3. The one exception is Dr. Arnold Hutschnecker, a psychotherapist who visited President Richard Nixon twice in the White House and possibly secretly elsewhere. Their relationship will be discussed at length later in this chapter.

4. Bert Park, in *Presidential Disability: Papers, Discussions and Recommendations on the Twenty-fifth Amendment and Issues of Inability and Disability in Presidents of the United States*, ed. James F. Toole and Robert J. Joynt (Rochester, NY: University of Rochester Press, 2001), 89.

5. C. Knight Aldrich, "Personal Grieving and Political Defeat: The Case of Calvin Coolidge," in *Papers on Presidential Disability and the Twenty-fifth Amendment*, vol. 3, ed. Kenneth W. Thompson (Lanham, MD: University Press of America, 1996), 92.

6. Robert E. Gilbert, "The Genius of the Twenty-fifth Amendment: Guarding Against Presidential Disability but Safeguarding the Presidency," in *Managing Crisis: Presidential Disability and the 25th Amendment*, ed. Robert E. Gilbert (New York: Fordham University Press, 2000), 31, 48.

7. Herbert L. Abrams, *"The President Has Been Shot": Confusion, Disability, and the 25th Amendment in the Aftermath of the Attempted Assassination of Ronald Reagan* (New York: W.W. Norton, 1992), 222–225.

8. Birch Bayh, "Reflections on the Twenty-fifth Amendment as We Enter a New Century," in *Managing Crisis*, 61–62; Jerrold Post; "Broken Minds, Broken Hearts, and the Twenty-fifth Amendment: Psychiatric Disorders and Presidential Disability," in *Managing Crisis*, 111–112.

9. Jerrold Post, *Presidential Disability: Papers, Discussions, and Recommendations on the Twenty-fifth Amendment and Issues of Inability and Disability in Presidents of the United States* (Rochester, NY: University of Rochester Press, 2001), 53.

10. Lawrence C. Mohr, *Presidential Disability*, 370.

11. Bert A. Park, "Reform: Yes," in *Presidential Disability*, 141–155.

12. Marjorie Hunter, "Senate Unit Backs Ford, 9 to 0; Approval on Floor Is Expected," *New York Times*, 21 November 1973.

13. "Is Barry Goldwater psychologically Fit to Be President of the United States," advertisement, *New York Times*, 12 September 1964.

14. "Doctors Deplore Goldwater Poll," *New York Times*, 2 October 1964.

15. Sally Satel, "The Perils of Putting National Leaders on the Couch," *New York Times*, 29 June 2004.

16. Geoffrey Barker, "Dukakis labeled 'an invalid'; Reagan sets tone for dirty campaign," *Advertiser*, 5 August 1988; Alex Brummer, "Therapy no bar to U.S. presidency," *Guardian* (London), 6 August 1988.

17. "Reagan jokes that Dukakis is an 'invalid,'" *Toronto Star*, 4 August 1988; Alex Brummer, "Reagan gaffe puts Dukakis in the spot; Furore over 'invalid' remark despite swift apology," *Guardian* (London), 3 August 1988; Stewart Fleming; "Dukakis Doctor Denies Depression," *Financial Times* (London), 5 August 1988.

18. *New York Times*, 2 August 1972.

19. *New York Times*, 28 July 1972; 31 July 1972; 2 August 1972.

20. *New York Times*, 26 July 1972; 27 July 1972.

21. *New York Times*, 1 August 1972; The Republican ticket of Nixon/Agnew swamped the reconstituted Democratic ticket of McGovern/Shriver in the 1972 presidential election with a 61 percent–38 percent margin in the popular vote and a 520–17 score in the electoral vote. William A. Degregorio, *The Complete Book of U.S. Presidents: From George Washington to Bill Clinton* (New York: Wings Books, 1993), 591.

22. *New York Times*, 28 July 1972.

23. Thomas Francis Eagleton, http://www.bioguide.congress.gov/scripts/biodisplay.pl?index=E00004 (accessed November 11, 2005).

24. Marjorie Hunter, "Ford Denies That He Was Treated by a New York Psychotherapist," *New York Times*, 17 October 1973; Marjorie Hunter,

"Senate Unit Backs Ford, 9 to 0; Approval on Floor Is Expected," *New York Times*, 21 November 1973.

25. Eve Bender, "With Politics and Mental Illness, The More Things Change..." *Psychiatric News* 37(1) (November 1, 2002): 10. This article did point out that at least one congressman had been successfully reelected after an admission of antidepressant therapy.

26. Rosemary Stevens, *American Medicine and the Public Interest: A History of Specialization* (Berkeley: University of California Press, 1971, 1998), 222–225.

27. Henry A. Bunker, "American Psychiatry as a Specialty," in *One Hundred Years of American Psychiatry*, ed. J.K. Hall, Gregory Zilboorg, Henry Bunker (New York: Columbia University Press, 1944), 480–481.

28. Marvin Stein, "The Establishment of the Department of Psychiatry in the Mount Sinai Hospital: A Conflict between Neurology and Psychiatry, *Journal of the History of the Behavioral Sciences* 43(3) (Summer 2004): 285–309.

29. Jonathan R.T. Davidson, Kathryn M. Connor and Marvin Swartz, "Mental Illness in U.S. Presidents between 1776 and 1974: A Review of Biographical Sources," *Journal of Nervous & Mental Disease* 194(1) (January 2006): 47–51. In this seminal article the authors reviewed biographical sources regarding mental illness in the 37 presidents who served up to 1974. Material was extracted by one of the authors and given to experienced psychiatrists for independent review of the correspondence of behaviors, symptoms, and medical information in source material to Diagnostic and Statistical Manual of Mental Disorders, fourth edition, criteria. Levels of confidence were given for each diagnosis.

30. David McCullough, *John Adams* (New York: Simon & Schuster, 2001), 285.

31. John Ferling, *John Adams: A Life* (New York: Henry Holt and Company, 1992), 381. George Washington and Thomas Jefferson both absented themselves from the nation's capital during their presidencies, but never approaching the length of Adams' absence.

32. Paul C. Nagel, *Descent from Glory: Four Generations of the John Adams Family* (New York: Oxford University Press, 1983), 78–80.

33. Paul C. Nagel, *John Quincy Adams: A Public Life, a Private Life* (Cambridge, MA: Harvard University Press, 1997), 155.

34. *Ibid.*, 259.

35. *Ibid.*, 304, 305, 308.

36. *Ibid.*, 315.

37. *Ibid.*, 329. George Washington Adams probably committed suicide while traveling by boat to Washington in April 1827. His mission was to assist the departing president and the family return to Massachusetts.

38. Roy Franklin Nichols, *Franklin Pierce: Young Hickory of the Granite Hills* (Philadelphia: Pennsylvania University Press, 1931, 1969), 225–6.

39. *Ibid.*, 284. Warren G. Harding III and J. Mark Stewart, *Mere Mortals: The Life and Health Histories of American Presidents* (Worthington, OH: Renaissance Publications, 1991), 70–75; Rudolph Marx, *The Health of Presidents* (New York: G.P. Putnam's Sons, 1960), 160–168; Bumgarner, *The Health of Presidents*, 80–84, all focus on Pierce's alcohol addiction. He died from liver cirrhosis. Davidson et al. designated Pierce's mental illnesses as alcohol dependence and major depressive disorder.

40. Robert E. Gilbert, *The Tormented President: Calvin Coolidge, Death, and Clinical Depression* (Westport, CT: Praeger, 2003), 3.

41. *Ibid.*, 250.

42. *Ibid.*, 250–254. Davidson et al. also characterized Coolidge's problem as a major depressive disorder. In addition, the authors applied the diagnoses of social phobia and hypochondriasis.

43. Aldrich, 92.

44. *Presidential Disability*, Toole and Joynt, eds., 72. Davidson et al.'s diagnosis is major depressive disorder, recurrent with psychotic features.

45. Joshua Wolf Shenk, *Lincoln's Melancholy: How Depression Challenged a President and Fueled His Greatness* (Boston: Houghton Mifflin, 2005)

46. *Ibid.*, 8.

47. *Ibid.*, 179.

48. *Ibid.*, 186.

49. *Ibid.*, 193.

50. *Ibid.*, 177–178.

51. *Ibid.*, 57.

52. Norbert Hirschhorn, Robert G. Feldman, and Ian A. Greaves, "Abraham Lincoln's Blue Pills," *Perspectives in Biology and Medicine* 44(3) (Summer, 2001): 315–332.

53. Richard W. Hudgens, "Mental Health of Political Candidates: Notes on Abraham Lincoln," letter to the editor, *Am J Psychiatry* 130(1) (January 1973): 110.

54. See the introduction to this chapter for an example of abnormal behavior.

55. Vamik D. Volkan, Norman Itzkowitz, Andrew W. Dod, *Richard Nixon: A Psychobiography* (New York: Columbia University Press, 1997). Woodrow Wilson was also "honored" by a psychobiography, written by Sigmund Freud and William C. Bullitt, *Thomas Woodrow Wilson: A Psychological Study* (Boston: Houghton Mifflin, 1966 reissue).

56. Volkan, 129.

57. *Ibid.*, 131–135.

58. "Personality Disorders," http://www.psyweb.com/Mdisord/jsp/personalityDis.jsp (accessed February 28, 2006).

59. Jerrold Post, in *Presidential Disability*, 55.

60. Jonathan Aitken, *Nixon: A Life* (London: Weidenfeld and Nicolson, 1993), 304–305.

61. Anthony Summers, *The Arrogance of Power: The Secret World of Richard Nixon* (New York: Viking, 2000), 376.

62. Vamik D. Volkan, "The Three Faces of Richard Nixon," in *Papers on Presidential Disability and the Twenty-fifth Amendment*, vol. 3, ed. Kenneth W. Thompson (Lanham, MD: University Press of America, 1996), 165–177.

63. Bob Woodward and Carl Bernstein, *The Final Days* (New York: Simon and Schuster, 1976), 104.
64. *Ibid.*, 104.
65. *Ibid.*, 170.
66. *Ibid.*, 32.
67. Davidson, 49.
68. Summers, 21.
69. *Ibid.*, 144–145.
70. *Ibid.*, 351.
71. *Ibid.*, 268–269.
72. John Erlichman, *Witness to Power: The Nixon Years* (New York: Simon & Schuster, 1982), 37.
73. Summers, 449.
74. *Ibid.*, 369.
75. Kenneth R. Crispell, in *Papers on Presidential Disability and the Twenty-fifth Amendment*, vol. 3, 93.
76. Richard Reeves, *President Nixon: Alone in the White House* (New York: Simon & Schuster, 2001), 92.
77. Summers' wife, Robbyn Swan, interviewed the 97-year-old Dr. Arnold Hutschnecker for three days in the mid-1990s.
78. Erica Goode, "Arnold Hutschnecker, 102, Therapist to Nixon," *New York Times*, 3 January 2001.
79. Summers, 88–90.
80. *Ibid.*, 95.
81. *Ibid.*, 90–91, 366. On page 366 Summers wrote that there was one unverified report that Hutschnecker visited Nixon in Key Biscayne, Florida, in 1970 in order "to piece together Nixon's shattered ego."
82. Goode.
83. Summers, 90–91.
84. *Ibid.*, 91.
85. See Chapter 8.
86. Summers, 88–89. Rita Hayworth, Celeste Holm and novelist Erich Marie Remarque reportedly were his patients.
87. Goode; Arnold Hutschnecker, "The Lessons of Eagleton," *New York Times*, 30 October 1972.
88. Arnold Hutschnecker, "A Suggestion: Psychiatry at High Levels of Government," *New York Times*, 4 July 1973.
89. Arnold Hutschnecker, "The Stigma of Seeing a Psychiatrist," *New York Times*, 20 November 1973.
90. Summers, 94.
91. See Chapter 8.
92. Jerome D. Levin, *The Clinton Syndrome: The President and the Self-Destructive Nature of Sexual Addiction* (Rocklin, CA: Forum, 1998).
93. Cathy Lynn Grossman, "Coming to Clinton's spiritual aid; Pair who will counsel Clinton have helped guide him before," *USA Today*, 16 September 1998.
94. Karen Tumulty, *The Triumph of Nancy Reagan* (New York: Simon & Schuster, 2001), 532.
95. *Ibid.*, 536–7
96. Mariano, personal correspondence with the author, 6 January 2006.
97. Rob Darling and Sean Conley, personal interviews with author, August 2023.

Chapter 15

1. William Degregorio, *The Complete Book of U.S. Presidents* 3rd ed. (New York: Barricade Books, 1991), 268. Schuyler Colfax, Grant's first term vice president (1869–1873), had been dumped from the national ticket because of his involvement in the Credit Mobilier scandal.
2. Ernest McKay, *Henry Wilson, Practical Radical: A Portrait of a Politician* (Port Washington, NY: Kennikat Press, 1971), 239–240.
3. T. Burton Smith, "The Presidential Physicians and the Reagan Presidency," in *Papers on Presidential Disability and the Twenty-fifth Amendment*, ed. Kenneth W. Thompson (Lanham, MD: University Press of America, 1991), 68, 81. Former presidential physician Smith recalled, "The President, Vice President Bush, Mrs. Reagan, and Mrs. Bush were my four sole responsibilities. As I say, Vice President Bush was never given a doctor until after the March 1981 shooting."
4. John P. Kaminski, *George Clinton: Yeoman Politician of the New Republic* (Madison, WI: Madison House, 1993), 290.
5. George Clinton's life is the subject of two good biographies: E. Wilder Spaulding, *His Excellency George Clinton: Critic of the Constitution* (New York: Macmillan, 1938) and Kaminski, *George Clinton: Yeoman Politician of the new Republic*. Jules Witcover has written a chatty, interesting, and often critical book that provides many useful anecdotes about the selection and competence of American vice presidents: Jules Witcover, *Crapshoot: Rolling the Dice on the American Vice Presidency* (New York: Crown, 1992).
6. Spaulding, 128, writes: "In spite of his chronic rheumatism..." in regard to his gubernatorial duties in 1779.
7. Spaulding, 216.
8. *Ibid.*, 301.
9. Kaminski, 275.
10. Spaulding, 302–303. See also Kaminski, 290.
11. *History of the Medical Society of the District of Columbia, 1817–1909* (Washington, D.C.: Medical Society of the District of Columbia, 1909), 1.
12. George Athan Billias, *Elbridge Gerry: Founding Father and Republican Statesman* (New York: McGraw-Hill, 1976), 324. This may be the only recent biography of Gerry. A second useful source is the chapter on Elbridge Gerry that appears in Mark O. Hatfield, *Vice Presidents of the United States, 1789–1993* (Washington: U.S. Government Printing Office, 1997), 61–70.
13. Billias, 329; Hatfield. The nature of Gerry's stoke is not documented in either account.
14. Billias, 329. See also Hatfield.
15. Ralph Ketcham, *James Madison: A Biography* (Charlottesville: University Press of Virginia, 1971, 1990 edition), 592, has a second version: Gerry died of a lung hemorrhage while riding in his carriage to the Senate chamber.
16. Mark O. Hatfield, "William Rufus King (1853)," in *Vice Presidents of the United States*,

179–190. Fortunately for contemporary researchers of vice-presidential trivia, a dedicated doctoral candidate had written a well-researched thesis that has lifted some of the darkness that had obscured King's life. John M. Martin's thesis, "Rufus King: Southern Moderate," was submitted as partial fulfillment of the Ph.D. degree by the University of North Carolina in 1955.

17. See Chapter 12.
18. Martin, 353.
19. *Ibid.*, 356.
20. "Hon. William R. King," *New York Times*, 27 January 1853. In Martin.
21. Martin, 357.
22. *Ibid.*
23. "The Vice-President: His Landing and Death, *New York Times*, 20 April 1853.
24. Mark O. Hatfield, "William Rufus King."
25. Martin, 60, 247.
26. Tom Bailey, *William Rufus King: Alabama's U.S. Vice President* (Hartselle, AL: Seacoast Publishing, 2022), 95.
27. Martin, in 1823 (81), in 1840 (178), in 1847–48 (269–270), 1849 (305).
28. Three biographies of Wilson are readily available: Elias Nason and Thomas Russell, *The Life and Public Services of Henry Wilson, Late Vice-President of the United States* (Boston: B.B. Russell, 1876), Ernest McKay, *Henry Wilson, Practical Radical: Portrait of a Politician* (Port Washington, NY: Kennikat Press, 1971) and Richard H. Abbott, *Cobbler in Congress: The Life of Henry Wilson, 1812–1875* (Lexington: University Press of Kentucky, 1972). Mark O. Hatfield, "Henry Wilson (1873–1875)," 231–240, again provides an excellent summary of Wilson's personal and political life.
29. Nason and Russell, 418.
30. McKay, 234.
31. "Vice President Wilson"; *New York Times*, 5 August 1873.
32. "Obituary of Edward Hammond Clarke," *The Chicago Medical Journal* 37 (1877): 111; "Obituary of Edward Hammond Clarke," *The Transactions of the American Medical Association* 29 (1878): 624–627.
33. McKay, 234.
34. Abbott, 249.
35. Hatfield; Abbott, 249–251; Nason and Russell, 419.
36. Hatfield.
37. Hatfield; Nason and Russell, 422; Abbott, 255–256.
38. Hatfield; McKay, 239–240; Abbott, 256; Nason and Russell, 422–424.
39. See Chapter 4.
40. William A. Hammond, "On the Causes of Vice-President Wilson's Death," *The Boston Medical and Surgical Journal*: 93(25) (December 16, 1875): 693–704.
41. See Chapter 4.
42. Hammond.
43. John W. Holcombe and Hubert M. Skinner, *Life and Public Services of Thomas A. Hendricks* (Indianapolis: Carlon and Hollenbeck, 1886), 373.
44. "Hendricks Dead; The Country Shocked by His Sudden Taking Off," *Indianapolis News*, 26 November 1885.
45. Hatfield, "Thomas Andrews Hendricks," 259–266.
46. Holcombe and Skinner, 389–390; "Governor Hendricks Dead," *Indianapolis News*, 25 November 1885; "Hendricks Dead," *Indianapolis News*, 26 November 1885.
47. See Chapter 5.
48. Presley Marion Rixey, "Guarding the Health of Our Presidents," *Better Health Magazine*, reproduced in William Braisted and William Bell, *The Life Story of Presley Marion Rixey, Surgeon General, U.S. Navy, 1902–1910* (Strasburg, VA: Shenandoah Publishing, 1930), 455.
49. Hatfield, "Garret A. Hobart (1897–1899)," 287–294.
50. David Magie, *Life of Garret Augustus Hobart* (New York: G.P. Putnam's Sons, 1910), 203.
51. *Ibid.*, 202–208, 212–214.
52. "Mr. McKinley by the Sea," *New York Times*, 26 August 1899.
53. Magie, 215.
54. "Vice President Hobart Dead," *New York Times*, 22 November 1899.
55. *Ibid.*; Magie, 216–217. Magie attributed Hobart's death to myocarditis, an inflammation of the heart muscle. The true nature of arteriosclerotic heart disease and heart attacks was not defined until twenty years later.
56. "William Kelly Newton, M.D.," Obituary, *JAMA* 54(1) (January 8, 1910): 152.
57. "Sherman Is Dead, Hurt by Speech," *New York Times*, 31 October 1912.
58. *Directory of Deceased American Physicians*, vol. 2 (Chicago: American Medical Association, 1993), 1209.
59. *Ibid.*; Hatfield, "James Schoolcraft Sherman," 323–334.
60. Hatfield, "Daniel D. Tompkins," 71–80; Ray W. Irwin, *Daniel D. Tompkins: Governor of New York and Vice President of the United States* (New York: The New York Historical Society, 1968), 223.
61. Hatfield.
62. Irwin, 234.
63. Irwin, 252.
64. Hatfield.
65. Hatfield; Irwin, 264, 280, 283.
66. Dr. Dan Ruge, interview with Bradley H. Patterson, Jr., October 11, 1986. Ruge increased the scope of the White House physician's responsibilities by an arrangement to serve the medical needs of the vice president. Bush took up perhaps forty percent of the medical staff's time.
67. T. Burton Smith, "The Presidential Physicians and the Reagan Presidency," in *Papers on Presidential Disability and the Twenty fifth-Amendment*, vol. 2, ed. Kenneth W. Thompson (Lanham, MD: University Press of America, 1991), 68.
68. *Ibid.*, 81.
69. Dr. Connie Mariano, interview with the author, 18 July 2003.

70. Dr. Robert Darling, telephone interview with the author, 27 January 2006.
71. Sean Conley, personal conversation with the author, 9 August 2023.
72. John Files, "Cheney Has Annual Physical," *New York Times*, 9 July 2005.
73. Susan Page, "Gore's Condition 'Outstanding Overall,' Doctor Says," *USA Today*, 16 December 1999; "Doctors Say Gore's Health Is Good, Despite Cholesterol," *Saint Louis Post-Dispatch*, 16 December 1999; Timothy J. Burger, "Gore's Health Is Called Superb," *Daily News (New York)*, 16 December 1999.
74. Rick Weiss, "Tipper Gore Has Lump Removed; Vice President's Wife Goes Home as Nodule Is Tested," *Washington Post*, 30 December 1999.
75. Dick Cheney and Jonathan Reiner, *Heart: An American Medical Odyssey* (New York: Scribner, 2013), 85.
76. Tumulty, *The Triumph of Nancy Reagan*, 274.
77. Robert Darling, M.D., personal correspondence with the author, 9 February 2006.
78. John D. McKinnon and Greg Hitt, "Fallout from Cheney Incident Besets White House," *Wall Street Journal*, 15 February 2006; Anne E. Kornblut, "Cheney Shoots Fellow Hunter in Mishap on a Texas Ranch," *New York Times*, 13 February 2006.
79. Connie Mariano, M.D., personal correspondence with the author, 15 February 2006.
80. Cheney and Reiner, *Heart*, 157.
81. Lawrence K. Altman, "Doctors Say Republican Candidates Are in Good Health," *New York Times*, 2 November 2000; Avery Comarow, "Cheney's Health: Does he have the heart?" *U.S. News & World Report*, 8 August 2000; Ron Fournier, "Doctor: Cheney OK After Heart Attack," Associated Press, 22 November 2000; Eric Schmitt, "Cheney Complains of Pains in Chest; Artery is Cleared," *New York Times*, 6 March 2001; Statement from Mary Matalin (Counselor to the Vice President), 29 June 2001; David E. Sanger and Lawrence K. Altman, "Doctors Implant Heart Regulator in Cheney's Chest," *New York Times*, 1 July 2001.
82. "Jonathan Reiner Biography," Medical Association of George Washington University.
83. Sam Levenback, "Cheneys donate 2.7 mil to new GW heart center," *GWU Daily Colonial*, 7 March Note 2006:
84. Cheney and Reiner, *Heart*.
85. *Ibid.*: 180–185
86. *Ibid.*: 244–252.
87. *Ibid.*: 315–318.
88. Statement from Denton A. Cooley, M.D., surgeon-in-chief, Texas Heart Institute, regarding Richard Cheney," 24 July 2000.
89. Lawrence Altman, *New York Times*, 24 July 2000; Lawrence Altman, "Doctors Say Republican Candidates Are in Good Health,"
90. *New York Times*, 2 November 2000.
91. Burton J. Lee III, "The Role of the Presidential Physician," in *Papers on Presidential Disability and the Twenty-fifth Amendment*, vol. 3, ed. Kenneth W. Thompson (Lanham, MD: University Press of America, 1996), 35.
92. Sheryl Gay Solberg, "Cheney Drops Doctor with Drug Addiction; Hospital Deemed Physician Unable to Care for Patients, Put Him on Leave," *New York Times*, 5 July 2004.
93. Rick Weiss, "Internist's Relapse into Drug Use Undetected," *Washington Post*, 8 July 2004.
94. *Ibid.*
95. Tony Leys, "Ex-Iowa health director admits pain killer addiction," *Des Moines Register*, 13 February 2006. The article discussed the addiction to narcotic pain medicines by the former director of the Iowa Department of Public Health and chief of staff to Governor Tom Vilsack.
96. Patrick G. O'Connor and Anderson Spickard, Jr., "Physician Impairment by Substance Abuse; http://www.mc.vanderbilt.edu/root/vumc.php?site=cph&doc=1088 (accessed February 13, 2006).
97. Eugene V. Boisaubin and Ruth E. Levine, "Identifying and Assisting the Impaired Physician," *The American Journal of the Medical Sciences* 322(1) (July 2001): 31–36.
98. Jennifer Pena, personal interview with author, 27 February 2022.
99. Kaitlin Collins and Manu Raju, "A doctor resigns after reports of concerns about Jackson's conduct," CNN Politics, 4 May 2018.
100. Jennifer Pena, personal correspondence with the author, 13 December 2023.
101. Vaughn Hillyard and Dartumorro Calrk, "Mike Pence's White House doctor quits amid fallout over Dr. Ronny Jackson," NBC News, 4 May 2018.
102. Jennifer Pena, personal correspondence, 12 December 2023.

Chapter 16

1. Burton J. Lee III, "The Stain of Torture," *Washington Post*, 1 July 2005.
2. Burton Lee, phone interview with the author, 16 May 2006.
3. Bill McAllister, "Looking Out for Number 1: The Precarious Role of the President's Physician," *Washington Post*, 9 February 1988; T. Burton Smith, *White House Doctor* (Lanham, MD: Madison Books, 1992), 4.
4. See Chapter 8.
5. Andrew Ferguson: "Bush's Exercise Guru," *The Weekly Standard* (May 7, 2001): 12–14.
6. Ferguson; "Kenneth Cooper: Dr. Aerobics," *The Baptist Standard*, 8 April 2002.
7. "Bush in 'Outstanding' Health, Doctors Say," Reuters, 4 August 2001; Jennifer Loven, "Bush Given Clean Bill of Health," Associated Press, 6 August 2002; "Bush Said 'Fit for Duty' after Physical," Associated Press, 11 December 2004; Jim VandeHei, "Doctors Pronounce Bush Fit, a Bit Heavier," *Washington Post*, 12 December 2005.
8. Robert H. Ferrell, *The Strange Deaths of*

President Harding (Columbia, MO: University of Missouri Press, 1996), 48.

9. Carl Sferrazza Anthony, *Florence Harding* (New York: William Morrow, 1988), 515–516.

10. Anthony; Stuart J. Koblentz, *Images of Marion* (Charleston, SC: Arcadia, 2004), 59–72.

11. Anthony, 65, 102–103.

12. *Ibid.*, 102–103, 490.

13. *Ibid.*, 517–521, 525.

14. *Ibid.*, 494, 517–525.

15. Stuart Koblentz, telephone interview with the author, 7 June 2006.

16. "Reagan Physician Begins Job," *New York Times*, 4 January 1985; "Appointments & Nominations, January 4, 1985," http://www.reagan.utexas.edu/archives/speeches/1985/10485a.htm (accessed May 9, 2006).

17. "Daniel Ruge, Former White House Physician," *Rocky Mountain News*, 7 September 2005.

18. Mark Zustovich (media relations associate, Recording for the Blind and Dyslexic), personal

19. *History News Network*, "Daniel Ruge Dies, Cared for Reagan after Shooting," 12 April 2023.

20. Daniel Ruge participated in the previously cited working group meetings on presidential disability held at the Carter Center, Atlanta, June 26–28, 1995, and at Wake Forest University, November 10–12, 1985. He was also interviewed by Dr. Kenneth Crispell for the Miller Center's *Papers on Presidential Disability and the Twenty-fifth Amendment*, vol. 4, ed. Kenneth Thompson (Lanham, MD: University Press of America, 1997), 132–134; Lawrence K. Altman, "Daniel Ruge, 88 Dies; Cared for Reagan After Shooting," *New York Times*, 6 September 2005.

21. F. Krisiloff, M.D., telephone interview with the author, 30 May 2006. Dr. Krisiloff, a urologist, knew Burton Smith for many years as a urology colleague on the St. John's staff. Interestingly, Krisiloff was one of four physicians selected by the Reagans to manage their medical care upon their return to Los Angeles in 1989. Since the three other doctors of the selected quartet retired, Mrs. Reagan used the urologist's advice in the selection of replacement physicians.

22. Lawrence K. Altman, "A President Falls into a World Apart," *New York Times*, 5 October 1997.

23. F. Krisiloff, M.D. After the retirement of the other local physicians, Krisiloff became the conduit for recommendations for specialty care outside urology. Nancy Reagan would inevitably turn to trusted medical confidant John Hutton to approve Krisiloff's suggestions.

24. T. Burton Smith, *White House Doctor* (Lanham, MD: Madison Books, 1992), xi.

25. *Ibid.*, 177; Nancy Reagan, *My Turn* (New York: Random House, 1989).

26. *Ibid.*

27. Lonnie R. Burton, "Distinguished Service Award to T. Burton Smith, Jr., M.D."; Janet Taylor (staff member USUHS Board of Regents), personal correspondence with the author, 31 May 2006.

28. T. Burton Smith, "The Presidential Physician and the Reagan Presidency," in *Papers on Presidential Disability and the Twenty-fifth Amendment*, vol. 2, ed. Kenneth Thompson (Lanham, MD: University Press of America, 1991), 65–87.

29. Krisiloff.

30. Burton Lee III, telephone interview with the author, 16 May 2006.

31. *Ibid.*

32. Burton Lee III, telephone interview with the author, 16 May 2006; Burton J. Lee III, "The Stain of Torture," *Washington Post*, 1 July 2005.

33. See Chapter 10 for the narration of Dr. Lee's term as presidential physician.

34. Sam Roberts, "Dr. Burton J. Lee, 86, Reagan AIDS panelist and Bush's White House Physician Dies," *New York Times*, 1 December 2016.

35. Janet Travell, *Office Hours Day and Night* (New York: World Publishing, 1968), 451; Virginia P. Wilson, "Janet G. Travell, M.D.: A Daughter's Recollection," *Texas Heart Institute Journal 2003* 30(1): 8–12.

36. Travell, *Office Hours Day and Night*. Please refer to Chapter 9 for alternative and critical accounts of Travell's presidential care.

37. Virginia P. Wilson, "Janet G. Travell, M.D.: A Daughter's Recollection," *Texas Heart Institute Journal 2003* 30(1): 8–12.

38. Janet G. Travell and David G. Simons, *Myofascial Pain and Dysfunction: The Trigger Point Manual*, vols. 1 and 2 (Media, PA: Williams & Wilkins, 1983).

39. David G. Simons, Janet G. Travell and Lois S. Simons, *Travell and Simons' Myofascial Pain and Dysfunction: The Trigger Point Manual* (New York: Lippincott Williams & Wilkins, 1998).

40. Wilson; David G. Simons, "Cardiology and Myofascial Trigger Points: Janet G. Travell's Contribution," *Texas Heart Institute Journal 2003* 31(1): 3–7.

41. Travell, *Office Hours*, 459.

42. Thomas D. Webber, "Travell's Myofascial Trigger Points and the Osteopathic Lesion," *Journal of the American Osteopathic Association* 77(4) (December 1977): 308–312; J.M. McPartland, "Travell trigger points—molecular and osteopathic perspectives," *Journal of the American Osteopathic Association* 104(6) (June 2004): 244–249.

43. Janet G. Travell, "A Trigger Point for Hiccup," *Journal of the American Osteopathic Association* 77(4) (December 1977): 308–312.

44. David G. Simons, Janet G. Travell, Lois S. Simons, "Protecting the Ozone Layer," *Arch. Phys. Med. Rehabil.* 71 (January 1990), letter to the editor; Janet G. Travell, *Washington Post*, 8 May 1990.

45. Gelman Library, "The President's Physician: The Life and Legacy of Dr. Janet G. Travell," http://www.gwu.edu/gelman/archives/exhibits/travell/credits.html (accessed May 9, 2006).

46. "Janet Travell Obituary," *Boston Herald*, 3 August 1997.

47. James E. Bagg, Jr., "The President's Physician," *Texas Heart Institute Journal 2003* 30(1): 1–2.; Gelman Library.

48. *Texas Heart Journal 2003* 30(1): 1–12; http://

www.search.barnesand noble.com/booksearch/results.aasp?WRD=Trigger+Point&z=y (accessed June 2, 2006).

49. Georgeanna Kavanaugh, personal communication with the author, 24 June 2006.

50. Alice Stock, "Getting to the Point: Myotherapy Targets 'Triggers' on Muscle Tissue to Relieve Pain," *Pittsburgh Post-Gazette*, 7 October 1997; Michele M. Macomber, "Janet Travell, Medical Pathfinder," *Washington Post*, letter to the editor, 12 August 1997.

51. "Walter Tkach, 72: Served as the Doctor to Three Presidents," *New York Times*, 9 November 1989.

52. James S. Nanney (historian, air force surgeon general's office), personal correspondence with the author, 12 June 2006.

53. Nanney, personal correspondence with the author, 13 June 2006.

54. "Dr. George G. Burkley," *The San Francisco Chronicle*, 7 January 1991, and George Burkley, http://www.arlingtoncemetery.net//ggburkle.htm (accessed July 21, 2003) are obituaries that provide modest information on Burkley's death. Reference copy, JFK Collection: HCSA (RG 233); http:www.geocities.com/jfkinf03/testimony/burkaff.htm (accessed August 7, 2003) and Henry Hurt, *Reasonable Doubt: An Investigation into the Assassination of John F. Kennedy* (New York: Holt, Rinehart, and Winston, 1985), 49, both refer to later investigations into Kennedy's assassination.

55. Richard Auld, William Lukash and Gerald Bordon, "Heterotopic Sebaceous Glands in the Esophagus," *Gastrointestinal Endoscopy* 33(4) (August 1987): 332–333.

56. Wolfgang Saxon, "William Lukash, 66, Doctor Who Watched Over Presidents," *New York Times*, 7 February 1998; Louie Estrada, "William Lukash Dies at 66; Chief Presidential Physician," *Washington Post*, 7 February 1998.

57. John Hutton, telephone interview with the author, 2 May 2006.

58. Lawrence K. Altman, "Reagan's ex-doctor: 'He did not know me.'" *New York Times*, 8 June 2004.

59. Salander, Janes, Norman Rich and Eric Rich: "Dr. John E. Hutton, Jr., physician to President Reagan, buried April 1," https://bul;etiin.facs.ord/20i5/06-john-hutton-jr-physician-to-president-reagan, accessed 16 April 2023.

60. Mayo Clinic Program Details, http://www.mayoclinic.org/executive-health/details.html (accessed June 10, 200

61. Center for Executive Medicine, http://www.drcmariano.com/index.html (accessed June 10, 2006).

62. *Ibid.*

63. *Ibid.*

64. Society for Innovative Medical Practice Design, http://www.simpd.org/conference.php (accessed June 10, 2006).

65. Connie Mariano, *The White House Doctor* (New York: St. Martin's Press, 2010).

66. "Richard Tubb. Board Member Lexis/Nexis Special Services: https.//www.linkedin.com/in/Richard-Tubb, accessed 31 March 2023.

67. Dr. Jeff Kuhlman, personal interview with the author, 25 February 2022.

68. *Ibid.*; Ronny Jackson, *Holding the Line*, (New York: Post Hill Press, 2022), 156.

69. Michael Curviello, "Election results: Jackson wins reelection by a landslide," *Amarillo Globe-News*, 9 November 2022.

70. Tyler Olson, "Ex-White House doctor Ronny Jackson demands Biden take cognitive test or drop out of 2024 race," Fox News, 25 April 2023.

71. Jackson, *Holding the Line*, 112–113.

72. Dr. Jennifer Pena, personal communication with the author, 12 December 2023.

73. Cameron Langford, "Report: Former Presidential Doctor Was a 'Toxic Leader' of the White House Medical Staff." Courthouse News Service, 15 January 2023; Ronny Jackson, personal interview with the author, 3 April 2023.

74. Jackson: Holding the Line, 156.

75. Kevin O'Connor, personal interview with tha author, December 28, 2023.

76. Sean Conley, personal interview with the author, August 9, 2023.

77. *Ibid.*

78. Sean Conley, personal interview with the author, 2021.

Chapter 17

1. William A. Degregorio, *The Complete Book of U.S. Presidents*, 4th ed. (New York: Wings Books, 1993). As of this writing (October 2023), Jimmy Carter is 99 years, 1 month; Bill Clinton is 77 years, 2 months; Barack Obama is 62 years, 2 months; and Donald Trump 77 years, 4 months. Ronald Reagan died in 2004 at the age of 93 years, 3 months; Gerald Ford died in 2006 at 93 years, 5 months: and George H.W. Bush passed on November 30, 2018, at the age of 94 years 5 months.

2. Denise Whitfield, M.D., personal conversation with the author, 15 May 2023.

3. Jan Herman (naval historian), correspondence with Andre Sobocinski, 25 January 2006; Connie Mariano and Robert Darling, ex–White House physicians, personal communications with the author, multiple dates, substantiate the absence of women doctors in the WHMU other than Travell and Mariano; "NavHosp Camp Pendleton Cardiologist Chosen for Clinton," *The Navy Public Affairs Library: Naval Service Medical News* (December 2003). Plastic surgeon Diane Colgan, who operated on Ronald Reagan's face, is the only female physician to serve as a medical consultant to a president.

4. "Clinton's nose lesion removed," *Associated Press*, 25 May 1996; *Reuters*, 4 September 1996.

5. *Ibid.*

6. Norman Gevitz, *The DOs: Osteopathic Medicine in America* (Baltimore: Johns Hopkins University Press, 2004), 152.

7. Gevitz, 152–154.

8. *Ibid.*, 176. The most recent school data was obtained from "The History of Osteopathic Medicine Virtual Museum," http://www.history.aoanet.org/Education/college hist.htm (accessed 20 March 2006).

9. Gewitz., 171–173. The 2005 numbers are from "Fact Sheet 2005," American Osteopathic Association.

10. Gewitz, 171–173.

11. *Ibid.*, 180–181.

12. *Ibid.*, 190–191.

13. "Fact Sheet 2005," American Osteopathic Association, August 2005.

14. "Critical Challenges: Revitalizing the Health Professions for the Twenty-first Century," Third Report of the Pew Health Professions Commission, December 1995; Sarah Brotherton, Paul Rockey and Sylvia Etzel, "U.S. Graduate Medical Education, 2004–2005: Trends in Primary Care Specialties," *JAMA* 294(9) (September 7, 2005): 1075–1082, analyzes population trends in hospital residency programs. Its definition of primary care as opposed to subspecialty residency programs includes family medicine, internal medicine, obstetrics/gynecology, pediatrics and combined internal medicine/pediatric programs.

15. "About AMOPS," Association of Military Physicians and Surgeons, http://www.amops.org/, accessed 20 March 2006).

16. Brotherton.

17. AAMC.org. "Active Physicians who are International Medical Graduates (IMGs) by specialty, 2019"

18. See Chapter 7. Both Woodrow Wilson and Franklin Roosevelt suffered significant losses of executive functioning during crucial times of their respective presidencies.

19. See Chapters 7 and 9.

20. See Chapters 4 and 9.

21. Sean Conley, personal interview by author, 8 August 2023; Sean Conley, personal interview by author, 29 August 2023.

22. Joanna Jackson/Sean Conley (Chapters 14, 17).

23. Ronny Jackson/Jennifer Pena (Chapters 15, 16).

Bibliography

Books

Abbott, Richard. *Cobbler in Congress: The Life of Henry Wilson, 1812–1875.* Lexington: University Press of Kentucky, 1972.

Abrahams, Harold. *Extinct Medical Schools of Nineteenth-Century Philadelphia.* Philadelphia: University of Pennsylvania Press, 1966.

Abrams, Herbert. *The President Has Been Shot: Confusion, Disability, and the 25th Amendment in the Aftermath of the Attempted Assassination of Ronald Reagan.* New York: W.W. Norton, 1992.

Aitken, Jonathan. *Nixon: A Life.* London: Weidenfeld and Nicolson, 1993.

Aldrich, C. Knight. "Personal Grieving and Political Defeat." In *Papers on Presidential Disability and the Twenty-fifth Amendment,* edited by Kenneth Thompson. Vol. 3. Lanham, MD: University Press of America, 1996.

Allen, Anne Beiser. *An Independent Woman: The Life of Lou Henry Hoover.* Westport, CT: Greenwood Press, 2000.

Ambrose, Stephen. *Eisenhower: The President.* New York: Simon & Schuster, 1984.

Ammon, Harry. *James Monroe: The Quest for National Identity.* New York: McGraw-Hill, 1971.

Anthony, Carl Sferrazza. *Florence Harding.* New York: William Morrow, 1988.

Ashburn, P.M. *A History of the Medical Department of the United States Army.* Boston: Houghton Mifflin, 1929.

Atkinson, William, ed. *A Biographical Dictionary of Contemporary American Physicians and Surgeons.* Philadelphia: D.G. Brinton, 1880.

Axson, Stockton, and Arthur Link. *Brother Woodrow: A Memoir of Woodrow Wilson.* Princeton, NJ: Princeton University Press, 1993.

Bailey, Tom, *William Rufus King Alabama's US Vice President.* Hartselle, AL: Seacoast Publishing, 2022.

Barkley, Alben. *That Reminds Me.* Garden City, NY: Doubleday, 1954.

Barton, David. *Benjamin Rush: Signer of the Declaration of Independence.* Aledo, TX: Wallbuilder Press, 1999.

Bassett, John, ed. *Correspondence of Andrew Jackson.* 7 vols. Washington: Carnegie Institute of Washington, 1926–1935.

Batchelor, John. *Father's Day.* New York: St. Martin's Paperbacks, 1994.

Bauer, K. Jack. *Zachary Taylor: Soldier, Planter, Statesman of the Old Southwest.* Baton Rouge: Louisiana State University Press, 1985.

Bayh, Birch. "Reflections on the Twenty-fifth Amendment as We Enter a New Century." In *Managing Crisis: Presidential Disability and the 25th Amendment,* edited by Robert Gilbert. New York: Fordham University Press, 2000.

Billias, George Athan. *Elbridge Gerry: Founding Father and Republican Statesman.* New York: McGraw-Hill, 1976.

Bishop, Jim. *FDR's Last Year.* New York: William Morrow, 1974.

Blanton, Wyndham. *Medicine in Virginia in the Eighteenth Century.* Richmond: Garrett & Massie, 1931.

Bonner, Thomas. *American Doctors and German Universities: A Chapter in International Intellectual Relations, 1870–1914.* Lincoln: University of Nebraska Press, 1963.

_____. *Iconoclast: Abraham Flexner and a Life in Learning.* Baltimore: Johns Hopkins University Press, 2002.

_____. *To the Ends of the Earth: Women Search for Education in Medicine.* Cambridge, MA: Harvard University Press, 1992.

Bowley, Arthur. *Wages in the United Kingdom in the Nineteenth Century.* Cambridge: University Press, 1900.

Braisted, William, and William Bell. *The Life Story of Presley Marion Rixey.* Strasburg, VA: Shenandoah Publishing, 1930.

Brant, Irving. *James Madison: Commander in Chief.* New York: G.P. Putnam's Sons, 1960.

Brodsky, Alyn. *Benjamin Rush: Patriot and Physician.* New York: St. Martin's, 2004.

Brody, Harold. "The Physician-Patient Relationship." In *Medical Ethics,* edited by Robert Veatch. 2nd ed. Sudbury, MA: Jones and Bartlett, 1997.

Brooks, S.M. *Our Murdered President: The Medical Story.* New York: Frederick Fell, 1966.

Brown, Harry, and Frederick Williams, eds. *The Diary of James A. Garfield.* Vol. 1, 1848–1871. Lansing: Michigan State University, 1967.

_____ and _____. *The Diary of James A. Garfield.*

Vol. 2, *1872–1874*. Lansing: Michigan State University Press, 1967.

_____ and _____. *The Diary of James A. Garfield.* Vol. 4, *1878–1881*. Lansing: Michigan State University Press, 1981.

Browne, Harvey. *The Medical Department of the United States Army from 1775 to 1787*. Part 3, *From the Revolution of the Corps in 1821 to the Declaration of the War against Mexico*. Washington: Surgeon General's Office, 1873.

Bumgarner, John. *The Health of the Presidents: The 41 United States Presidents through 1993 from a Physician's Point of View*. Jefferson, NC: McFarland, 1994.

Bunker, Henry. "American Psychiatry as a Specialty." In *One Hundred Years of American Psychiatry*, edited by J.K. Hall, Gregory Zilborg and Henry Bunker. New York: Columbia University Press, 1944.

Busey, Samuel. *Personal Reminiscences and Recollections of Forty-six Years Membership in the Medical Society of the District of Columbia*. (Philadelphia: Dornan, printer, 1895.

Bush, Barbara. *Barbara Bush: A Memoir*. New York: Charles Scribner's Sons, 1994.

Carter, Jimmy. "Opening Address, January 26, 1995." In *Presidential Disability, Papers, Discussions and Recommendations on the Twenty-fifth Amendment*, edited by James Toole and Robert Joynt. Rochester, NY: University of Rochester Press, 2001.

Cheney, Dick, and Jonathan Reiner. *Heart*. New York: Scribner's, 2013.

Clark, James C. *The Murder of James A. Garfield: The President's Last Days and the Trial and Execution of His Assassin*. Jefferson, NC: McFarland, 1993.

Clarke, Jeanne Nienaber. *Roosevelt's Warrior: Harold Ickes and the New Deal*. Baltimore: Johns Hopkins Press, 1996.

Clinton, Hillary Rodham. *Living History*. New York: Scribner's, 2003.

Cowan, Frank. *Andrew Johnson, President of the United States: Reminiscences of His Private Life and Character*. Greenesburgh, PA: Oliver Publishing, 1894.

Cresson, W.P. *James Monroe*. Chapel Hill: University of North Carolina Press, 1946.

Crispell, Kenneth, and Carlos Gomez. *Hidden Illness in the White House*. Durham: Duke University Press, 1988.

"Critical Challenges: Revitalizing the Health Professions for the Twenty-first Century." The Pew Health Professions Commission, December, 1995.

Curtis, George. *Life of James Buchanan, Fifteenth President of the United States*. Freeport, NY: Books for Libraries Press, 1883.

Dallek, Robert. *An Unfinished Life: John F. Kennedy*. Boston: Little, Brown, 2003.

Davidson, Jonathan, Kathryn M. Connor and Marvin Swartz. "Mental Illness in U.S. Presidents between 1776 and 1974: A Review of Biographical Sources." *Journal of Nervous and Mental Disease* 194(1) (January 2006): 47–51.

Davison, Kenneth. *The Presidency of Rutherford B. Hayes*. Westport, CT: Greenwood Press, 1972.

Decatur, Stephen, Jr. *Private Affairs of George Washington, from the Records and Accounts of Tobias Lear, Esquire, His Secretary*. Boston: Houghton Mifflin, 1933.

DeGregorio, William. *The Complete Book of U.S. Presidents*. 3rd ed. New York: Barricade Books, 1991.

_____. *The Complete Book of U.S. Presidents*. 4th ed. New York: Wings Books, 1993.

Derbyshire, Robert. *Medical Licensure and Discipline in the United States*. Westport, CT: Greenwood Press, 1978.

Directory of Deceased American Physicians. Vol. 2. Chicago: American Medical Association, 1993.

Drake, Daniel. *Practical Essays on Medical Education and the Medical Profession in the United States, 1832*. Baltimore: Johns Hopkins Press, 1953.

Earle, A. Scott, ed. *Surgery in America from the Colonial Era to the Twentieth Century*. 2nd ed. New York: Praeger Scientific, 1965.

Erlichman, John. *Witness to Power: The Nixon Years*. New York: Simon & Schuster, 1982.

"Fact Sheet 2005." American Osteopathic Association, August 2005.

Feerick, John. *The Twenty Fifth Amendment. Its Complete History and Application*. Third edition. New York. MIT Books, 2014.

Feis, R.S-B. *Mollie Garfield in the White House*. Chicago: Rand McNally, 1963.

Ferling, John. *John Adams: A Life*. New York: Henry Holt, 1992.

Ferrell, Robert H. *The Dying President: Franklin Roosevelt, 1944–1945*. Columbia: University of Missouri Press, 1998.

_____. *Ill-Advised: Presidential Health and the Public Trust*. Columbia: University of Missouri Press, 1992.

_____. *The Presidency of Calvin Coolidge*. Lawrence: University of Kansas Press, 1998.

_____. *The Strange Deaths of President Harding*. Columbia: University of Missouri Press, 1996.

_____, ed. *Off the Record: The Private Papers of Harry S. Truman*. New York: Harper & Row, 1980.

Fitzpatrick, John, ed. *The Writings of George Washington from the Original Manuscript Sources, 1745–1786*. Vol. 30, *The George Washington Papers of the Library of Congress, 1741–1799*.

Flexner, Abraham. *Medical Education in the United States and Canada: A Report to the Carnegie Foundation for the Advancement of Teaching, 1910*. Bulletin 4. Boston: D.B. Updike, Merrymount Press, 1960.

Flexner, James Thomas. *George Washington: Anguish and Farewell, 1793–1799*. Boston: Little, Brown, 1972.

Flynn, Vince. *Transfer of Power*. New York: Simon & Schuster, 2000.

Foltz, Charles. *Surgeon of the Seas: The Adventurous Life of Surgeon General Jonathan M. Foltz in the Days of Wooden Ships*. Indianapolis: Bobbs-Merrill, 1931.
Forsyth, Frederick. *The Negotiator*. New York: Bantam Books, 1990.
Freeman, Douglas. *Washington*. New York: Simon & Schuster, 1992.
French, John. *Celebration of the Sesquicentennial of the Medical and Chirurgical Faculty of Maryland, 1799–1949*. Baltimore: Waverly Press, 1949.
Freud, Sigmund, and William Bullitt. *Thomas Woodrow Wilson: A Psychological Study*. Boston: Houghton Mifflin, 1966 reissue.
Friedel, Frank. *Franklin Roosevelt: A Rendezvous with Destiny*. Boston: Little, Brown, 1990.
Garrison, Fielding. *An Introduction to the History of Medicine*. 4th ed. Philadelphia: W.B. Saunders, 1963.
Gevitz, Norman. *The DOs: Osteopathic Medicine in America*. 2nd ed. Baltimore: Johns Hopkins University Press, 2004.
Gilbert, Robert. "The Genius of the Twenty-fifth Amendment: Guarding Against Presidential Disability but Safeguarding the Presidency." In *Managing Crisis: Presidential Disability and the 25th Amendment*, edited by Robert Gilbert. New York: Fordham University Press, 2000.
_____. *Mortal Presidency: Illness and Anguish in the White House*. New York: Basic Books, 1992.
_____. *The Tormented President: Calvin Coolidge, Death, and Clinical Depression*. Westport, CT: Praeger, 2003.
_____, ed. *Managing Crisis: Presidential Disability and the 25th Amendment*. New York: Fordham University Press, 2000.
Gillett, Mary. *The Army Medical Department, 1865–1917*. Washington: U.S. Government Printing Office, 1994.
Goodwin, Doris Kearns. *No Ordinary Time*. New York: Simon & Schuster, 1994.
Graham, Wallace H. *Wallace H. Graham: The Man Who Became President Truman's Physician*. Columbia, MO: Compass Flower Press, 2019.
Grayson, Cary. *Woodrow Wilson: An Intimate Portrait*. Washington, D.C.: Potomac Books, 1960.
Haldeman, H.R. *The Haldeman Diaries: Inside the Nixon White House*. New York: G.P. Putnam's Sons, 1994.
Hamilton, Holman. *Zachary Taylor: Soldier in the White House*. Indianapolis: Bobbs-Merrill, 1951.
Hamilton, Stanislaus, ed. *The Writings of James Monroe*. New York: G.P. Putnam's Sons, 1901.
Harding, Warren G., II, and Mark Stewart. *Mere Mortals: The Lives and Health Histories of American Presidents*. Worthington, OH: Renaissance, 1992.
Harrison, John. *Oure Tounis College: Sketches of the History of the Old College of Edinburgh*. Edinburgh: William Blackwood and Sons, 1884.
Harvey, A. McGehee, et al. *A Model of Its Kind*. Vol. 1, *A Centennial History of Medicine at Johns Hopkins*. Baltimore: Johns Hopkins University Press, 1989.
Hatfield, Mark. *Vice Presidents of the United States, 1789–1993*. Washington: U.S. Government Printing Office, 1997.
Heitman, Francis. *Historical Register and Dictionary of the United States Army*. Washington: U.S. Government Printing Office, 1903.
Heller, Milton F., Jr. *The Presidents' Doctor: An Insider's View of Three First Families*. New York: Vantage Press, 2000.
Hersh, Seymour. *The Dark Side of Camelot*. Boston: Little, Brown, 1997.
Heymann, C. David. *A Woman Named Jackie*. London: Heinemann, 1989.
Holcombe, John, and Hubert Skinner. *Life and Public Services of Thomas A. Hendricks*. Indianapolis: Carlon and Hollenbeck, 1886.
Holmes, John. *Thomas Jefferson Treats Himself*. Fort Valley, VA: Loft Press, 1997.
Hoover, Herbert. *The Ordeal of Woodrow Wilson*. New York: McGraw-Hill, 1958.
Horn, D.H. *A Short History of the University of Edinburgh, 1556–1889*. Edinburgh: University of Edinburgh Press, 1967.
Hunt, Roger, and Jack Brown. *Brevet Brigadier Generals in Blue*. Gaithersburg, MD: Lode Soldier Books, 1990.
Hurst, J. Willis, and James Cain. *LBJ: To Know Him Better*. Austin, TX: LBJ Foundation, 1995.
Hurt, Henry. *Reasonable Doubt: An Investigation into the Assassination of John F. Kennedy*. New York: Holt, Rinehart, and Winston, 1985.
Irwin, Ray. *Daniel D. Tompkins: Governor of New York and Vice President of the United States*. New York: New York Historical Society, 1968.
Jackson, Donald, and Dorothy Twohig, eds. *The Diaries of George Washington*. Vol. 6. Charlottesville: University Press of Virginia, 1979.
Jackson, Ronny, *Holding the Line, A Lifetime of Defending Democracy and American Values*. New York: Post Hill Press, 2022.
Kalt, Brian C., *Unable*. New York: Oxford University Press, 2014.
Kaminski, John. *George Clinton: Yeoman Politician of the New Republic*. Madison, WI: Madison House, 1993.
Katz, Catherine Grace. *The Daughters of Yalta*. New York: Houghton Mifflin Harcourt, 2020.
Kaufman, Martin. *Homeopathy in America: The Rise and Fall of a Medical Heresy*. Baltimore: Johns Hopkins Press, 1971.
Kaufman, Martin, Stuart Galishoff and Todd Savitt, eds. *Dictionary of American Medical Biography*. Vol. 1. Westport, CT: Greenwood Press.
Kelly, Howard, and Walter Burrage. *American Medical Biographies*. Baltimore: Norman Remington, 1920.
_____ and _____. *Dictionary of American Medical Biography*. New York: D. Appleton, 1928.
Ketcham, Ralph. *James Madison: A Biography*. Charlottesville: University Press of Virginia, 1990.

King, W.H., ed. *History of Homeopathy and Its Institutions in America*. Vol. 3. New York: Lewis Publishing, 1905.
Kirschmann, Anne Taylor. *A Vital Force: Women in Homeopathy*. New Brunswick, NJ: Rutgers University Press, 2004.
Knorr, Norman, and Daniel Harrington. "Psychological Considerations." In *Papers on Presidential Disability and the Twenty-fifth Amendment*, edited by Kenneth Thompson. Lanham, MD: University Press of America, 1988.
Koblentz, Stuart. *Images of Marion*. Charleston, SC: Arcadia Publishing, 2004.
Langley, Harold. *A History of Medicine in the Early U.S. Navy*. Baltimore: Johns Hopkins University Press, 1995.
Langstaff, J. Brett. *Dr. Bard of Hyde Park*. New York: E.P. Dutton, 1942.
Lasby, Clarence. *Eisenhower's Heart Attack: How Ike Beat Heart Disease and Held on to the Presidency*. Lawrence: University Press of Kansas, 1997.
Leamer, Lawrence. *The Kennedy Men, 1901–1963: The Laws of the Father*. New York: William Morrow, 2001.
Lee, Bandy, editor. *The Dangerous Case of Donald Trump*. New York: St. Martin's Press, 2017.
Lee, Burton J., III. "The Role of the Presidential Physician." In *Papers on Presidential Disability and the Twenty-fifth Amendment*, edited by Kenneth Thompson. Vol. 3. Lanham, MD: University Press of America, 1996.
Leech, M., and H.J. Brown. *The Garfield Orbit*. New York: Harper & Row, 1978.
Leech, Margaret. *In the Days of McKinley*. New York: Harper and Brothers, 1959.
Levin, Jerome. *The Clinton Syndrome: The President and the Self-Destructive Nature of Sexual Addiction*. Rocklin, CA: Forum, 1998.
Link, Arthur, and James Carroll. *The Real Woodrow Wilson: An Interview with Arthur S. Link, the Editor of the Wilson Papers*. Bennington, VT: Images from the Past, 2001.
Lungren, John C., and John C. Lungren, Jr. *Healing Richard Nixon: A Doctor's Memoir*. Lexington: University Press of Kentucky, 2003.
Lynaugh, John. "From Respectable Domesticity to Medical Efficiency: The Changing Kansas City Hospital, 1875–1920." In *The American General Hospital: Communities and Social Contexts*, edited by Elizabeth Long and John Golden. Ithaca, NY: Cornell University Press, 1989.
MacMahon, Edward, and Leonard Curry. *Medical Cover-Ups in the White House*. Washington, D.C.: Farragut, 1987.
Magie, David. *Life of Garret Augustus Hobart*. New York: G.P. Putnam's Sons, 1910.
Mariano, E. Connie. "The Evolution of the White House Medical Unit." In *Managing Crisis: Presidential Disability and the 25th Amendment*, edited by Robert Gilbert. New York: Fordham University Press, 2000.
_____. *Press Briefing on the Occasion of the President's Annual Checkup* (January 12, 2001).
_____. *The White House Doctor*. New York: St. Mark's Press, 2010.
Marx, Rudolph. *The Health of the Presidents*. New York: G.P. Putnam's Sons, 1960.
McAllister, Bill. "The Precarious Role of the Presidential Physician." In *Papers on Presidential Disability and the Twenty-fifth Amendment*, edited by Kenneth Thompson. Vol. 4. Lanham, MD: University Press of America, 1997.
McCullough, *John Adams*. New York: Simon & Schuster, 2001.
_____. David. *Truman*. New York: Simon & Schuster, 1992.
McIntire, Ross. *White House Physician*. New York: G.P. Putnam's Sons, 1946.
McKay, Ernest. *Henry Wilson: Practical Radical: A Portrait of a Politician*. Port Washington, NY: Kennikat Press, 1971.
Medical Society of the District of Columbia. *History of the Medical Society of the District of Columbia, 1817–1890*. Washington, D.C.: Medical Society of the District of Columbia, 1909.
Mooney, James. *Dictionary of American Fighting Ships*. Vol. 6. Washington: Navy Dept., Office of the Chief of Naval Operations, 1976.
More, Ellen. *Restoring the Balance: Women Physicians and the Profession of Medicine*. Cambridge, MA: Harvard University Press, 1999.
Morrell, J.B. "Medicine and Science in the Eighteenth Century." In *Four Centuries of Edinburgh University Life, 1583–1983*, edited by Gordon Donaldson. Edinburgh: Edinburgh University Press, 1983, 38–39, 47.
Morris, Edmund. *Theodore Rex*. New York: Random House, 2001.
Nagel, Paul. *Descent from Glory: Four Generations of the John Adams Family*. New York: Oxford University Press, 1983.
_____. *John Quincy Adams: A Public Life, a Private Life*. Cambridge, MA: Harvard University Press, 1997.
Nason, Elias, and Thomas Russell. *The Life and Public Services of Henry Wilson, Late Vice President of the United States*. Boston: B.B. Russell, 1876.
Nevins, Allan. *Grover Cleveland: A Study in Courage*. New York: Dodd, Mead, 1948.
_____, ed. *The Diary of John Quincy Adams, 1794–1845*. New York: Charles Scribner's Sons, 1951.
Nichols, Roy Franklin. *Franklin Pierce: Young Hickory of the Granite Hills*. Philadelphia: Pennsylvania University Press, 1931.
Ogelsby, Paul. *"Take Heart."* Boston: Harvard University Press, 1986.
Palmer, Michael, Robert Weiss and Lilli Sentz. "Dr. Roswell Park and the McKinley Assassination." In *Medical History in Buffalo, 1846–1996*, edited by Lilli Sentz. Buffalo, 1996.
Park, Bert. *Aging, Ailing, Addicted: Studies of Compromised Leadership*. Lexington: University Press of Kentucky, 1994.

_____. *The Impact of Illness on World Leaders*. Philadelphia: University of Pennsylvania Press, 1986.

Parmet, Herbert. *JFK: The Presidency of John F. Kennedy*. New York: Dial Press, 1983.

Parton, James. *The Life of Andrew Jackson in Three Volumes*. New York: Mason Brothers, 1860.

Patterson, Bradley H. *The White House Staff: Inside the West Wing and Beyond*. Washington: Brookings Institution Press, 2000.

Paul, Oglesby. *Take Heart: The Life and Prescription for Living of Dr. Paul Dudley White*. Boston: Harvard University Press, 1986.

Peskin, Allan. *Garfield*. Kent, OH: Kent State University Press, 1978.

Pilcher, James. *The Surgeon Generals of the Army of the United States*. Carlisle, PA: Association of Military Surgeons, 1905.

Post, Jerrold. "Broken Minds, Broken Hearts and the Twenty-fifth Amendment: Psychiatric Disorders and Presidential Disability." In *Managing Crisis: Presidential Disability and the 25th Amendment*, edited by Robert Gilbert. New York: Fordham University Press, 2000.

_____, and Robert Robins. *When Illness Strikes the Leader: The Dilemma of the Captive King*. New Haven, CT: Yale University Press, 1993.

Puzo, Mario, *The Fourth K*. New York: Ballantine Books, 1990.

Quaife, Mile Milton, ed. *The Diary of James K. Polk during His Presidency, 1845 to 1849*. Chicago: A.C. McClurg, 1910.

Reagan, Nancy. *My Turn: The Memoirs of Nancy Reagan*. New York: Random House, 1989.

Reeves, Richard. *Alone in the White House*. New York: Simon & Schuster, 2001.

_____. *President Kennedy: A Profile of Power*. New York: Simon & Schuster, 1993.

Reeves, Thomas. *A Question of Character: A Life of John F. Kennedy*. New York: Free Press, 1991.

Reich, W.T., ed. *Encyclopedia of Bioethics*. New York: Macmillan, 1995.

Remini, Robert. *Andrew Jackson*. Vol. 1, *The Course of American Empire*. Baltimore: Johns Hopkins University Press, 1977.

_____. *Andrew Jackson*. Vol. 2, *The Course of American Freedom*. Baltimore: Johns Hopkins University Press, 1981.

Rosenberg, Charles. *The Care of Strangers: The Rise of America's Hospital System*. New York: Basic Books, 1987.

Ross, Ishbel. *Grace Coolidge and Her Era*. New York: Dodd, Mead, 1962.

Rothstein, William. *American Physicians in the 19th Century: From Sects to Science*. Baltimore: Johns Hopkins University Press, 1985.

Russell, Francis. *The Shadow of Blooming Grove: Warren G. Harding and His Times*. New York: McGraw-Hill, 1968.

Safire, William. *Full Disclosure*. New York: Ballantine Books, 1977.

Schwartz, Susan. *Into the Unknown: The Remarkable Life of Hans Kraus*. New York: iUniverse, 2005.

Serling, Robert, *"The President's Plane Is Missing."* London: Cassell and Company, 1968.

Shenk, Joshua Wolf. *Lincoln's Melancholy: How Depression Challenged a President and Fueled His Greatness*. Boston: Houghton Mifflin, 2005.

Shyrock, Richard. *Medical Licensing in America, 1650–1965*. Baltimore: Johns Hopkins Press, 1967.

Sievers, Harry. *Benjamin Harrison: Hoosier President*. Newton, CT: American Political Biography Press, 1996.

Simons, David, Lois Simons and Janet Travell. *Travell and Simons Myofascial Pain and Dysfunction*. 2 vols. New York: Lippincott Williams & Wilkins, 1999.

Smith, T. Burton. "The Presidential Physician and the Reagan Presidency." In *Papers on Presidential Disability and the Twenty-fifth Amendment*, edited by Kenneth Thompson. Vol. 2. Lanham, MD: University Press of America, 1991.

_____. *White House Doctor*. Lanham, MD: Madison Books, 1992.

Socolofsky, Homer, and Allan B. Spetter. *The Presidency of Benjamin Harrison*. Lawrence: University of Kansas Press, 1987.

Spaulding, E. Wilder. *His Excellency George Clinton: Critic of the Constitution*. New York: Macmillan, 1938.

Speakes, Larry, and Robert Pack. *Speaking Out: The Reagan Presidency from Inside the White House*. New York: Charles Scribner's Sons, 1988.

Starling, Edmund. *Starling of the White House*. Chicago: People's Book Club, 1946.

Starr, Paul. *The Social Transformation of American Medicine*. New York: Basic Books, 1982.

Stevens, Rosemary. *American Medicine and the Public Interest: A History of Specialization*. Updated ed. Berkeley: University of California Press, 1998.

_____. *In Sickness and in Wealth: American Hospitals in the Twentieth Century*. Baltimore: Johns Hopkins University Press, 1999.

Stewart, William. "McIntire, Ross." *Dictionary of American Biography*. Supplement 6, *1956–1960* (1980): 413–414.

Styron, Arthur. *The Last of the Cocked Hats: James Monroe and the Virginia Dynasty*. Norman: University of Oklahoma Press, 1945.

Summers, Anthony. *The Arrogance of Power: The Secret World of Richard Nixon*. New York: Viking, 2000.

Thomas, Lately. *The Three Lives of the Seventeenth President of the United States of America*. New York: Morrow, 1968.

Thompson, John, and Grace Goldin. *The Hospital: A Social and Architectural History*. New Haven, CT: Yale University Press, 1974.

Thompson, Kenneth W., ed. *Papers on Presidential Disability and the Twenty-fifth Amendment by Six Medical, Legal and Political Authorities*. Lanham, MD: University Press of America, 1988.

_____, ed. *Papers on Presidential Disability and*

the *Twenty-fifth Amendment by Six Medical, Legal and Political Authorities*. Vol. 2. Lanham, MD: University Press of America, 1991.

_____, ed. *Papers on Presidential Disability and the Twenty-fifth Amendment by Medical, Historical and Political Authorities*. Vol. 3. Lanham. MD: University Press of America, 1996.

_____. ed. *Papers on Presidential Disability and the Twenty-fifth Amendment by Dr. Kenneth Crispell and other Medical, Legal and Political Authorities*. Vol. 4. Lanham, MD: University Press of America, 1997.

Thompson, Loyd, and Winfield Downs, eds. *Who's Who in American Medicine*. New York: Who's Who Publications, 1925.

Thor, Brad. *The Lions of Lucerne*. New York: Pocket Star Books, 2002.

Toole, James, and Robert Joynt, eds. *Presidential Disability: Papers, Discussions and Recommendations on the Twenty-fifth Amendment and Issues of Inability and Disability in Presidents of the United States*. Rochester, NY: Rochester University Press, 2001.

Trani, Eugene, and David Wilson. *The Presidency of Warren G. Harding*. Lawrence: University of Kansas Press, 1977.

Travell, Janet. *Office Hours Day and Night: The Autobiography of Janet Travell, M.D.* New York: World Publishing, 1968.

_____, and David G. Simons. *Myofascial Pain and Dysfunction: The Trigger Point Manual*. 2 vols. New York: Lippincott, 1983.

Trefousse, Hans. *Andrew Johnson: A Biography*. New York: W.W. Norton, 1989.

Truman, Margaret. *Harry S. Truman*. New York: William Morrow, 1973.

Tumulty, Karen, *The Triumph of Nancy Reagan*. New York: Simon & Schuster, 2021.

Unger, Irwin, and Debi Unger. *LBJ: A Life*. New York: John Wiley & Sons, 1999.

Volkan, Vamik. "The Three Faces of Richard Nixon." In *Papers on Presidential Disability and the Twenty-fifth Amendment*, edited by Kenneth Thompson. Vol. 3. Lanham, MD: University Press of America, 1996.

_____, Norman Itzkowitz and Alfred Dod. *Richard Nixon: A Psychobiography*. New York: Columbia University Press, 1997.

Walsh, James. *History of Medicine in New York: Three Centuries of Medical Progress*. Vol. 3. (New York: National Americana Society, 1919.

Walsh, Mary. *"Doctors Wanted, No Women Need Apply": Sexual Barriers in the Medical Profession, 1835–1975*. New Haven, CT: Yale University Press, 1977.

Weinstein, Edwin. *Woodrow Wilson: A Medical and Psychological Biography*. Princeton: Princeton University Press, 1981.

Welch, Richard D., Jr. *The Presidencies of Grover Cleveland*. Lawrence: University Press of Kansas, 1988.

White, Paul Dudley. *My Life and Medicine*. Boston: Gambit, 1971.

Who Was Who in America. Vol. 1, *1897–1942*. Chicago: Marquis, 1966.

Whorton, James. *Nature Cures: The History of Alternative Medicine in America*. New York: Oxford University Press, 2002.

Williams, T. Harry, ed. *Hayes: The Diary of a President, 1875–1881*. New York: David McKay, 1964.

Wilson, Edith Bolling Galt. *My Memoir*. Indianapolis: Bobbs-Merrill, 1939.

Witcover, Jules. *Crapshoot: Rolling the Dice on the Vice Presidency*. New York: Crown, 1992.

Woodward, Bob, and Carl Bernstein. *The Final Days*. New York: Simon & Schuster, 1976.

Periodical Articles

Adler, Selig. "The Operation on President McKinley." *Scientific American* 208(3) (March 1963): 118–130.

American Association of Medical Colleges. "Active Physicians who are International Medical Graduates (IMGs) by specialty 2019.

American Institute of Homeopathy. "Deaths: Susan A. Edson, M.D." In *Transactions of the 54th Session of the American Institute of Homeopathy* (1899).

American Medical Association. "James C. Hall." *Transactions of the American Medical Association* 32 (1881): 506–513.

American Medical Association. "Obituary of Edward Hammond Clarke." *Transactions of the American Medical Association* 29 (1878): 624–627.

American Osteopathic Association. Fact Sheet 2005 (August 2005).

Auld, Richard, William Lukash and Gerald Bordon. "Heterotopic Sebaceous Glands in the Esophagus." *Gastrointestinal Endoscopy* 33(4) (August 1987): 332–333.

Baehrs, Oliver. "The Medical History of President Ronald Reagan." *Journal of the American College of Surgeons* 178 (January 1994): 86–96.

Bagg, James, Jr. "The President's Physician." *Texas Heart Institute Journal 2003* 30(1): 1–2.

Barzansky, Barbara, and Sylvia Etzel. "Educational Programs in US Medical Schools, 2003- 2004." *Journal of the American Medical Association* 293(9) (September 1, 2004): 105–1031.

Bell, Whitfield J., Jr. "Some American Students of 'That Shining Light of Physic,' Dr. William Cullen of Edinburgh, 1755–1766." *Proceedings of the American Philosophical Society* 94(3) (1950): 275–278.

Bender, Eve. "With Politics and Mental Illness, The More Things Change…" *Psychiatric News* 37(1) (November 1, 2002): 10.

"A Biographical Sketch of the Late Henry Huntt, M.D. *The Medical Examiner* 1 (1838): 363–365.

Blinderman, Andrew. "George Washington's Health in Peace and War." *New York State Journal of Medicine* (January 1975): 122–132.

Bliss, D.W. "Report of the Case of President

Garfield." *The Medical Record* 20(15) (October 8, 1881): 393–402.

Boisaubin, Eugene, and Ruth E. Levine. "Identifying and Assisting the Impaired Physician." *The American Journal of the Medical Sciences* 322(1) (July 2001): 31–36.

Breo, Dennis. "Tough Talk from the President's Physician." *Journal of the American Medical Association* 262(9) (November 17, 1989): 2742–2745.

Brotherton, Sarah, Paul Rockey and Sylvia Etzel. "US Graduate Medical Education, 2004- 2005: Trends in Primary Care Specialties." *Journal of the American Medical Association* 294(9) (September 7, 2005): 1075–1082.

Bruenn, Howard. "Clinical Notes on the Illness and Death of President Franklin D. Roosevelt." *Annals of Internal Medicine* 72 (1970): 579–591.

Bryant, Joseph. "A History of Two Hundred and Fifty Cases of Excision of the Superior Maxilla." *Transactions of the Medical Society of the State of New York* (1890): 63–76.

"Camp Pendleton Cardiologist Chosen for Clinton," *The Navy Public Affairs Library: Naval Service Medical News* (December 2003).

Coblens, K., et al. "American College of Physicians Ethics Manual." 3rd ed. *Annals of Internal Medicine* 117 (1992): 947–960.

Comarow, Avery. "Cheney's Health: Does he have the heart?" *U.S. News & World Report* (August 8, 2000).

Coucher, Shane. "Trump's Mental Impairment Means He Cannot Think Strategically or Abstract Terms." *Newsweek* (October 24, 2019).

Crellin, J.K. "Robert King Stone, M.D., Physician to Abraham Lincoln." *Illinois Medical Journal* (February 1979): 97–99.

"Critical Challenges: Revitalizing the Health Professions for the Twenty-first Century," *Third Report of the Pew Health Professions Commission.* (December 1995).

Davidson, Jonathan R.T., Kathryn M. Connor and Marvin Swartz, "Mental Illness in U.S. Presidents between 1776 and 1974: A Review of Biographical Sources," *Journal of Nervous & Mental Disease* 194(1) (January 2006): 47–51.

"Death of President McKinley." *Journal of the American Medical Association* 37 (September 21, 1901): 779–787.

Deppisch, Ludwig M. "Andrew Jackson and American Medical Practice: Old Hickory and His Physicians." *Tennessee Historical Quarterly* 62(9) (Summer 2003): 130–151.

_____. "Homeopathic Medicine and Presidential Health: Homeopathic Influences upon Two Ohio Presidents." *Pharos* 60(4) (Fall 1997): 5–10.

_____. "President Cleveland's Secret Operation: The Effects of the Office upon the Care of the President." *Pharos* 58(3) (Summer 1995): 11–16.

DeToledo, John, Brian DeToledo and Meredith Lowe. "The Epilepsy of First Lady Ida Saxton." *Southern Medical Journal* 93(3) (March 2000): 267–271.

Duncan, Louis. "The Days Gone By—The Strange Case of Surgeon Hammond." *Military Surgeon* 64(1) (January, 1929): 98–100; 64(2) (February 1929): 252–262.

"FDA authorizes REGEN-COV antibody therapy for post-exposure prophylaxis (prevention) for Covid-19," www.fda.drugs (August 10, 2021.

Ferguson, Andrew. "Bush's Exercise Guru." *The Weekly Standard* (May 7, 2001): 12–14.

Francis, Samuel. "Biographical Sketch of General R.C. Wood." *The Medical and Surgical Reporter* 20 (April 10, 1969): 275–276.

Hammond, William A. "On the Causes of Vice-President Wilson's Death." *The Boston Medical and Surgical Journal* 93(25) (December 16, 1875): 693–704.

Hirschhorn, Norbert, Robert Feldman and Ian Greaves. "Abraham Lincoln's Blue Pills." *Perspectives in Biology and Medicine* 44(3) (Summer 2001): 315–322.

Howard, John Tilden. "The Doctors Gustavus Brown, Father and Son, of Charles County, Maryland. *Annals of Medical History* 9 (1937): 437–448.

Hudgens, Richard. "Mental Health of Political Candidates: Notes on Abraham Lincoln." *American Journal of Psychiatry* 130(1) (January 1973): 110.

Jackson, Edward. "Obituary of George E. de Schweinitz." *American Journal of Ophthalmology* 21(3) (1938): 1285–1287.

"John Jones (1729-1791), Physician to Washington and Franklin." *Journal of the American Medical Association* 202(1) (October 2, 1967): 152–153.

"Jonathan Reiner Biography," Medical Association of George Washington University. *Medical Sciences* 322(1) (July 2001): 31–36.

Kidder, J.H. "Foltz, Jonathan Messersmith." *Transactions of the American Medical Association* 33 (1882): 555–558.

King, James. "In Memoriam: Matthew Derbyshire Mann." *Transactions of the American Gynecological Society* 46 (1921): 386–389.

Kopperman, Paul. "Venerate the Lancet: Benjamin Rush's Yellow Fever Therapy in Context." *Bulletin of the History of Medicine* 78 (2004): 539–574.

"The Late Dr. Hall." *The Boston Medical and Surgical Journal* 102 (1880): 621–622.

Lloyd, James. "Obituary of Francis X. Dercum." *Archives of Neurology and Psychiatry* 25 (1931): 1333–1335.

Lundberg, George. "Closing the Case in *JAMA* on the John F. Kennedy Autopsy." *Journal of the American Medical Association* 268(13) (October 7, 1992): 1736–1738. "Major General Howard McCrum Snyder, USA (Ret.)." *Military Medicine* (1970): 1180–1181.

Markin, Tim. "Democrat Suggest Invoking 25th Amendment Against Donald Trump." *Newsweek* December 23, 2018.

Mayo Clinic. "The Medical History of George Washington (1732-1799) I, II, III." *Staff*

Proceedings of the Mayo Clinic (February 11, 18, 25, 1942): 82–96, 107–112, 116–123.

McLean, Robert. "Leonard Heaton—Military Surgeon." *Military Medicine* 147 (September 1982): 717–727.

McPartland, J.M. "Travell's trigger points—molecular and osteopathic perspectives." *Journal of the American Osteopathic Association* 104(6) (June 2004): 244–249.

Miller, Thomas. "A Biographical Sketch of the Professional Life and Character of the Late Henry Huntt, M.D., of Washington, D.C." *The Medical Examiner* 1 (1938): 363–365.

Miller, Virginia. "Dr. Thomas Miller and His Times." *Records of the Columbia Historical Society* 3 (1900): 303–323.

Moreels, C.L., Jr. "New Historical Information on the Cleveland Operations." *Surgery* 62 (1967): 542–551.

Morens, David. "The Death of a President." *New England Journal of Medicine* 341(4) (December 9, 1999): 1845–1849.

"Obituary of Bailey Washington." *Journal of the American Medical Association* 28 (1897): 431.

"Obituary of Charles H. Mayo." *Journal of the American Medical Association* 112 (April–June 1939): 2342.

"Obituary of Dr. Charles E. Sawyer." *J. Am. Inst. Homeopathy* 17 (1924): 1020–1023.

"Obituary of Edward Hammond Clarke." *The Chicago Medical Journal* 37 (1877): 111.

"Obituary of Edward Hammond Clarke," *The Transactions of American Medical Association* 29 (1878): 624–627

"Obituary of James Francis Coupal, M.A., M.D. *Bulletin of the International Society of Medical Museums* 14 (March 1935): 114–116.

"Obituary, Roswell Park, M.D., LL.D." *The Lancet* (March 24, 1914): 780.

"The Official Report on the Case of President McKinley." *Journal of the American Medical Association* 37 (1901): 1029–1036.

Park, Roswell. "Emergency Hospital at the Pan-American Exposition." *Buffalo Medical Journal* (1901): 701–704.

_____. "Report of the Medical Department of the Pan-American Exposition, Buffalo, 1901." *Buffalo Medical Journal* (December 1901).

Parmenter, John. "The Surgery in President McKinley's Case: An Account of the Operation by One of the Surgeons." *Buffalo Medical Journal* 41 (1901): 205–206.

Pelisati, D., and G. Sperati. "George Washington." *Acta Otorhinolaryngol Ital* 25 (2005): 55–58.

Pillitteri, Adele. "OR Nursing 100 Years Ago: Nursing Care of President McKinley." *Today's OR Nurse* 12(12) (December 1991): 19–24.

Pritchard, Richard, and A.L. Herring. "The Problem of the President's Bullet." *Surgery, Gynecology and Obstetrics* 92 (1951): 625–633.

Radbill, Samuel. "The Autobiographical Ana of Robley Dunglison, M.D." *Transactions of the American Philosophical Society* 53(8) (December 1963): 1–212.

Reyburn, Robert. "Clinical history of the case of President James Abram Garfield." *Journal of the American Medical Association* 22 (1894): 411–417, 440–464, 578–582, 621–624, 664–669.

Riccards, Michael P. "The Presidency in Sickness and in Health." Presidential Studies Quarterly. (Summer 1977): 215–231.

Rixey, Presley, et al. "The Official Report on the Case of President McKinley." *Journal of the American medical Association* 37 (October 19, 1901): 1029–1036.

Roddis, Louis. "Thomas Harris, M.D., Naval Surgeon and Founder of the First School of Naval Medicine in the New World." *Journal of the History of Medicine* (Summer 1950): 236–250.

Roos, Charles A. "The Physicians to the Presidents and Their Patients: A Biobibliography." *Bulletin of the Medical Library Association* 49 (1961): 291–360.

"Samuel Bard (1742–1821) Colonial Physician." *Journal of the American Medical Association* 205(8) (August 19, 1968): 114–115.

Simons, David. "Cardiology and Myofascial Trigger Points: Janet G. Travell's Contributions." *Texas Heart Institute Journal 2003* 30(1): 3–7.

Simons, David, Janet G. Travell, and Lois Simons. "Protecting the Ozone Layer." *Arch. Phys. Med. Rehabil.* 71 (January 1990).

Stein, Marvin. "The Establishment of the Department of Psychiatry in the Mount Sinai Hospital: A Conflict between Neurology and Psychiatry." *Journal of the History of the Behavioral Sciences* 43(3) (Summer 2004): 285–309.

"Susan Edson, M.D." *Homeopathy Today* 17(19) (October 17, 1997).

Sutphin, Rebecca L. "Nurse Practitioner vs Physician Assistant: What's the Difference?" *Nurse Journal* (February 13, 2023).

Taylor, Blaine. "The Aftermath of the Wallace Shooting: A Maryland Medical Success Story." *MD State Medical Journal* (May 1976): 35–50.

_____. "An Exclusive Interview with William Lukash, M.D., Personal Physician to the President of the United States." *MD State Medical Journal* (November 1977): 35–71.

Travell, Janet G. "A Trigger Point for Hiccup." *Journal of the American Osteopathic Association* 77(4) (December 1977): 308–312.

"Trigger Points," *Texas Heart Journal 2003* 30(1): 1–12.

Tyler, Lyon G. *Tyler's Historical Quarterly and Genealogical Magazine* 5 (1924): 18, 21, 22, 23.

"A Violation of Medical Ethics." *Walsh's Retrospect: A Quarterly Compendium of American Medicine and Surgery* (1881): 457–459.

Webber, Thomas. "Travell's Myofascial Trigger Points and the Osteopathic Lesion." *Journal of the American Osteopathic Association* 77(4) (December 1977): 308–312.

Wesson, Miley. "Hugh Hampton Young." *The Journal of Urology* 57 (1957): 203–208.

"William Kelly Newton, M.D., Obituary." *Journal of the American Medical Association* 54(1) (January 8, 1910): 152.

Wilson, Nelson. "Details of President McKinley's Case, Narrated by the Recorder at the Operation." *Buffalo Medical Journal* 41 (1901): 207–225.

Wilson, Virginia P. "Janet G. Travell, M.D.: A Daughter's Recollection." *Texas Heart Institute Journal* 2003 30(1): 8–12.

Wotherspoon, A.S. "Some Cases of a Rare Form of Exanthem." *American Periodical Series* II(ii) (1844): 203–217.

Newspapers and Magazines

Advertiser, 1988.
Amarillo Globe News, 2022.
Associated Press, 1986–2004, 2021.
Atlanta Business Chronicle, 2004.
Baptist Standard, 2002.
Boston Herald, 1997.
Daily News (New York), 1999.
Des Moines Register, 2006.
Financial Times (London), 1988.
Guardian (London), 1988–1992, 2018.
GWU Daily Colonial, 2006.
Independent (London),
Indianapolis News, 1885.
Naval Service Medical News, 1993.
New York Post, 2022–3.
New York Times, 1853–2006, 2016, 2021.
Niles National Register, 1841.
Ottawa Citizen, 2004.
Pittsburgh Post-Gazette, 1997.
Reuters, 1996–2001.
Rocky Mountain News, 2005.
Saint Louis Post-Dispatch, 1999.
St. Petersburg Times, 2002.
San Francisco Chronicle, 1991.
Seattle Times, 2004.
Toronto Star, 1988.
Town Hall, 2022.
US News & World Report, 2000.
USA Today, 1984–1999, 2013.
Wall Street Journal, 1991–2006, 2022.
Washington Examiner, 2021.
Washington Free Beacon, 2020.
Washington Globe, 1832.
Washington Post, 1988–2005, 2021.
Washington Times, 2000, 2021.
Weekly Standard, 2001.
Youngstown Vindicator, 1997.

Internet and Cable News Channels

"Biden Removes Dr. Sean Conley, Trump Physician Accused of Misleading the Public About Trump's Covid-19 Diagnosis," Yahoo News, January 27, 2021.

Coles, Nick. "New book claims Rod Rosenstein thought John Kelly and Jeff Sessions would back use of 25th Amendment against Trump," Fox News, October 8, 2019.

Collins, Kaitlan, and Manu Raju. "A doctor resigns after reports of concerns about Jackson's conduct," CNN Politics, May 4, 2018.

Givas, Nick. "New book claims Rod Rosenstein thought John Kelly and Jeff Sessions would back use of 25th Amendment against Trump," Fox News, October 8, 2019.

Herb, Jeremy, and Kevin Liptak: "Trump's White House doctor facing fresh scrutiny over Covid test timeline," CNN Politics, February 3, 2021.

Hillyard, Vaughn, and Dartumorro Calrk: "Mike Pence's White House doctor quits amid fallout over Dr. Ronny Jackson." NBC News, May 4, 2018.

Hoft, Jim. "Deep State Rod Rosenstein Now Admits He Talked with Andrew McCabe About Recording President Trump—After Lying During Senate Testimony." The Gateway Pundit, March 6, 2021.

Johnstone, Caitlin. "Stop Calling It a Stutter: Dozens of Examples Show Biden's Dementia Symptoms," Consortium News, March 6, 2020.

Langford, Cameron. "Report: Former Presidential Doctor Was a "Toxic Leader" of the White House Medical Staff," *Courthouse News Service*, January 15, 2023.

"Man Sets Himself Ablaze at White House," http://www.foxnews.som/story/0,2933,138621,00.html, accessed November 15, 2004.

Martin-Joy, John. "Donald Trump and the 25th Amendment: Errors of judgement and lack of popularity do not constitute an inability," Psychology Today; https://psychologytoday/.com/us/blog/politics, accessed April 4, 2021.

McCarthy, Andrew: "McCabe, Rosenstein and the Real Truth About the 25th Amendment Coup Attempt," Fox News, February 16, 2019.

Olson, Tyler: "Ex-White House Doctor Ronny Jackson demands Biden take cognitive test or drop out of 2024 race," Fox News, April 25, 2023.

Rall, Ted: "Joe Biden Obviously Has Dementia and Should Withdraw, Political Commentary, Rasmussen Reports, March 14, 2020.

"Ronny Jackson, House Republicans September 20.2021; Call for Joe Biden's Cognitive Assessment, Breitbart, June 18, 2021.

"Transcript: President Trump's Doctors Provide Saturday Update on His Health, "NPR playlist as viewed on YouTube, October 3, 2020.

Interviews and Correspondence

Carnejo, Frank, PA, LCDR (former WHMU administrator), telephone conversation with author, April 18, 2021.

Cimino, Francesca, Captain USN (former WHMU physician), telephone conversation with author, June 5, 2023.

Conley, Sean, M.D., Captain USN (former presidential physician), telephone interviews with author, March 14, 2021; 2022; August 8, 29, 2023.

Conley, Sean, M.D., Captain USN (former presidential physician), personal correspondence with the author, November 2023.
Cox, Gerard R. (former White House physician), telephone interview with the author, June 16, 2006.
Culbertson, Tom (Spiegel Grove curator), personal correspondence with the author, June 7, 2001.
Darling, Robert, M.D. (former White House physician), telephone interviews with the author, December 29, 2005; January 27, 2006; February 14, 2006.
Greenwood, John (chief, Office of Medical History), Office of the Army Surgeon General, telephone interview, February 4, 2005.
Hoth, David (assistant editor of the papers of Andrew Jackson), personal communication, September 8, 1998.
Hurst, J. Willis (President Lyndon Johnson's consulting cardiologist), personal correspondence with the author, June 25, 2004.
Hutton, John (former physician to President Ronald Reagan), telephone interview with the author, May 2, 2006.
Jackson, Carl, personal correspondence with the author, September 15, 2004.
Jackson, Joanna, M.D., (former WHMU physician), telephone interview with author, April 15, 2021.
Jackson, Ronny, M.D., (Congressman and former presidential physician), interviews with author, December 12, 2020; April 3, 2023.
Kavanaugh, Georgeanna (LCMT, neuromuscular therapist), personal correspondence with the author, June 26, 2006.
Koblentz, Stuart (Marion, Ohio, historian), June 7, 2006.
Krisiloff, F. (Santa Monica urologist), telephone interview with the author, May 30, 2006.
Kuhlman, Jeffrey (former presidential physician), interviews with author, November 24, 2020, February 25, 2022.
Law Library of Congress, personal communication with author, October 7, 2022.
Lee, Burton, III (former physician to President George H.W. Bush), telephone interview with the author, May 31, 2006.
Lewis, Frank (executive director of the American Board of Surgery), personal correspondence with the author, September 7, 2004.
Mariano, E. Connie, interview by the author, Scottsdale, AZ, July 18, 2003.
Mariano, E. Connie, interview by the author, Tempe, AZ, August 27, 2005.
Mariano, E. Connie, personal correspondence with the author, September 8, 2003; March 19, 2004; January 6, 2006; February 15, 2006; May 1, 2006, October 10, 2022.
Molan, Kate (National Archives), personal communication with author, October 26, 2022.
Nanney, James S. (historian, air force surgeon general's office), personal correspondence with the author, June 12, 2006; June 13, 2006.
O'Connor, Kevin (presidential physician), text message to author, November 2, 2023.
O'Connor, Kevin (presidential physician to Joe Biden) telephone interviews, December 15, 2023; December 28, 2023.
Odum, Lisa (associate librarian, Mount Vernon Ladies' Association), telephone interview, July 1, 2002.
Pena, Jennifer (former WHMU vice presidential physician), personal interview with author, February 25, 2022.
Pena, Jennifer (WHMU physician to vice president Pence), personal correspondence, December 12, 2023.
Smith, Hugh, M.D. (former student of Dr. Ruge at Northwestern School of Medicine), interview by author, Tucson, AZ, September 5, 2005.
Sobocinski, Andre (archivist BUMED), personal communications with author, April 21, 2021; January 2022.
Socha, Patricia (American Board of Medical Specialties), personal correspondence with the author, November 15, 2004; November 23, 2005.
Socha, Patricia (American Board of Medical Specialties), telephone interview with the author, June 29, 2005.
Stanish, Julia (Washington Hospital Center), personal correspondence with author, February 25, 2005.
Syler, Heidi (reference librarian, Sewanee University), personal correspondence with the author, August 2, August 16, 2004.
Taylor, Janet (staff, USUHS Board of Regents), personal correspondence with the author, May 31, 2006.
Tubb, Richard M.D. (Brigadier General, former presidential physician), interview with author, December 16, 2001.
Tubb, Richard, M.D. (Brigadier General, former presidential physician) written summary to author, December 14, 2023.
Ullman, Dana (Homeopathic Educational Services), personal correspondence with the author, June 2, 2006.
Whitfield, Denise, M.D. (former WHMU physician), interview with author, May 15, 2023.
Whitfield, Denise, M.D. (former WHMU physician), personal correspondence with the author, November 8, 2023.
Zustovich, Mark (media relations associate, Media Recording for the Blind and Dyslexic), personal correspondence with the author, June 23, 2006.

Internet

AAMC org: 2022 Facts. Applicants and matriculants data (accessed June 20, 2023)
"About AMOPS," http://www.amops.org (accessed March 26, 2006).
"American Board of Emergency Medicine," http://www.abem.org/rainbow/portal/alias (accessed December 5, 2005).

"American Board of Medical Genetics," http://www.abmg.org/genetics/abmg/general.htm: December 7, 2005.

"American Board of Medical Specialties," http://www.abms.org (accessed May 11, 2005).

"American Board of Physical Medicine and Rehabilitation," http://www.abpmr.org.about/ (accessed June 10, 2005).

"Appointments & Nominations, January 4, 1988," http://www.reagan.texas.edu/archives/speeches/1985/10485a.htm (accessed May 9, 2006).

"Biden tests positive for Covid 19 again," www.foxnews.com.politics. (Accessed August 3, 2022)

"Blockley: The Memory Lingers On," http://www.uchs.net/Rosenthal/Blockley.html (accessed January 12, 2005).

"Bureau of Medicine and Surgery Administrative Activities." http://www.navalmedicine.mid.navy.mil/bumedindex.cfmocid (accessed February 11, 2005)

"Burkley, George," http://www.arlingtoncemetery.net//ggburkle.htm (accessed July 21, 2003); Reference copy, JFK Collection: HCSA (RG 233); http:www.geocities.com/jfkinf03/testimony/burkaff.htm (accessed August 7, 2003).

"Cary Travers Grayson," http://www.lupinfo.com.encyclopedia/E/E-GraysonC.html (accessed July 7, 2003).

"Center for Executive Medicine," http://www.drcmariano/com/index.html (accessed June 10, 2006).

"Chiefs of the Bureau of Medicine and Surgeons General of the Navy Medical Department," http://www.navymediicne.med.nay.mil/bumed/index.cfm?docid=10328 (accessed February 11, 2005).

Crumley, Cheryl. "Is Joe Biden Mentally Fit for the Presidency? No, and these 10 Gaffes Show Why." https://genzconservative,com/is-joe-biden-mentally-fit-for-the-presidency (accessed December16, 2020).

"Dr. Diane Colgan Elected to Suburban Hospital Board of Trustees," http://www.suburbanhospital.org/publications/pr0526056.html (accessed April 5, 2006).

"Dr. John E. Hutton, Jr., physician to President Reagan, buried April 1," https://bulletin.facs.ord/20i5/06-john-hutton-jr-physician-to-president-reagan (accessed April 16, 2023).

"Donald Trump's Medical Exam full transcript." The Guardian (January 17, 2018) The Guardian, guardian.com/us-news/2018/jan/17/donald-trump (accessed February 16, 2022)

"Dwight Eisenhower Administration of White House," http://www.americanpresident.org/history/dwighteisenhpwer/staffactivities/administration (accessed August 18, 2023)

"Eagleton, Thomas Francis," http://www.bioguide.congress.gov/scripts/biodisdplay.pl?index=E00004 (accessed November 11, 2005).

"Edinburgh and Medical Schools in North America," http://www.ed.ac.uk/history/note11.tmm (accessed December 16, 2004).

"The Edinburgh Medical School," http://www.mvm.ed.ac.uk/history/index/htm (accessed December 16, 2004).

Everett's Thesis, http:///www.franklin.library.upenn.edu/cgi-in/Pwebrecon.egi?Search_Arg_Everett%2C+Ch (accessed February 4, 2005).

"The Foundation of the Faculty of Medicine," http://www.mvm.ed.ac.uk/history2.htm (accessed December 16, 2004).

"FP Reflects on Service on Front Lines of Family Medicine," https://wwwaafp.org/news/family-doc-focus/20190603fdf-oconnor.html, accessed December 9, 2023.

"George F. Fuller: White House Medical Support," http://www.afip.org/Departments/legalmed/legmed2003?Fuller.pdf (accessed July 30, 2004).

"George G. Burkley," http://www.geocities.com/jfkinf03/tetsimony/burkley.htm (accessed August 7, 2003).

"George Gregory Burkley," http://www.arlingtoncemetary.net/ggburklle.htm (accessed August 7, 2003).

"History of Osteopathic Medicine Virtual Museum," http://www.history.aoa-net.org/Education/college.hist.htm (accessed March 20, 2006).

"History of the Washington Navy Yard," http://www.history.navy.mil/faqs/faq52-1.htm (accessed February 11, 2005).

"In the Line of Fire," http://www.filipinasmag.com/magazine/issues/nov2000/eature.html (accessed May 12, 2001).

"Jedediah Hyde Baxter," http://www.arlingtoncemetary.com/jhbaxter.htm (accessed June 8, 2001).

"Joel Thompson Boone: The Maverick Physician," http://www.joelboone.com/ (accessed November 20, 2003).

"Joseph K. Barnes," http://www.history.amedd.army.mil.tsgs/Barnes.htm (accessed April 3, 2005).

"Joseph K. Barnes," http://www.virtualmuseumofhistory.com/josephbarnes (accessed May 27, 2001).

"Leiden University Medical Center History," http://www.145.88.210.153/englishj/geranl/history.html (accessed December 18, 2004).

"Kuhlman: Transform Healthcare," httpss://jeffreykuhlman.com.about (accessioned November 24, 2020).

"Lukash WM," http://www.pubmed.gov (accessed January 10, 2006).

"Man Sets Himself Ablaze at White House," http://www.foxnews.som/story/0.2933.138621.00.html (accessed November 15, 2004).

"Mayo Clinic Program Details," http://www.mayoclinic.org/executive-health/details.html (accessed June 10, 2006).

"Mitchill, Samuel Latham," http://www.clements.umich.edu/Webguides/M/Miychill.html (accessed January 20, 2006).

"Montreal Cognitive Assessment," https://www.verywellhealth.com/alzheimers-ad-montreal-cognitive assessment,

"National Hotel Disease," http://www.everything2.com/index.pl?node-National1%20Hotel 1%disease (accessed August 22, 2005).

"Navy Bureau of Medicine and Surgery-History," http://www.navymedicine.med.navy.bil/bumed/index.cfm?docid+10259 (accessed February 11, 2005).

"Old Blockley," http://www.phila.gov/health/history/parts/part_5.html (accessed January 12, 2005).

"Old Naval Hospital Building," http://www.nlm.nih.gov/hmd/medtour/oldnavy.html (accessed February 19, 2005).

"O'Reilly" Military Office Records, National Archives, http://www.armymedicine.army.mil/history/O'Reilly.htm

"Osteopathic Medical Profession Report," osteopathic.org/about/aoa/statistics.

"Penn in the 18th Century," http://www.archives.upenn.eduhisty/features/1700s/people/kuhn _ adam.html (accessed April 17, 2006).

"Personality Disorders," http://www.psyweb.com/Mdisord/jsp/personalityDis.jsp (accessed February 28, 2006).

"Physician Impairment by Substance Abuse," http://www.mc.vanderbilt.edu/root/vumc.php?site=cph&doc=1088 (accessed February 13, 2006).

"The President's Physician: The Life and Legacy of Dr. Janet G. Travell," http://www.gwu.edu/gelman/archives/exhibits/travell/credits.html (accessed May 9, 2006).

"Procaine," http://www.en.wikipedia.org/umw/Procaine (accessed November 2, 2005).

"Propofol," https://en.wikipedia.og//wiki//Propofol (accesssed July 10, 2022).

Providence Hospital, http://www.provhosp.org/jistory&mission.htm (accessed May 23, 2004).

"Remdesivir," https://www.drugs.com/mtm/remdesivir.html

"Richard Tubb. Board Member Lexis/Nexis Special Services,' https://www.linkedin.com/in/Richard-Tubb (accessed March 31, 2023).

"Robert Maitland O'Reilly," http://www.armymedicine.army.mil/history/tsgs/O'Reilly.htm (accessed May 31, 2001).

"Say Goodbye to Back Pain Biographies," http://www.saygoodbyetobackpain.com/ biographies (accessed November 16, 2005).

"Sean Conley," https://enwikipedia.org/wiki/Sean Conley (accessed March 30, 2021; May 31, 2022)

"Society for Innovative Medical Practice Design," http://www.simpd.org/conference.php (accessed June 10, 2006).

"The Surgeon Generals of the U.S. Army and Their Predecessors, 1775–2000," http://www.history.amedd.army.mil.tsgs/defaylty.htm (accessed February 11, 2005).

"Tipper Gore and Thyroid Problems," http://www.hopkins.med.jhu.edu/news/thyroid/ (accessed May 11, 2001).

"US College of Osteopathic Medicine," www.aacom (accessed June 9, 2022).

"US Medical schools 2022 total graduates," www.aama.org/data/reports.americamed (accessed June 9, 2022).

"The USS *Boone*," http://www.joelboone.com.uss_boone.htm (accessed November 20, 2003).

Verdi, http://www.famousamericans.net/tulliosuzzaraverdi (accessed September 16, 2005).

Verdi, http://www.hoemeoint.org/history/cleave/v/verdits.htm (accessed September 16, 2005).

Verdi, http://www.hoemeint.org/phot/uv/verdits.htm (accessed September 16, 2005).

"Walter Robert Tkach," http://www.af.mil/bios/bio.asp?biolD-7401 (accessed August 8, 2005).

"Which First Lady Flies Highest? Michelle vs. Laura," July 9, 2013. https://www.ntu.org/publications/detail/which-firstladyflies-highest-michelle-vs-laura (accessed February 26, 2023).

"William Sternberg," http://www.arlingtoncemetary.com,gmrecords.htm (accessed July 2, 2001).

Collections of Correspondence and Personal Papers

Cleveland, Grover. Grover Cleveland Papers. Library of Congress.

Coolidge, Calvin. Calvin Coolidge Papers. Library of Congress.

Foltz, Jonathan Messersmith. Franklin & Marshall College Collection of Jonathan Messersmith Foltz Papers. Franklin & Marshall Library.

Garfield, James. James A. Garfield Papers. Western Reserve Historical Library.

Harding, Warren. Warren G. Harding Papers. Ohio Historical Society.

Jackson, Andrew. Andrew Jackson Correspondence. Library of Congress.

Norris, Basil. Basil Norris Military Records. National Archives and Records Administration.

O'Reilly, Robert. Robert O'Reilly Medical Officers Files. National Archives and Records Administration.

Rixey, Presley. Record of Service of Surgeon Presley M. Rixey. Naval Service Records, National Archives and Records Administration.

Washington, George. George Washington Papers. Library of Congress.

Wood, Robert C. Robert C. Wood's Medical Officer's Files. National Archives and Records Administration.

Speeches

Moore, Walton. "Dr. James Craik, Chief Physician and Surgeon of the Continental Army," Alexandria, VA (published in the Congressional Record, February 22, 1929, 1–8).

Oral Histories

Bruenn, Howard. Oral history.
Graham, Wallace, Truman Presidential Library, January 10, 1976.
Graham, Wallace. Truman Presidential Library. March 30, 1989.
Heaton, Leonard. Army War College. October, November, December 1978.

Unpublished Material

Griffen, Ward O., Jr. "The American Board of Surgery in the Twentieth Century—Then and Now." The American Board of Surgery (2004).
Martin, John M. "Rufus King: Southern Moderate." Ph.D. diss., University of North Carolina, 1955.
Peterson, Bradley. "Oral Interview with Daniel Ruge, M.D." (October 11, 1986).

White House Office

The White House Office of the Press Secretary; Summary of the President's Physical Examination August 4, 2001
The White House Office of the Press Secretary; Summary of President Barack Obama's Physical Examination June 12, 2014.

Congress

Miscellaneous Document #14. "Expenses of President Garfield's Illness and Death." House of Representatives. 47th Congress, 2d sess., 11 December 1882.
Public Law 89. Chapter 104, 4 April 1930.
Public Law 393. Chapter 573, 16 May 1928.
Statute 1. Chapter II. 27th Congress, 30 June 1841.
Statute 34. Title 10, 70A. Chapter 1041, 10 August 1956.
United States Code.1994 Edition: Containing the General and Permanent Laws of the United States in Force on January 3, 1995. Volume Three. Chapter 104: "That the officer of the Medical Corps, United States Army, or of the Medical Corps, United States Navy, below the rank of colonel or captain respectively, who is now, or hereafter may be assigned to duty as physician to the White House, shall have the temporary rank and the pay and allowances of a colonel, Medical Corps, United States Army, or of a captain, United States Navy, while serving.

Index

Numbers in *bold italics* indicate pages with illustrations

Aaron, Benjamin 167–168
abdominal surgery 59, 86–87
acute illnesses: health maintenance versus treatment 19, 65, 171, 181; medical attention reserved for 36; presidential physician focus on 3, 9
Adams, Charles 155
Adams, George Washington 155, 213n57
Adams, John 18, 19, 155
Adams, John Quincy 30, 155
Addison, Thomas 106
Addison's disease 106
administration officials, physicians serving 90
adrenal insufficiency 106
advanced life support capability 168
advanced trauma life support (ATLS) and advanced clinical life support (ACLS) certification 118
aerobic exercise 124
aging and the presidency 149–150, 159–160, 181, 182–183
Agnew, Spiro 144, 153, 154
AIDS commission 121, 175
AIDS vaccine 175
Air Force One 124, 134, 140
Air Force Reserves 89
Air Force Systems Command, command surgeon for 177
Airforce Two 168
alcoholism: in presidents 155, 156, 158, 160; in vice presidents 161, 166–167
Aldrich, C. Knight 151–152
allergy medicine 122
allopath (term) 42
allopathic medicine 66, 67, 183
allopathic school 44
almshouses 28, 35
alternative medicine 66
Altman, Lawrence 174
Alzheimer's disease 152, 159–160
AMA Council on Medical Education 61
American Board of Internal Medicine, certification by 102, 203n2

American Board of Medical Genetics 137
American Board of Medical Specialties (ABMS) 137
American Board of Neurological Surgery, certification by 102, 203n2
American Board of Physical Medicine and Rehabilitation, certification by 109
American Board of Psychiatry and Neurology 154
American Board of Surgery 87, 91, 102, 203n2
American Board of Urology, certification by 102, 203n2
American College of Physicians Ethics Manual 148
American College of Surgeons 91
American Gynecological Society 57
American Institute of Homeopathy 47
American Journal of Ophthalmology 28
American Medical Association: code of ethics 40, 43, 44; criticism 121; founding 26; health insurance, position on 91; osteopathic medicine, policies concerning 99, 100; polls criticized by 153; positions descriptions according to 141; presidents 49; women admitted to 47
American medicine: changes affecting 181; historic overview 3–4, 6–7; trends in 183
American Ophthalmologic Society 28
American Osteopathic Association (AOA) 99, 184
American Psychiatric Association 127, 153, 156
American Revolution 14–15
American School of Osteopathy 98–99
American Surgical and Gynecological Association 70
amphetamines 113, 155, 159
anatomy, study and teaching 23, 24

anesthesia 86–87
anesthetic techniques 59
anthrax 124
antisepsis, introduction 59
armed services, osteopaths in 100
Army, U.S., reorganization 51
Army Dispensary 39, 48
Army doctors 41, 66
Army Medical Department 56
Army Surgeon Generals: appointments and promotions *41*, 47, 51–52, *86*, 88; conferences 139; establishment of office 51; presidential physician dealings with 85; presidential physicians as 37, 38, 50–51, 56
army surgeons 51, 195n116
The Arrogance of Powers (Summers) 158
aseptic operating room technique 86–87
Ashburn, P.M. 51, 52, 195n126
Ashcroft, John 139
assassinations and assassination attempts 57–59, 101; *see also under name of president*
assistant White House physicians: military doctors as 106; promotion to presidential doctor 95; thyroid malfunction treated by 121
Association of Military Osteopathic Physicians and Surgeons (AMOPS) 184
atherosclerosis of the arteries 164
aural surgery 23

bacterial abscesses 15
Bailey, Tom 163
Baltimore General Hospital 35
Bard, John 14, 15–16
Bard, Samuel: career 14; as first presidential physician 1, 5, 9; as hospital founder 17; medical education 10–11, 13, 14; political views 14–15; as Washington, G.'s physician *11*, 15–16, 18, 26
Bard, William 14
Barkley, Alben W. 139, 210n46
Barnes, Joseph K.: as Army Surgeon General 51, 52;

233

assassinated presidents treated by 38, *39*; Garfield, J. treated by 42; homeopaths, association with 43; military doctors, views concerning 40; residency 61
Barton, William P.C. 51
Baruch, Bernard 77
Baxter, Jedediah: as Army Surgeon General *41*, 51–52, 54; Garfield, J. treated by 37, 42; Hayes, B. treated by 41, 42; homeopath-orthodox rivalry impact on 47; residency 61; as vice presidential physician 164
Bayh, Birch 152
Beahrs, Oliver 120
Beaumont, William 31
Bedford Springs, Pennsylvania, waters 29, 33
Bell, Whitfield J., Jr. 13, 188n18, 189n22
Bellevue Hospital 35, 58, 61
Bernstein, Carl 157–158
Bethesda Naval Hospital: cardiologists at 97; FDR at 73, 81, 86; inpatient suite at 140; Reagan, R. at 115, 116, 117, 120; as teaching hospital 94
Biden, Ashley 131
Biden, Beau 131
Biden, Hunter 131
Biden, Jill 131, 136, 138
Biden, Joe: background and family 130–131; colonoscopy 146; Covid infection 132; debates 129; dementia, suspicions 159, 182–183; dental surgery 132; disability claims made against 149–150; fitness for office 130; health challenges 131; health, state 171; inauguration 180; mental health and cognitive ability 150, 179; opponents 179; physician selected by 8; physician serving 1, 123, 131–132, 136, 138, 177; physician serving (as vice president) 123, 167; term 123; Twenty-fifth Amendment raised during administration 8
Bishop, Jim 81–82
black physicians
Blackwell Island hospital 61
bleeding, practice 18, 23, 24, 25, 44
Bliss, D.W.: controversies, involvement in *43*; District of Columbia medical society, expulsion and reinstatement in 42–43, 44; Edson, S., behavior toward 46; Garfield, J. treated by 37, 42, 45, 46, 52; internship training lacking for 61; professional behavior, questionable by 37, 44, 185
Blockley Hospital 27–28, 61
blue pills 157

board certification: attractiveness 88; development 7; physician's 91; as White House Medical Unit requirement 182; for White House physicians 137
Boerhaave, Herman 11
bone setting 98
Bonner, Thomas N. 61, 62, 197n75
Boone, George 66
Boone, Joel: career after White House post 72; FDR discharge 75; as first family physician 68–69; medal awarded to 67; medical education 66; as presidential physician 64, *65*, 70–71, 74, 76, 173, 183; White House physician office institutionalized by 63
Boone, Suzanne 64, 68, 197n2
Booth, John Wilkes 38
Boston Female Medical College 104
Boston Medical and Surgical Journal 26
Bowles, Chester 176
Boynton, Silas 44, 45–56, 66
Brady, Nicholas 102–103
Bright's disease 166
British army 10
broad osteopaths 99
Bronze Star 93
Brothers Mayo 87
Brown, Gustavus Richard 13
Bruenn, Howard 74, *80*, 81, 82, 185
Bryant, Joseph *48*, *49*, 49–50
Buchanan, James: correspondence 156; Foltz, Jonathan, relations with 33, *34*, 34–35, 52; military doctor selected by 36
Buffalo General hospital 58
Buffalo hospitals 58
bullets, extraction 23, 31, 51, 168
bullets, retained 25
Bullitt, William C. 157, 213n55
Bureau of Medicine and Surgery (BUMED): assignments to 67; chief 35, 52 (*see also* Navy Surgeon Generals); establishment 51
Burkley, George: as assistant White House physician 107, *107*, 108, 111, 112; as military doctor 103; post-presidential career 177; Travell, J., disputes with 109; as White House physician 98, 114, 177
Busey, Samuel C. 44
Bush, Barbara 167
Bush, George H.W.: atrial fibrillation 145; death 182, 218n1; health, state 171; Mariano, E.C., association with 178; medical emergencies 181; physicians serving 121–122, 139, 140, 172, 180; physicians serving (as vice president)

103; positions under 168; presidential power transfer, temporary to 115, 145; thyroid malfunction 121, 145; as vice president 116, 161, 167
Bush, George W.: back issues 123; cardiac collapse 102; colonoscopies 124, 145–146; health status 181; hospitalization 86; Mariano, E.C., association with 178; mental competence 146; orthopedic issues 131; physical examination 146; physicians serving (as president) 122, 123–124, 125, 126, 136, 173; treasury secretary 102–103; trips 103
Bush, Laura 138
Bush family pets 139
Bush family, physicians serving 103, 118, 123, 124
Byrnes, Jimmy 90

cabinet members' families 22
cabinet members, medical care for 139
Calhoun, John 51, 144
Calwalader, Thomas 16
Camp David 134, 140, 145, 146, 170, 185
Campolo, Tony 159
Capote, Truman 113
Carter, Jimmy: age 182, 218n1; physician-patient relationship ramifications raised by 147; physician serving 95, *95*, 96–97, 116, 122, 147; presentations 143, 211n4
Carter Center of Emory University 143
cats, presidential 42
Center for Executive Medicine 178
cerebral malaria 30
chain of command, fragmentation 141–142
Charlton, John 16
chemistry 99
Cheney, Dick: health challenges 171; heart problems 167–169, 181; physician dispatched by 138; physicians serving 161, 167; presidential power transfer, temporary to 145, 146
chiropractor, limiting prerogatives 66
cholera death 25
cholera epidemic 1832, 23, 36
cholera hospitals 36
cholera infantum 69–70
Christian Scientists 66
chronic illnesses: challenge posed by 101; during domestic political disputes 74; kidney problems 67–68
Churchill, Winston 82, 88
Cimino, Francesca 141
civilian doctors: compensation

for 9; in consultant roles 84; contributions 21; presidential treatment role 85; versus military *see* military versus civilian doctors; as White House physicians 3, 26, 172–173, 182; women as 103
Civil War: civilian practices during 40; doctors during 47; internships after 61; nurses 45; property expropriated during 55; Union Army during 43
Clarke, Edward H. 163, 164
Clay, Lucius 84
Cleveland, Grover: civilian-military doctor relations under 37; first term 48, 50; hospital care not given to 54; oral cancer and surgery 2, 47, **48**, 49, **49**, 50, 52, 86; presidential leverage used by 53; vice president under 164
clinical laboratory 87, 102
Clinton, Bill: age 182, 218*n*1; blood sample 134, 137; contingency meetings during administration 148–149; health status 181; impeachment 134, 136, 209*n*13; inauguration 102; knee surgery and rehabilitation 140; Mariano, E.C., association with 178; medical expenses 141; physical examinations 137; physician selected by 122; physician serving 72, 106, 125, **135**, 136, 139, 160, 177; precancerous lesion 183; sex addiction 155, 159; tendon tearing and repair 145; travels 137
Clinton, George 144, 161–162
Clinton, Hillary 138
The Clinton Syndrome (Levin) 159
coeducation 104
Cohen, Eugene 109, 110, 111
Colgan, Diane 120, **120**, 183, 218*n*3
colonial army medical department 10
colon polyps 124, 132, 146
colonoscopy, effects of anesthesia before 118, 119, 145–146
Columbia Hospital for Women and Lying In 36
Columbian College 23
Comey, James 149
commodities, trading in 91
common cold 176
concierge executive medicine (term) 139
concierge medicine 178
congestive heart failure 73, 74, 81, 86, 165, 168–169
Congress, Twenty-fifth Amendment and 147
Congressional Medal of Honor recipients 64, 67

congressmembers, doctors serving 41
Conley, Sean: as military officer 8; post-presidential career 180; as presidential physician 126, **128**, 128–130, 142, 177; press conferences 124, 129, 130
consultants *see* medical consultants
consultation 185
Consultation Clause 43
consultative boards 81
consultative groups 84
consumer food prices 91
contingency planning 181
continuous medical presence 25, 54, 61
"contraria" 42, 194*n*44
Cook County Hospital 61
Coolidge, Calvin: depression 68, 155, 156, 198*n*36; physician serving 64, **65**, 67, 68, 71–72, 173
Coolidge, Calvin, Jr. (president's son) 68, 71, 156
Coolidge, Grace 68–69, 71
Coolidge, John 68
Coolidge, Richard H. 32, 51, 61
Coolidge family 66
Coolidge sons 68, 69
Cooper, Ken (Kenneth H.) 124, 140, 173
Corbett, David W. 183
coronary artery stenting 124
corrective exercise 99
cortisone 106
Coupal, James 66, 68, 69, 71–72
Covid illness **128**, 132, 149, 182
Covid pandemic 128–129, 139
Cox, Christopher 43
Cox, Edward 151
Cox, Gerald 136
Craik, James: doctors assisting 13; Everett, C. compared to 22; medical education and career 10, 12; as presidential physician **10**; Washington, G., relations with 9
criminally indicted doctor 98
Crispell, Kenneth R. 5, 78, 158
Crohn's disease 73, 74–75, 87
Cullen, William 13, 188*n*18
Curie, Madam 68
Custis, George Washington 18
Czolgosz, Leon 57

Daniels, Josephus 78
Darling, Robert 125, 138, 210*n*32
Darman, Richard 117
Daugherty, Harry M. 68
Davis, Loyal 103, 115, 117
death in the family 151, 152, 153; loss of a child 55, 56, 57
death of presidents: line of succession in event 144; overview 29, 86; statistics 5, 21, 143; *see also* death *under name of president*; terms assassination *or*

Declaration of Independence 12, 18
Deep State 129
Delaney, Matthew 139
dementia 159
dementia screening exam 127
dental care 132, 139, 140
Department of Defense 136
depression 5, 153–154, 155, 156
Dercum, Francis X. 78
dermatology 61
dignitaries, medical care for 1, 90, 139
diphtheria 60
Director of the White House Medical Unit (title) 135
disability 5, 149, 152
disabled president 96, 147
disease prevention 65, 171
Distinguished Service Medal 94
District of Columbia, medical services in 162
District of Columbia Medical Society *see* Medical Society of the District of Columbia
doctor of osteopathy (D.O.) degree 99, 100, 128, 183
domestic political disputes, chronic illnesses during 74
Drake, Daniel 27
Dukakis, Michael 153
Dunglison, Robley 18–19
dysentery 10, 31, 34, 51

Eagleton, Thomas 153–154
ear, nose and throat (ENT) diseases 80, 200*n*64
ear, nose and throat (ENT) specialists 80
early disease detection 178
Edinburgh Infirmary 11–12
Edinburgh School of Medicine 182
Edison, Thomas 68
Edson, Susan A.: compensation 46; demotion **46**; female presidential physicians in addition to 103; as Garfield family physician 45; as homeopathic physician 44, 66; post-presidential career 47
Eisenhower, Dwight: assistant physician serving 92, **93**, 131; death 87; heart attack 2, 73, 75, 84, **85**, 87, 89, 182; hospitalization 85–86, 88; illnesses 85–86, 143, 181; illnesses, political and media management 74; medical history 75; physicians serving 74–75, 82, 83–85, 88, 92, 107; President's Council on Physical Fitness 110; stroke 87; surgery **86**; Vice President under 93
Eisenhower, Julie 96
Eisenhower, Mamie 82, 83, 88
Eisenhower Executive Office Building (EEOB) 138

Index

Eisenhower family 83
ejection fraction 169
electroconvulsive treatments 157
electro-shock therapy 153
emergency care 23, 138
emergency medicine 126, 137
Emergency Room doctors 8
Emmerglick, Leonard 148
Enemies Lists 157
epilepsy 56
Erdmann, John 50, 61
Erlichman, John 158
erysipelas 164
Esselman, John 23
ether anesthesia 26
Everett, Charles 22, 23, 31
ex-presidents: death 87, 182, 218n1; longevity 182; medical care 94, 186; physician treatment 96
Experiments and Observations on the Gastric Juice and the Physiology of Digestion (Beaumont) 31

family doctor, vice presidential physician replacing 167
Fauci, Anthony 139
Feerick, Robert 143
Ferrell, Robert 81, 83
Fielding, Fred 115, 145
financial panic, 1893 50
Finney, John 70
first families 1, 68
first ladies: malaria 42, 45, 47; mastectomies 120; medical needs (general) 67; physicians serving 118; trips outside Washington 138
Fisher, Eddie 113
Fitzsimmons Army Hospital 84, 85
flag rank billets 128–129
Flexner, Abraham, report on medical education 55, 62, 63, 66–67, 99–100, 104
Flexner, Simon 62
Foltz, Jonathan: Bedford Springs, Pennsylvania, writings on 29; as Navy Surgeon General 35, 51, 52; as presidential physician 33–35, **34**
food and diet 99
Ford, Gerald: death 182, 218n1; Nixon, R., pardoned by 94; physician serving 95, **95**, 96, 116, 122; positions under 168; presentations 143, 211n4; psychiatric treatment, alleged 153, 154; as vice president 144
foreign dignitaries, physicians serving 90, 139
foreign doctors 184–185
foreign legations, families 22
foreign policy, presidential illness affecting 185
foreign policy crises, chronic illnesses during 74

Forney, John 156
Fowler, H. 78
Fox, George A. 65
"fracture surgery" (term) 110
Franklin, Benjamin 16, 155
free medical care 40
French and Indian war 17
Freud, Sigmund 157, 213n55

Gaillard, C.A. 94
gall bladder removal 86, 201n114
Galt, Edith Bolling (Wilson's 2nd wife) 73–74, 77, 78
Gardner, Franklin A. 47
Garfield, James: autopsy 45–46; Boynton, S. relationship with 44–45; civilian-military doctor relations under 37, 182; emergency care 183; hospitalization, alternatives to 7; physicians serving **39**, 42, 46, 179
Garfield, James assassination: attending physicians 62, 66; Bliss-Baxter confrontation 37, 42, 133, 179, 185; care of president 52; death, location 86; overview and surgery following 57–58
Garfield, Lucretia 42, 45, 47
Garfield family, physician serving 41, 42, 45
Garfield Memorial Hospital 36
Garnett, A.Y.P. 41
gastroenterologist as presidential physician 94, 95
gender disparity in White House medicine 183
generalists 28, 122
George Washington Hospital (GWH) 117, 167–168, 169–170
George Washington Medical School 23, 28
George Washington University Hospital and School of Medicine 176
German universities, medical education at 61
Gerry, Eldridge 144, 162
Gilbert, Robert 143, 152, 156
Gillett, Mary 51, 52, 195n126
Goldwater, Barry 153, 176
"Goldwater Rule" 149, 153
Gomez, Carlos 5, 78
Gonzales, Alberto 145
Goodhue, Lemira 68
Gordan, Alice Gertrude 77
Gore, Albert 140, 145, 161, 167, 171
Gore, Tipper 140, 167
Gore family 138
Gout 50
government employees, presidential physicians as 6
government health insurance 141
government officials, doctors serving 41
Graham, James Walter 90
Graham, Wallace Harry:

criticism against 8; memoirs 91; political involvement **89**, 91, 121, 139; as presidential physician 89–91; as retired president's physician 94
Grant, Ulysses S.: civilian-military doctor relations under 37, 39–40; Foltz, J., appointment by 35, 52; health challenges 50; physician serving 38, 39, **40**; Rixey, P., appointment by 55; vice president under 161
Grayson, Cary: controversies during tenure 89; education and career 75–79; McIntire, Ross relations with 79–80; medical education 62; memoir 5, 75, 77; press and public misled 74, 106; as retired president's physician 94; as White House physician 60, 71, 73, 75, **76**, 185
Greenwood, John T. 52, 195n128
Gregory, Samuel 104
Grenada 140
grief over loss of loved one 151, 152
Griffin, Martin E. 85
Griffin, Robert 151
Guiteau, Charles 37, 42
gunfights 23, 31, 51

Haggerty, James 84, 87
Hahnemann, Samuel 44
Hahnemann Medical College 66, 70
Haiti 67
Halifax, Lord (Edward Wood) 90
Hall, James Crowdhill: career 27–28; compensation for services 39; future trends foreshadowed 22; medical education 23–25, 61; as Medical Society president 20, 21; as Pillar of the Profession **20**; as Polk family physician 33; as presidential physician 25, 26, 27; Taylor, Z., treated by 32
Halsey, William 72
Hamilton, Alexander 17
Hammond, William 164
Hanna, Mark 56
Harding, Florence 67, 68, 69, 70, 83, 173–174
Harding, Phoebe 69–70
Harding, Warren G.: death 67, 68, 71, 86, 173, 174; heart attack 182; homeopathic physicians supported by 70; medical team 69; parents 69; physician serving 64, **65**, **71**, 182; successor 156; terminal illness 69, 70
Harrington, Daniel 160
Harris, Kamala 146, 167, 171
Harris, Thomas 23, 31, **32**, 38, 51
Harrison, Benjamin 41, 47, 50, 51, 52

Harrison, Caroline 47
Harrison, William Henry: appointments **41**; hospitalization, alternatives 7; illness and death 26, 27, 29, 86, 144; medical expenses 26–27
Hatfield, Mark 164
Hay, John 56
Hayes, Rutherford B. 41–42
Hayes family, physician serving 41
health care: evolution 171; payment 3–4; specialist teams, past and present compared 17
health insurance 7, 91, 140–141, 183
health maintenance: commitment to 65; emphasis on 3, 19, 171, 182; promotion 178
health maintenance organization, White House Medical Unit as 130
Health of the Presidents (Marx) 5
Heart (Cheney and Reiner) 168
heart attack 97, 162, 182; *see also* Eisenhower, Dwight: heart attack
heart failure 165
heart surgery 167–168
Heaton, Leonard: Mattingly, T., remarks to press controlled by **84**, 85, 87; as medical consultant 92; Snyder, H., friendship with 88; surgery performed **86**, 87
Heller, Milton 64, 197–198n2
Henderson, Thomas 24–25
Hendricks, Thomas A. 164–165
Henry, Will 69
Hidden Illness in the White House (Crispell and Gomez) 5
Hinckley, John 116–117
Hobart, Garret 57, 144, 165
Hofmann, Lewis (Lew) 167, 168
Holding the Line (Jackson) 130, 134, 138–139, 179–180
holistic medicine 184
home health care, history 36
Homeopathic Free Dispensary 47
homeopathic-orthodox medicine conflict: AMA sanctions against homeopaths 43–44; homeopaths, professional ostracism 43, 44, 47; homeopathy challenge to orthodox practice 37–38; overview 3; presidential care impacted 183
homeopathic-orthodox medicine truce 47, 52, 67, 183, 194n87
homeopaths: influence 69; as presidential physicians 44, 45, 64, 66, 70, 103; restrictions on 45
homeopathy: education 99; patient preferences 42; rise and fall 7, 66–67; women attraction to 46–47, 104
Hoover, Herbert: medical treatment for visitors offered 68; physician not reappointed 72; physician serving 64, 65, **65**, 69; promotions granted 66; as Secretary of Commerce 70–71
Hoover, Lou 69
hospital interns 87
hospital internship 7, 59, 60–61
hospitalization: alternatives to 7, 17, 29–30, 35–36, 54, 58, 86; of ex-presidents 96; of presidents 7, 85–86, 90–91
hospitals: advent and growth 3, 63, 86–87; continuous care 61; development 35–36; expansion 59; first American 7; naval 30–31; past and present compared 17; for poor 58; underdevelopment 28
host nation, medical representatives 137
House, Edward 77
House of Representatives, Speaker of 144
house physician (term) 60
Howe, Mrs. Annie 77
hunting, trauma 168
Huntt, Henry: as District of Columbia medical society organizer 20; expertise, areas 28; medical education 182; Miller, T., apprenticeship under 25; Monroe, E., treated by 23; as presidential physician 21, 22, 25
Hurst, J. Willis 92, 97–98, 140, 173
Hussein, King of Jordan 139
Hutschnecker, Arnold 151, 154, 158–159, 212n3
Hutton, John: certification 102, 203n2; as doctors' advisor 174; Mayo physicians, dealings with 120; post-presidential career 177, 178; as presidential physician 177; as Smith, B.'s successor 103; in White House Medical Unit 118; as White House physician 119, 145, 160
hydrotherapy 99
hydroxychloroquine 129

Ibn Saud, King of Saudi Arabia 90
ileocolic bypass 87
impairments 152; assessment 147
independent practitioners, presidential physicians as 6
infectious diseases 10
infinitesimals, law 44
infirmaries 11–12, 17
influenza pandemic, 1918–1919 99
informed consent 185
in-hospital physician training 7, 59, 60–61
insurance companies, third party payment 7
international medical graduates (IMGs) 184–185
An Intimate Memoir (Grayson) 75
Iran/Contra episode 160
Iraq, doctors in 125
IV fluids 139

Jackson, Andrew: bullet extraction 31; medical challenges 23; physicians serving 8, 13, **15**, 25; Physick, P.S., consultation with 26; surgeon serving 38, 51
Jackson, Jesse 159
Jackson, Joanna 141, 142
Jackson, Ronny: cabinet appointment, opposition 127–128; imbroglio 182; Kuhlman, J., relations with 179; memoir 130, 134, 138–139, 179–180; as military officer 8; Pena, J., relations with 170, 171; post-presidential career 179; as presidential physician 95, 125, **126**, 126–127, 131, 141, 177; press conferences 124; resignation 8; as White House Medical Unit director 136, 185
Jackson, William 16, 17
Jacobson, Max ("Doctor Feelgood"): free services offered 140; as German emigre 159, 185; as presidential physician 112–113; unorthodox therapies 108, 185
Janeway, Edward 50, 58, 60, 61
Jefferson, Thomas: absence from capital 155, 213n31; correspondence 13, 188n19; medicine, attitudes concerning 18–19, 27; vice president under 162
Johns Hopkins School of Medicine 104
Johnson, Andrew: campaign, 1960 106; civilian-military doctor relations under 37; kidney stones 38–39; physicians serving 38, **40**
Johnson, Lady Bird 113
Johnson, Lyndon: accession to presidency 113; administration 122; cardiac status 92; heart attack 97; physician serving 97–98, 114; surgery performed on 86
Johnson (Lyndon) family 113
Johnston W.W. 58
Jones, John 16–17
Joyce, James 110
Joynt, Robert 149

Kalt, Brian 143
Kansas City, hospitals 59
Kaufman, Martin 42, 194n44
Keen, William Williams 50, 61
Kelly, John 170
Kennedy, Jackie 107
Kennedy, John F.: Addison

disease 2; amphetamine and steroid misuse 155, 159; assassination 103, 108, 143, 177; assistant physician serving 92, 93; autopsy 106; back pain and therapy 102, *105*, *107*, 108–110, *109*, 111–112, 176; health and medical cover-ups 5, 107, 110–111, 187n3; health care, delivery to 108; hospitalization 107; inauguration 102; medical emergencies 181; physical therapy 109–110, 111; physicians serving 102, 105–113, 177; as senator 105
Kennedy, Robert 113
Kennedy family 105, 107
Khrushchev, Nikita 113
kidney problems: chronic 67–68, 69; failure 74, 166, 168; kidney extraction 70; stones 38; terminal 173–174, 185
King, William Rufus 162–163
King's College School of Medicine (*later* Columbia School of Medicine): Bard, S. ties to 15; founding 14, 17
Kirschmann, A.T. 46
Kissinger, Henry 100, 158
Knorr, Norman J. 160
Kraus, Hans: free services offered 140; as German emigre 159, 185; as presidential physician 108, *109*, 109–111, 112; selection *107*; Travell, J., dealings with 102
Krisloff, F. 174, 217n21, 217n23
Kuhlmann, Jeff: Jackson, R., relations with 179–180; as military officer 8; post-presidential career 177; as presidential physician 125, 131, 177, 178–179
Kuhn, Adam 12, 17–18

laboratory departments, hospital 59
Lamont, Daniel S. 49–50
Langstaff, J. Brett 5
Lasby, Clarence 83, 84
Lawson, Thomas 31–32
League of Nations 89
Leale, Charles A. 38
Lear, Tobias 15, 16
Lee, Bandy 127, 149
Lee, Burton, III: clinical laboratory use 102; connections and relationships 102–103; interviews conducted 136; post-presidential life 172, 175–176; presidential disability issues discussed 148; as presidential physician 121–122; press, comments regarding 169; Quayle, D., disliked by 167; specialty 102; successor 103; tradition of duties, rebellion against 103

Leech, Margaret 57
Left Ventricular Assist Device (LVAD) 169
Lerner, Allan Jay 113
lesion (defined) 98
lesion osteopaths 99
Levin, Jerome D. 159
Lewinsky, Monica 137, 159
licensing laws, state 24
licensing, medical, requirements 25
lieutenant general, physician as 88
life-threatening emergencies 17
life-threatening illnesses *11*
limb amputation, accidental 24
Lincoln, Abraham: depression 155, 156–157; hospital chartered 36; physicians serving 27, *39*
Lincoln, Abraham assassination: autopsy results 20; death 21, 37; death, location 29, 86; doctors at deathbed 27, 28, 52; military doctors as responders 38
Lincoln, Robert Todd 42
Lincoln family, physician serving 20
Link, Arthur 77
Living History (Clinton) 138
Livingstone, Robert 155
Long, John D. 54, 55–56
Long family 54
loss of a child 155, 156, 157
Lowell, Joseph 51
Lukash, William: as assistant White House physician 92; career 94–97; on civilian doctors as White House physicians 172; post-presidential career 177–178; as presidential physician *95*; as White House physician 116, 122, 136, 177
Lungren, John C. 96

MacDonald, Gordon 159
MacKnight, Charles 16
Madison, Dolley 162
Madison, James: correspondence 22; inauguration 21; physician serving 13; vice president under 162
magnetic healing 98
Malakoff, Gary 168, 169–170
malaria: first ladies 42, 45, 47; Jackson, A. 23; Monroe, J. 22, 30; Taylor, Z. 31; Washington, G. 10
Malone, Tracy 119
management by committee: origin of tradition 18; overview 16; in times of crisis 9, 26
Mann, Matthew 57, 58, 61
Mariano, Eleanor C. (Connie): foreign dignitaries served 139; medical consultants, dealings with 140, 160; medical disability, role in determining 143; memoir 178;

post-presidential career 177, 178; Twenty-fifth Amendment, discussions concerning 148–149; as White House Medical Unit director 136, 185; White House Medical Unit transformed 134, 137; as White House physician 72, 103, 106, 125, *135*, 136, 141, 177, 183
Martin, John 162–163
Marx, Rudolph 5
Maryland (battleship) 76
Massachusetts General Hospital 26, 35
massage tables 107
massage therapy 177
Materia medica 99, 163
Mattingly, Thomas 84, *84*, 85, 87, 92
May, Francis 23
May, Frederick 20, 26
Mayflower (presidential yacht) 67, 76
Mayo, Charles 70, 78
Mayo Clinic 78, 120
Mayo Clinic, Phoenix, Arizona 178
McBurney, Charles 58
McCurry, Mike 140–141
McEnany, Kayleigh 129
McGovern, George 153, 154
McIntire, Ross: as Bruenn, H.'s commanding officer *80*; controversies during tenure 89; Grayson, C. relations with 79–80; medical education 63; memoir 5, 75, 82; press and public misled 74, 106; press, dealings with 73; reward system impact on 52; as White House physician 73, 75, *79*, 79–82, 185; White House physician, first regular identified by 35
McKinley, Ida: physician accompanying 57; physician serving 54, 56, 83, 95
McKinley, William: assassination 57–59; death, location 86; physician serving 54, 76; Rixey, P., appointment considered by 59–60; surgery performed on 86; travels, physician accompaniment during 56, 57; vice president under 165
McKinley family: physician serving 29, 37; travels, physician accompaniment during 54, 57
McNamara, Robert 100
M.D. degree 100, 184
Meadows, Mark 129, 130
media, White House doctor dealings with 1
Medical and Chirurgical Faculty, Maryland 13
medical apprenticeship 22, 23, 24–25

medical attention, episodic nature 36
medical committees 81
medical consultants: assembly 26; definition and overview 136; German emigres as 159; impairment assessment, role 147; president's care, association with 88, 92, 116, 140; psychiatrists as 160; for vice presidents and their families 167; women as 183, 218n3
Medical Corps 72
medical crisis, management by committee in times 9
medical degree 12
medical education: apprenticeships as part 24–25; continuing 137; development 12–13, 21, 23–25, 183; historic overview 6–7; presidential care and 3, 182; reforms and reorganization 61–63; reports on 55, 62, 66–67, 99, 104; U.S. students abroad 11, 61, 182
medical emergencies: causes 182; challenges posed 101, 181; conflict during 69; doctor competitiveness and professional arrogance unmasked 182; overview 102
medical ethical codes 185
medical expertise standard, urban and rural areas compared 23
medical information, press and public demands 3
Medical Inquiries and Observations upon the Disease of the Mind (Rush) 154
medical insurance 7, 91, 140–141, 183
medical internship 7, 54–55, 59, 60–61
medical licensing, requirements 25
medical records, secrecy 81
medical release from prison, appeal 139
Medical Reserve Corps 69
Medical School of the College of Philadelphia *12*, 13
medical schools, American: closure and consolidation 104; coeducational training 104; colleges, decrease 55; first 11, 12, 13; graduates, presidents treated by 27; historic overview 6–7; poor quality 25, 27; psychiatry taught 155; recommendations 62; women 103, 104; women graduates 183
Medical Society of the District of Columbia: code of ethics 37, 39, 40, 41; founding 20; hospitals organized 36; interpersonal and institutional conflicts within 44; leaders 21; members 22, 30, 42–43; military-civilian doctor dispute within 38, *40*; military doctor civilian practices, policy on 56
Medical Society of the State of New York 49
medical specialization: advent 22; certification 102; growth 87–88; rise 3, 28
medical students, gender breakdown 104
medical subspecialists 178
medical therapeutics 99
medically disabled president, replacement against will 96
Medicare 100, 108, 120
medicines and medications, delivery 139
menstruation, dissertations on 22, 190n12
mental disability, political effects 152
mental disorders 154
mental health certificates 159
mental health consultant 160
mental illness: causes and treatment 19; neurologist approach to 154–155; in presidents 155, 158; as sensitive matter 151; signs, difficulty of detecting 152
mental institutions 35, 59
mentally disabling conditions 152
Meredith, James 112
Mexican-American War 29, 33
microscopic anatomy 23
midwifery 12, 24
Milburn, John G. 57, 58
military chain of command 147, 182
military doctors: as assistant White House physicians 106; chain of command 87; after Civil War 3, 47–48; civilian practices 40–41, 54, 55–56; compensation paid to 33; in consultant roles 84; disease information, limited disclosed by 88–89; duration of service 136; importance 36; management by committee, participation 27; medical emergencies managed by 73; osteopaths as 100; presidential patients, relations with 37; presidential physicians as *30*, 64, 65–66, 135, 147, 177, 182; presidential shootings, response to 38; promotions granted to 114; relations between 88; varying roles 92; White House rotation 116
military medical staff, White House assignment 116
military versus civilian doctors: civilian doctor advantages 131; conflicts between 37, 39–40, *40*, 41, *43*, 52; death watches, participation 28; medical disputes 101; military doctor advantages 29, 31, 51, 103; overview 6; post–Civil War to present 3; post-presidential careers 172, 177–178; presidential preferences 23, 36, 41; reconciliation between 52; through Civil War 21
Miller, Thomas: as D.C. district board of health president 23; Harrison, W.H., treated by 26; medical education 25; as Medical Society president 20; as Polk family physician 33; presidential medical care, involvement 21, 22
Miller Center for Public Affairs 143
minimalist approach toward treatment 44
Mitchill, Samuel Latham 13–14, *16*
Mohr, Lawrence 103, 122
Monro, Alexander 11
Monroe, Elizabeth (James M.'s wife) 22, 23
Monroe, James: correspondence 13, 188n19; illnesses in office 22, 23, 29, 30; medical society approval signed 20; physicians serving 30, 31; presidential heir apparent 162; vice president under 166
Montreal Cognitive Assessment 127, 149
mood disorder 154
Moore, Joseph B. 40–41
Morgan, John 12
My Turn (Reagan) 175
Mynter, Herman 57, 58
Myofascial Pain and Dysfunction (Travell and Simons) 105, 176

nasal polyps 34
National Aeronautics and Space Administration (NASA) 123
National Board of Examiners in Otolaryngology 80, 200n64
national health insurance program 91
national health policy 121
National Homeopathic Hospital 47
National Hotel (Washington, D.C.) 34
National Hotel Disease 34
National Medical College (*later* George Washington Medical School) 23, 28
national security concerns 140
national security, presidential illness affecting 185
Naval Examination Board 60
naval medical corps 31
Naval Medical Institute 31

Naval Observatory 139–140
Navy Dispensary (Washington) 55, 56, 57, 79
Navy doctors: civilian practices 40; commanders 128; legislation applying to 66; surgeon's staff 51, 195*n*116
Navy, reorganization 51
navy ships named after presidential physicians 60, 72
Navy Surgeon Generals: appointments and promotions **34**, 35, 52, **55**; civilian practices 40; conferences 139; first 51; friendships 67; presidential physicians as 37, 50–51, 59–60, 75, 78–79, 80
neurologic dyspepsia 42
neurological disability 78
neurologists 152, 154–155
neurology 151, 154, 163
New England Journal of Medicine 26, 96
New York City: hospitals 35; infirmaries 17; medical school 11; as nation's first capital 9
New York College of Osteopathic Medicine 100
New York Hospital 14, 17
Newton, William 165–166
9/11 attack 124
Nixon, Pat 94, 158
Nixon, Richard: alcoholism 151, 157, 158; assistant physician 96, 122; debates 112; hospitalization 86, 96; impeachment drama 151; medical consultants serving 183; mental problems 151, 155, 157–158; musculoskeletal problems 92; physician serving 92, **93**, 93–94, 95, 96, 98, 100, 116, 131; physician serving (as vice president) 177; psychotherapy 158, 159; resignation 94, 122, 144; urgent care clinic location selected 138; as vice president 106; vice presidential pick 144, 154
nongovernmental physicians 101
nonmedical consultants, role in impairment assessment 147
Norris, Basil 38–39, **40**, 40–41
nurse practitioners 126, 135, 141
nurses: increase 87; as White House Medical Unit director 136; on White House Physician's Office staff 90
nursing schools 59

Oath of Hippocrates 148
Obama, Barack: advisor to presidential physicians serving 178; age 182, 218*n*1; health status 181; presidential physicians serving 124, 125, 126, **126**, 131, 136, 139, 179, 207*n*9; smoking cessation 124, 207*n*9; terms 123; vice president under 130
Obama, Michelle 125
Obama family 125
obstetrics 61, 99
O'Connor, Kevin: as civilian doctor 8; imbroglio 182; Jackson, R. criticism 179; as presidential physician 1, 123, 131–132, 136, 138, 177; Twenty-fifth Amendment, approach to 124, 146; as vice presidential physician 167
Odria, Manuel 90
Office Hours Day and Night (Travell) 103, 176
Old Executive Office Building 138, 140
O'Leary, Dennis 117
ophthalmic and aural surgery 23
ophthalmology **21**, 28, 61, 80, 200*n*64
Oquendo, Maria 149
O'Reilly, Robert Maitland: as Army Surgeon General 51, 52; education and career 47–48; internship training lacking 61; as presidential physician **48**, 49, 50; VIPs treated by 57
organized medicine, rules and regulations 42–43
orthodox doctors, prescriptions by 42, 44, 194*n*44
orthodox medicine 67, 99
orthopedics 110
osteopathic medicine: advances 183–184; current conditions 99–100; influence 4; overview 98–100; rise 7; trigger point therapy compared to 176
osteopaths: prerogatives, limiting 66; presidents treated by 98; in White House Medical Unit 8; as White House physicians 128
Ostrow, M. 154
otology 61
outpatient clinic 140

Pan American Exposition 57; dispensary 58
pancreatitis 57
paranoid personality disorder 155, 157
Paris Peace Conference, 1919 77
Park, Roswell 58, 61, 63
Parks, Daniel 139
Pathologic Anatomy (Rokitansky) 33
patient care, work forces 59
patient confidentiality: erring on side 185; lifting veil 148; limits 146; misuse 6; versus press and public demands for medical information 3, **49**
patient-physician contract 109–110
Peck, Fayette H. 166
pejorative terms 152
Pena, Jennifer: as first woman practitioner in White House 141; imbroglio 182; Jackson, R., relations with 127, 170–171, 179; Pence, K., treated by 142; resignation 128, 171; as vice presidential physician 138, 167, 183
Pence, Karen 142, 170
Pence, Mike: health, state 171; physician serving 127, 141, 161, 167, 183
Pence family, physician serving 127, 128, 138, 183
Pennsylvania Hospital 7, 17
Pennsylvania waters 29, 33
Pepper, Claude 113
Peritonitis 58
personality evaluations 159
Peters, John Charles 33
pets, first family 68
pharmacology 99
pharmacology department, Cornell 105
Philadelphia: first American medical school 7, 11, **12**; hospitals 35
Philadelphia College of Medicine 62
Philadelphia College of Osteopathic Medicine 100
Philadelphia General Hospital 35
physical examination 124, 125, 140, 146, 167, 173
physical fitness 182
physical therapy 109–110, 111, 141
physician access, presidents and constituents compared 182
physician assistants (PAs): recruitment 8; in White House Medical Unit (WHMU) 126, 135, 141; as White House Medical Unit director 136
physician associates, WHMU 127
physician compensation: changes 183; consultants 88; early, records lacking 26–27; ethics rules concerning 39; from ex-presidents 96, 120; failure to report 98, 100–101; fee for service 9, 15–16, 18, 22, 28, 33; by government 29, 45–46, 140; government employment 106; health insurance role 140–141, 183; institutionalization 7; for military physicians 37, 38; waiving 97, 112, 113, 140, 205*n*104
physician-consultants *see* medical consultants
physician cooperation at president's bedside 57–58
physician deference 6
physician-educators, professional formation 12
physician-patient confidentiality **49**
physician-patient deference 53
physician-patient relationship:

changes to 3, 6, 89; close relations, lack 116; doctor secrecy characterizing 112–113; falling out 33, 34, 35, 52; friendships 49–50, 59, 69, 77, 80–81, 83–84, 89, 90, 94, 96–97; historic overview 5; physician opinion affected by 182; presidency leverage impact on 53; presidential patient dominance 37; professional detachment impacted 74; psychiatric nature 158; rewards stemming from 54; trust-based 123, 148; Twenty-fifth Amendment and 146, 147
"Physician to the Executive Mansion" (term) 56
Physician to the President (defined) 135, 136
physicians: hospital-affiliated 86; prescription drugs, addiction to 169–170, 171; training 6, 23, 62 (see also medical internship)
Physick, Philip Syng 13, *13*, 26
physiology 23
Pierce, Franklin 151, 155, 156, 162
Pilcher, J.E. 48
Pillars of the Profession 20, 21, *21*, 28, 61, 103
Pillitteri, Adele 58
plastic surgeons 120, *120*, 183, 218n3
"plausible deniability" (term) 74
Plumer, William 162
pneumonia 26, 85–86
political career, former White House doctors pursuing 128, 179
political interference 18
political leaders, proposals 159
political pressures, physician acquiescence in face 6
political subterfuge 101
political talk, confidentiality regarding 134
politically correct criteria for clinical laboratory use 102
politics: doctors entangled *89*, 91, 93–94; medical practice based on 2, 3
Polk, James 33, *34*
Polk family physicians 33
polyps 34, 124, 132, 146
poorhouses (term) 35
Post, Jerrold 69, 157
postgraduate training: advent 22, 63; discrimination 104; in Europe 61; in-hospital, rarity 28
Potsdam, Germany, war conference 90
Powell, Louis 38
Powers, Charles 63
preceptors 24
prescription drugs, addiction to 169–170, 171
president: cabinet (see cabinet members); as commander-in-chief 29; death 5, 21, 29, 86, 143, 144 (see also terms assassination or death under name of president); disabled 96, 147; hospitalization 183; physical examinations 65; physician proximity to 140; staff, medical care to members 138–139; vice presidents running 167
president pro tempore of the Senate 144, 146–147
presidential candidates 153, 181–182
presidential care: bureaucratization 142; continuous 25, 54 (see also presidential trips outside Washington); factors affecting 181; innovations 118; politicizing 8
presidential disability: considerations 151; determining 143, 149–150; discussions concerning 148; laws concerning 3; secrecy concerning 78, 79, 144; statistics 5; transfer of power during 124; see also 25th Amendment
presidential illnesses: coverage 6; disability resulting from, 5
presidential illnesses, secrecy concerning: disease diagnoses, masking 106; doctor consultations 17; examples 74; information withheld from patient 74–75, 87; informed consent versus 185; literature on 5; mental illness 152; political versus medical concerns 88–89; precedent set 9, 18; by president's demand 50; wartime 81–82, 87
presidential medical care, historic overview 6
presidential patient-physician relationships see physician-patient relationship
presidential patients, information withheld from 74–75, 87
presidential physicians: attacks on 8; authority over 141–142, 147; challenges, lack of preparedness 101; conflicts among 3; hostility toward 133; internship training lacking 61; literature on 5–6; long-distance monitoring of patients 173; medical education 12, 21–22, 62–63; memoirs 5, 96, 103, 130 (see also under name of individual); political considerations imposed on 9; post-presidential careers 172; professional opinions 106–107; psychiatry and neurology training lacking 151; public policy matters and 108, 121, 139; selection 8, 9, 18, 25, 26, 28, 33, 48, 49, 102, 136; ships named after 60, 72; with specialty certification 80; Twenty-fifth Amendment, responsibility for invoking 143, 147–148; women as 7, 46–47, 120, *135*, 141, 183; working conditions 141
presidential power transfer, temporary 115, 145–146
presidential retirees see ex-presidents
Presidential Succession Act, 1947 144
presidential trips outside Washington: abroad 82, 100, 113, 118, 132, 137–138; domestic 25, 33, 57, 107, 122, 132; medical assistance to others during 138; medical attendance lacking 42, 103; military doctors on 29, 31–32, 36, 54
president's advisors, mental illness concealed 152
President's Committee for Employment of the Physically Handicapped 82
President's Council on Physical Fitness 110
president's health care, evolution 3
president's health, leaks concerning 2
presidents, mental illness 155, 158
press conferences, post exam 124, 127
press corps, management of relations with 169
press pool members, physician responsibility 1
press, questions from 2
preventive care 3
preventive medicine 124
primary care 178, 184; specialties 137, 209n17
Pritchett, Henry S. 62
procaine 108, 109, 111
Proctor, Redfield 47, 52
professional decisions, personal attachments influencing 69
professional deference, controversies over 89, 182
professional detachment 74
professional ethics 185
Providence Hospital 36
psychiatric treatment 153–154
psychiatrists: appointment, recommended 152; stigma of seeing 153, 159, 160
psychiatry: board examination 154; development of American 152, 154–155; as pejorative term 152; presidential physicians lacking training 151
psychoactive drugs, use 152
psychobiographies 157

psychological evaluation 150
psychotherapists: duties 148; Nixon, R., visited by 151, 212n3
psychotherapy 153–154, 156
public disclosure, controversies over 89
Public Health Service, surgeon general 108, 121

Quayle, Dan 145, 161, 167, 171
quinine 10

Rayburn, Sam 176
Reagan, Nancy: mastectomy 120; medical consultations, decisions regarding 122; medical information controlled by 119, 120; memoir 175; physicians serving 167, 174–175; stepfather 103, 115
Reagan, Ronald: age in office 126, 130; Alzheimer's disease 159–160, 174, 178; assassination attempt 102, 116–117, 145, 161, 168; bladder and prostate problems 117; colon surgery 102, 115, 118, 119, 145; death 182, 218n1; Dukakis, M., statements concerning 153; inauguration 95; medical crises 174, 181; mental acuity test 102; physicians serving 8, 83–84, 102, 115, 117–122, 140, 167, 177, 203n2; skin cancer 119, 120; surgery performed on 86, 183, 218n3; vice president medical coverage extended by 103, 167
Reeves, Richard 108
Regan, Don 115, 118, 119, 145
Reiner, Jonathan 168–169
representatives, families 22
residency training 7, 61, 87
resident physician (term) 60
Revolutionary War 15, 17, 23, 161
Reyburn, Robert 42, 61, 62
rheumatism 41–42
Riland, Kenneth 92, 98, 100–101, 183
Rivers, Mendel 88
Rixey (hospital ship) 60
Rixey, John Franklin 60
Rixey, Presley: civilian practice 40, 54, 55–56; first ladies treated 83; as first White House physician 37, **55**, 56–57, 59–60, 63, 69, 74, 95; Grayson, C. relations with 76, 77, 78–79; McKinley family treated 29; at McKinley, W.'s fatal shooting aftermath 58; as Navy Surgeon General 51; reward system impact on 52; ship named after 72; White House medical practice reformed 61, 64; White House physician responsibilities described 165; White House responsibilities, full-time assumed 6

Rixey, Samuel 55
Robins, Robert 69
Rockefeller, Nelson 100, 144
Rokitansky's *Pathologic Anatomy* 33
Roos, Charles 21, 38
Roosevelt, Anna 81, 82
Roosevelt, Archie 60
Roosevelt, Eleanor 82
Roosevelt, Franklin Delano: as Allied leader 89; death 74, 81, 82, 86, 90; disability 85; executive functioning, loss 185, 219n18; health challenges 73, **79**, 182; heart disease 2, 74, **80**, 82, 185; inaugural committee chairman 79; physician discharged 72, 75; physicians serving 8, **79**, 79–82, 84; secrecy over health matters 86; stroke 81
Roosevelt, Theodore: Grayson, C. relations with 76; physician serving **55**, 76, 95; Rixey, P., relations with 59
Roosevelt (Theodore) family 54, 60
Rosenberg, Charles E. 36
Rosenstein, Rod 149
round-the-clock house staff (hospital) 87
Ruffin, Sterling 78
Ruge, Dan: connections and relationships 103; Hutton, J., recruited by 118; Reagan, N., attitude concerning 119; retirement 174; specialty 102; as vice presidential physician 103; on White House Medical Unit doctors away from public eye 121; as White House physician 115–117, 172
Rush, Benjamin
as father of psychiatry 154
house physician position advocated by 60–61
influence and legacy 19
Jefferson, T. friendship with 18, 19
medical education 12
as medical educator **18**, 21
Russell, Francis 70
Rutgers Medical College 14

Salinger, Pierre 111, 113
Savage, Ronald 118
Sawyer, Carl 173, 174
Sawyer, Charles: as civilian physician 103; first ladies treated 83; on Harding, W.G.'s medical team 69; as homeopathic physician 66; post-presidential career 173–174; as White House physician 67, 70–71, **71**, 172; work area 64
Sawyer Sanitorium 173–174
scarification 44
Schanno, Joseph 96
Schweinitz, George 78

scientific medicine 67
Scripps Clinic and Research Foundation, preventive medicine section at 95
second opinions 185
sectarian medicine 7
self-immolation, attempted 138
semi-bureaucratic health care organizations 6
Senate, president pro tempore 144
senators, doctors serving 41
senators' families 22
Senior White House Physician (defined) 135
septicemia 45–46
Seward, William H. 38, 43
sex addiction 155, 159
sexism 46
Sharpe, John 117
Shaw, Mark 112, 113
Shenk, Jonathan 156–157
Sheridan, Philip 48
Sherman, James S. 144, 166, 168
Shippen, William, Jr. 12
Shriver, Sargent 106
Siam (cat) 42
Sim, Thomas: as District of Columbia medical society organizer and leader 20, 21; Monroe, J., treated by 23, 30; as presidential physician 22; professional reputation 25
similars, law 67
"similia" 42, 44, 194n44
Simmons, Josh 167
Simons, David 105, 176
skeletons for examination 27
slaves at Mount Vernon, medical care 24
smallpox 10, 23
Smith, Burton: departure 121; memoir 5, 118, 174–175; presidential doctor-patient relationships described by 83–84; as presidential physician 115, 117–119, 140, 145; on presidential physicians and Reagan presidency 161, 214n3; retirement 174–175; Ruge, D. dealings with 116; specialty 102; successor 103; on vice presidential medical care 167; as White House physician 172–173
Smith, Jess 68
Snyder, Howard: controversies during tenure 89; death 87; Heaton, L., friendship with 88; information withheld from patient 74–75, 87; press and public misled 74, 87; unfinished book project 75; White, P.D., selected by 85; as White House physician 73, 82–84, 92
Society for Innovative Medical Practice Design 178
Spalding, Charles 112

Index

Spanish American War, 1898 55, 56
Speaker of the House of Representatives 144, 146–147
Speakes, Larry: mental acuity test, role in devising 115; physician compensation discussed 120; Smith, B., criticized by 118–119; statements released to media 117; Twenty-fifth Amendment discussion, participation 145
specialists 122, 152
specialization, development 7
specialties among White House doctors 126, 137
specialty board, certification 94
spinal cord injury and disability, texts on 115
spiritual versus psychiatric counseling 159
sports medicine 110
Spot (dog) 139
Stanton, Edwin 52
Starling, Edmund 77
state department 137
stereotypes of women 103
Sternberg, George M. 56
Sternberg, William 61
steroids 113, 150, 155
Stevenson, Adlai 50
Still, Andrew Taylor 98–99
Stitt, Edward 67
Stitt, E.R. 78
Stockton, Charles 58
Stone, Eugene 57
Stone, Robert King: as D.C. district board of health president 23; future trends foreshadowed 22; as Lincoln family physician 20, 28, 38; as Pillar of the Profession *21*; presidential medical care, involvement 21
strokes 73, 162, 163, 164, 182
sub-Saharan Africa 137
Summers, Anthony 158
Supreme Court justices, families 22
surgeon general 29, 139
Surgeons General, Offices of 37
surgeons, osteopaths as 100
surgery/ies: bullets, extraction 23, 31, 51, 168; in or out of hospitals 59; increase 86–87; osteopathic medicine, integration into 99; texts on 16, 49
surgery/ies on presidents: disability resulting from 5; in hospital 86; ileitis operation 87; key actors *86*; post-shooting 57–59; Truman, H. 90
Sutherland, Charles 41, 51

Taft, Charles S. 38
Taft, William Howard 76, 139, 166

Talmadge, John 127
Taylor, Zachary: illness and death 27, 29, 32, 51, 86; military doctors preferred 31–32, 36
Tester, John 127, 128
Thompson, Dr. 164, 165
Thompson, William 33
thyroid function tests 121
thyroid gland tumors 167
thyroid malfunction 145
thyroid surgery 140
Tkach, Walter: as military doctor 177; post-presidential career 177; as vice presidential physician 177; vouchers signed 101; as White House physician 92–94, *93*, 98, 123, 131
Tompkins, Daniel 166–167
Toole, James 149
torture, condemnation 172
Tracy, Benjamin 55
Travell, Janet: correspondence 72; Jacobson, M., accosted by 113; Johnson, L., cardiac exam urged 97; after Kennedy administration 113; Kennedy, J., health management control, loss 108; Kennedy travels, absence during 103; Kraus, H. antipathy toward 102; memoir 5, 103, 111; post-presidential career and legacy 176–177; routine 116; successor 103; successor, potential 97, 98; unorthodox therapies 185; as White House physician 93, 103, *105*, 105–109, 110, 111–112, 141, 172, 183
treadmill tests 124
treatment outcomes, negative, *apologia* 22
Trigger Point Manual (Travell and Simons) 176
"trigger point" theory 108
trigger point therapy 176, 177
Truman, Bess 90
Truman, Harry: hospitalization 7, 85–86, 90–91, 183; physician serving *89*, 89–91, 139; terminal illness 90
Truman, Ralph 90
Truman family doctor 90
Trump, Barron 127
Trump, Donald: advisor to presidential physicians serving 178; age 182, 218n1; cognitive function test 149; Covid infection 129–130, 149, 180, 181, 182; dementia, suspicions 159; disability claims made against 149; hospitalization 86, 129, 130, 180, 181; physicians serving *126*, 126–130, *128*, 136, 142, 179, 129, 179; term, first 123; Twenty-fifth Amendment raised during administration 8
Trump, Melania 127, 129

Trump family 127
Tubb, Richard: interviews conducted 136, 209n13; Jackson, R. relations with 179–180; as military officer 8, 134; post-presidential career 178; Twenty-fifth Amendment, involvement with 145–146; as vice presidential physician 138, 167; as White House Medical Unit director 136, 185; as White House physician 123–124, 125, 131, 141, 173, 177
tuberculosis 47, 69, 163; sanitoriums 59
Tucker, Thomas Tudor 13, *14*
Tumulty, Joseph 78
25th Amendment: aberrant interpretation 115; compliance with, responsibility 139; disability provisions 140; discussions regarding 119, 149, 174; historic overview 143–144; implementation 3, 117, 142, 152; implementation contingency planning 6; invoking 8; invoking, theoretical 96; meetings concerning 149; misuse or nonuse 102; passage 75, 79; physician's role 1, 186; presidential power transfer under 145–146; protocols, adherence to 124; provisions 144; terms of, attention paid to 122; vice presidents and 161
25th Amendment Section 2 154
25th Amendment Section 3: application 151; disregard 144–145; failure to invoke 116, 118, 145; implementation 124, 132, 133, 146; invoking 8, 144, 152
25th Amendment Section 4: discussions concerning 8, 146–148, 151, 152; failure to invoke 116, 118; implementation 144; invoking 127, 143
Tyler, John 51, 144

undergraduate medical education, reorganization 61–62
Union Army 40, 43
U.S. Capitol Building, January 6, 2021, occupation 149
U.S. representative, former White House doctor as 128, 130
United States Steel Corporation 100
University of Edinburgh medical school 11, 12, *12*, 21
University of Leiden school of medicine 11
University of Maryland School of Medicine 13
University of Mississippi 112
University of Pennsylvania 19
University of Pennsylvania Medical School 21

University of Rheims 16
University of the South (Sewanee) medical school 62, 76
urgent care clinic 138

Vaughn, Harry 90
Verdi, Tullio Suzarra 43
Versailles, Treaty of 89
veterinary medicine 42, 139
vice presidential trips outside Washington: medical assistance to others during 138; medical staff serving on 167; physicians serving on 138, 168
vice presidents: as acting president 147; alcoholism 161; care 185; deaths 143–144, 161–166; duties 166; health 150; medical care 161, 171; physical examinations 167; physicians serving 97, 103, 116, 141; presidency, elevation to 143, 144; resignations 143–144; spouses 167, 170
Vietnam, military operations 93
VIPs (very important persons)/VIP medicine: amphetamines 113; management by committee 16; physician-physician deference and 53; standing up to VIPs 122; White House physician involvement 48, 57, 68, 90, 185

Wake Forest University 143
Wallace, George 96
Walter Reed National Military Medical Center: cardiologists from 84; inpatient suite at 140; presidential wives at 88; staff at 90; surgeries performed at 87; Truman, H. at 91; Trump, D. at 129, 130; vice presidential wives at 170
Walter Reed National Military Medical Center: emergency medicine department 180; psychiatrists at 160
The War History of Homeopathic Doctors 70
War of 1812 26, 30, 31
war related illness and injury 87–88
Warren, Gustavus Richard 13
Warren, John Collins **15**, 25–26
Washington, Bailey 23, **30**, 30–31
Washington, George: absence from capital 155, 213n31; death 10; hospitalization, alternatives to 7; medical history 9–10, 17; medical knowledge advances since era 7; mortal illness 13; physicians serving 5, **11**, 15–16, 18, 25; residences (Manhattan) 9
Washington Asylum 35
Washington, D.C.: births, record keeping 23; climate 29; doctors' meetings 20; as nation's capital 18
Washington Hospital Center 36

Washington Naval Hospital 79
Washington Navy Yard 56
Washington Navy Yard and Marine Barracks 30, 33
Watergate 96, 157–158, 160
Webster, Daniel 26
Weinstein, Edwin 74
White, Paul Dudley 84–85, **85**, 87, 88, 92, 140
White House dispensary 107, 140
The White House Doctor (Mariano) 178
White House Doctor (Smith) 174–175
White House doctors: consecutive presidents treated 95; first regular 34–35; health and medical cover-ups, complicity 81–82, 144; informal role 59; mental health consultant recommended to assist 160; osteopaths as 128; overnight stays 22, 26; as permanent position 75; position defined 60; press anonymity 119, 124, 125, 132; press, dealings with 73, 74; promotions granted to 75; public policy matters and 108, 121, 139; relations between 1; reputation 2; responsibilities 6, 69, 89, 103, 142; at urgent care clinic 138; White House Physicians (defined) 135; women as 183
White House medical care providers 6
White House medical practice, reform 61
White House medical presence, changes to 54, 63
White House medical space, establishment 59
White House medical staff 8, 65
White House Medical Unit (WHMU): bureaucratization 118; conflict among members 8; current conditions 122, 134–142; designation 134; directorship 72, 136, 139, 141–142, 185; doctor longevity 123; evolution 8; expanded role 116; facilities staffed 139–140; funding 140; growth 3; as health maintenance organization 130; internal complaints from 127; physical therapy through 141; professionalization 148; public profile, low 121; responsibilities and structure 181; selection to 136–137, 182, 183; as semi-bureaucratic health care organization 6; staff 106–107, 118, 125, 126, 127, 134–135; structure and organization 186; tours **93**; Twenty-fifth Amendment dilemmas

affecting 143; vice presidents served 161; women doctors 8
White House medicine, institutionalization **65**
White House Military Office (WHMO): command structure 131; current conditions 122; members, medical care 138, 181; persons reporting to 185; units under command 134; White House Medical Unit funded through 116, 140
White House Military Office of Security 136
White House occupants, health care 3
White House Physician (McIntire) 75, 82
"White House Physician" (title) 6, 72, 135
White House Physician's Office: bureaucratization and transparency 89; duties and responsibilities 103; institutionalization 63; respect lacking 117–118; staffing 77–78, 90, 103; standard order of procedure lacking 116; women 46, 90
White House physician's office (physical space) 64, 65, 72, 139
White House press office 119, 132
White House press, partisanship 133
White House staff, visitors, and tourists, medical care 138
Whitfield, Denise 141
Whittington, Harry 168
widows, compensation paid to 27
The Will to Live (Hutschnecker) 158
Willamette medical school 63
Williams, Tennessee 113
Wilson, Edith Bolling (Galt) (Wilson's 2nd wife) 73–74, 77, 78
Wilson, Ellen 74, 77
Wilson, Henry 144, 161, 163–164
Wilson, Woodrow: Boone, J. awarded medal 67; disability 78, 79, 85; executive functioning, loss 185, 219n18; health and medical cover-ups 5, 187n3; hospitalization, alternatives to 7; physician serving 60, 62, 73–74, **76**, 79, 185; psychobiography 157, 213n55; stroke 2, 74, 78, 182; treaty negotiations, involvement 89
Winslow, Carolyn 47
Witherspoon, John 12
women as patients 23, 41; Garfield, L. 42, 45
women doctors: first in Washington, D.C. 45; historic overview 7; as presidential

physicians 7, 46–47, 120, *135*, 141, 183; United States and Europe compared 103, 104; White House and U.S. population compared 8; White House Medical Unit, role 141

women in medicine: acceptance 52; admission to medical school 42, 103; historic overview 103–105; rise 37–38; role 4, 7

Wood, Robert Crooke 31–32, 33, 51, 52

Wood, W.W. 32
Woodward, Bob 157–158
Woodward, Joseph 42
Work, Hubert 70
Working Group on Presidential Disability 143, 147, 148
World War I: end 77, 89; German medical education prior to 61; German medical training after 159; Liberty bond drives 78; Switzerland during 110; U.S. entry into 67, 79
World War II: end 75, 89; hospital ships during 60; Navy during 51, 80; practical experiences 87
Worthington, Nicholas 20, 26
Wotherspoon, Alexander S. 32, 33, 51

X-rays 87; departments 59; equipment 107

Yalta Conference, 1945 82
yellow fever 17, 31
Young, Hugh 78

www.ingramcontent.com/pod-product-compliance
Ingram Content Group UK Ltd.
Pitfield, Milton Keynes, MK11 3LW, UK
UKHW050535150426
5217IPUK00026B/1944